The Midwife's Labour and Birth Handbook

The Midwife's Labour and Birth Handbook

Third Edition

Edited by

Vicky Chapman
RGN, RM (Dip), MA

Cathy Charles
RGN, RM, BA (Hons), BSc (Hons)

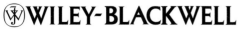
WILEY-BLACKWELL

A John Wiley & Sons, Ltd., Publication

This edition first published 2013
© 2004 and 2009 by Blackwell Publishing, Ltd, 2013 by John Wiley & Sons, Ltd

Wiley-Blackwell is an imprint of John Wiley & Sons, formed by the merger of Wiley's global Scientific, Technical and Medical business with Blackwell Publishing, Ltd.

First published 2004
Second edition 2009
Third edition 2013

Registered office: John Wiley & Sons, Ltd, The Atrium, Southern Gate, Chichester,
West Sussex, PO19 8SQ, UK

Editorial offices: 9600 Garsington Road, Oxford, OX4 2DQ, UK
The Atrium, Southern Gate, Chichester, West Sussex, PO19 8SQ, UK
2121 State Avenue, Ames, Iowa 50014-8300, USA

For details of our global editorial offices, for customer services and for information about how to apply for permission to reuse the copyright material in this book please see our website at www.wiley.com/wiley-blackwell.

Library of Congress Cataloging-in-Publication Data

The midwife's labour and birth handbook / edited by Vicky Chapman,
Cathy Charles. – 3rd ed.
        p. ; cm.
    Includes bibliographical references and index.
    ISBN 978-0-470-65513-9 (pbk. : alk. paper)
    I. Chapman, Vicky.   II. Charles, Cathy.
    [DNLM: 1. Midwifery–methods–Handbooks.   2. Labor, Obstetric–Handbooks.
3. Parturition–Handbooks.   4. Prenatal Care–Handbooks. WQ 165]
    618.2–dc23
                                                        2012031334

A catalogue record for this book is available from the British Library.

Wiley also publishes its books in a variety of electronic formats. Some content that appears in print may not be available in electronic books.

Cover photo by Kali Shanti Park, www.mamamatters.com
Cover design by Steve Thompson

Set in 9.5/12pt Palatino by Aptara Inc., New Delhi, India
Printed in Singapore by Ho Printing Singapore Pte Ltd

2   2014

Contents

Preface

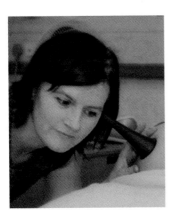

Vicky Chapman

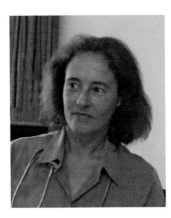

Cathy Charles

We have been delighted at the success of *The Midwife's Labour and Birth Handbook*, now in its third edition.

We have continued our collaboration in writing and editing a handbook for midwives and students. Our aim is to make the book easy to read, grounded in research (both anecdotal and quantitative) with a strong woman-centred perspective.

This edition has some useful new additions. Twelve per cent of the population are left-handed, as is Vicky herself, so she addresses the difficulties that left-handed midwives may face in her chapter on suturing: this edition includes some diagrams specifically to assist left-handed midwives.

This edition includes photographs for the first time. Vicky herself has donated photographs from the birth of her twins (pages 90, 205, 216, 247 and 248). We thank all the mothers and fathers who gave permission for photographs of their very private experiences to be shared in this book.

We have been lucky to obtain some superb birth photographs, including an amazing face presentation. Thank you to Brittany for allowing us to see this extraordinary photograph of her baby's birth, taken by doula and birth photographer Kali Shanti Park (page 141). Also we have a wonderful kneeling vaginal breech home birth sequence (page 230) from independent midwives Joy Horner (www.birthjoy.co.uk) and Sally Randle; we thank Jacqui for allowing these photos of her breech birth to be shared. We feel strongly that the skills of assisting at an upright spontaneous vaginal breech birth should not be lost, and proudly reproduce these fascinating photographs.

Thank you to Tor and Steve (and baby Daisy) for their home VBAC water birth photos (page 124): these photos have an intensity that shines out from their experience ...

you can see the exhaustion too! Also to Sue, with baby Amber, for sharing her home birth photos (pages 87, 94 and 110).

Thank you to Adrienne Price for allowing us to take photos on the delivery suite at Frimley Park Hospital. We thank Debbie Gagliano-Withers for the clean crisp photos which resulted, and of course our 'model mum' Stacey who posed for the photos. Kali Shanti Parks provided our cover photograph and we are grateful to the Johnson family for letting us see this special moment in their lives.

We are grateful to Jane Evans, a very experienced midwife and supporter of breech birth, for advice and review of the breech chapter.

Once again we thank our great team of writers for their patience and hard work.

Cathy Charles and Vicky Chapman

Contributors

The editors

Vicky Chapman *RGN, RM(Dip), MA*
As a midwife Vicky has worked in a variety of hospital settings and as a caseload midwife. She has a particular interest in normal birth, as well as an interest in the politics of childbirth and their impact on women's birth experiences. Vicky has recently returned to midwifery practice in Surrey, having had a break in order to be at home with her four children, the last three of which were born at home, including twins.

Cathy Charles *RGN, RM, BSc(Hons), BA(Hons)*
Cathy is a midwife and ventouse practitioner, practising in acute and community settings in Wiltshire and Somerset. She has lectured and written on the subject of practising as a midwife ventouse practitioner in a stand-alone birthing centre. Like Vicky, Cathy has an interest in water birth and home births. She also gained experience in investigating adverse events as a clinical audit/risk management coordinator and has been a supervisor of midwives. She teaches aquanatal classes.

The contributors

Charlise Adams *BSc*
Charlise qualified as a midwife in 2003 and has practised in a consultant-led unit and the private sector but currently works in a Wiltshire birthing centre. She has been published in various midwifery journals and facilitates teaching obstetric emergencies. She is involved with a local university, interviewing and clinically assessing students. Charlise is married with two small cats.

Annette Briley *SRN, RM, MSc*
Annette is a clinical trials midwifery manager within the Maternal and Fetal Research Unit at St Thomas' Hospital, London. She was a clinical midwife for many years, working in all areas of maternity provision, including obstetric ultrasound. Annette joined the St Thomas' research team in 1997 and was involved in a major study on vitamins in pre-eclampsia. She has since worked on numerous pregnancy-related research projects. Annette has worked with Tommy's, the baby charity, and Parentalk, a charity that aims to inspire and aid parents, and has written a book with Tim Mungeam, Parentalk's CEO, about the first six weeks of parenthood.

Nick Castle *MSc(Dist), DipIMC, RCS(Ed), RGN, SRParamedic ENB 100 & VS300*
Nick is an Honorary Research Fellow at the Durban University of Technology (South Africa) and Consultant Nurse in Resuscitation and Emergency Care in a large district hospital. He has twin daughters.

Jo Coggins *Dip HE (Midwifery) (Dist), BSc(Hons), MSc*
Jo is a community midwife in Wiltshire where she lives with her husband Mark and two children. She previously practised in both acute and community settings in Bath. Her role incorporates caring for women giving birth at the local birthing centre and being on call for homebirths. In addition she provides antenatal and postnatal care in the local community. Jo also enjoys writing and has published articles in various midwifery journals.

Julie Davis *RGN, RM*
Julie qualified as a midwife in 1994. She is a mother of three children. She works as a community midwife at Frimley Park NHS Foundation Trust and is actively involved in the Baby Friendly Initiative.

Mary-Lou Elliott *RM, Dip HE (Midwifery), BA(Hons)*
Mary-Lou qualified as a midwife in 1998 and is currently developing a private midwifery business as well as working as an NHS bank midwife. Her experience is varied, having worked in the acute unit in Bath, with the community teams in the city, and in a community birthing centre. She has also worked as a supervisor of midwives and assistant risk manager, and visiting practice educator/student support midwife for the University of the West of England.

Janet Gwillim *RGN, RM, ADM*
Janet trained as a general nurse in 1968 and a midwife in 1969. After suspending her career to have two children, she returned to midwifery and completed the Advanced Diploma in Midwifery and the Supervisor of Midwives course. Janet attended the first woman to have a water birth in East Kent, and she has been an enthusiastic teacher and resource on water and homebirths. Following the Changing Childbirth Report in 1993, Janet helped to change the way midwives work in south-east Kent by gaining funding for a pilot scheme for a midwifery group practice called JACANES, which provided choice and continuity for midwives and women. Janet retired from midwifery in February 2002 and now is thoroughly enjoying being a grandparent.

Barbara Kavanagh
Barbara is married with two daughters. She is a nurse and midwife with an interest in bereavement issues. She spent 5 years as a Cruse counsellor and has a Diploma in Bereavement Counselling.

Sheila Miskelly *RGN, RM, Dip HE*
Sheila is a practice development midwife, teaching skills drills and other clinical skills. Previously she worked in a stand-alone midwifery-led unit for eight years, enjoying all the pleasures of woman-centred care and home births. Sheila is married with three children.

Bryony Read *RM, BA(Hons)*
Bryony completed her midwifery degree from Oxford Brookes in 2001 and worked at the John Radcliffe Hospital until 2003. Since then she has worked at the Princess Royal University Hospital in Kent, working for six years mainly on the delivery suite, until

after the birth of her first child when she joined the Young Parents Team. This is a caseloading team looking after all under-21-year-olds in the borough of Bromley and parts of Bexley. This has been the most inspiring and exciting job in her career so far as it has so many different aspects. There is never a dull moment and is also a flexible and supportive way to work, due to a great team!

Caroline Rutter *RM, Cert Ed, Dip(HEM), BSc(Hons)*
Caroline was an NCT teacher prior to becoming a midwife in 1993 and has worked as a midwife in stand-alone midwifery units in Wiltshire until 2009. Whilst continuing to work as a bank midwife Caroline is now a full-time lecturer at the University of the West of England, where she shares her passion for empowerment through education, effective communication and promotion of woman-centred values.

Lesley Shuttler *NCT Antenatal Teacher and Assessor, RN, Dip RM, BSc(Hons)*
Pregnancy and birth have always held a fascination for Lesley. She has been involved with the NCT for over thirty years, as a mum, teacher, tutor and study day facilitator and has been a midwife for 20 years. She has two daughters and is enjoying the honour of becoming a grandmother.

'I feel blessed that I can work in a manner that supports so many of my beliefs and values as a woman and as a mother. The women I have met both as a midwife and as an NCT specialist worker have been inspiring and have provided numerous challenges along the way. The day that I cease to feel challenged or inspired, the day I feel I have nothing to learn, is the day I will hang up my pelvis: I hope that is a long way in the future.

1 Labour and normal birth

Cathy Charles

Introduction

> *'Undisturbed birth ... is the balance and involvement of an exquisitely complex and finely tuned orchestra of hormones'* (Buckley, 2004a).

The most exciting activity of a midwife is assisting a woman in labour. The care and support of a midwife may well have a direct result on a woman's ability to labour and birth her baby. Every woman and each birthing experience is unique.

Many midwives manage excessive workloads and, particularly in hospitals, may be pressured by colleagues and policies into offering medicalised care. Yet the midwifery philosophy of helping women to work with their amazing bodies enables many women to have a safe pleasurable birth. Most good midwives find ways to provide good care, whatever the environment, and their example will be passed on to the colleagues and students with whom they work.

Some labours are inherently harder than others, despite all the best efforts of woman and midwife. A midwife should be flexible and adaptable, accepting that it may be neither the midwife's nor the mother's fault if things do not go to plan. The aim is a healthy happy outcome, whatever the means.

The Midwife's Labour and Birth Handbook, Third Edition. Edited by Vicky Chapman and Cathy Charles.
© 2013 John Wiley & Sons, Ltd. Published 2013 by John Wiley & Sons, Ltd.

This chapter aims to give an overview of the process of labour, but it is recognised that labour does not simplistically divide into distinct stages. It is a complex phenomenon of interdependent physical, hormonal and emotional changes, which can vary enormously between individual women. The limitation of the medical model undermines the importance of the midwife's observation and interpretation of a woman's behaviour.

Facts and recommendations for care

- Women should have as normal a labour and birth as possible, and medical intervention should be used only when beneficial to mother and/or baby (DoH, 2004, 2007).
- Midwife-led care gives the best outcomes worldwide: more spontaneous births, fewer episiotomies, less use of analgesia, better breastfeeding rates. Women use less analgesia, and report that they feel more in control of their labour (Hatem *et al.*, 2008).
- Women should be offered the choice of birth either at home, in a midwife-led unit or in an obstetric unit (NICE, 2007), although only 83% report being offered any sort of choice (CQC, 2010). While an obstetric unit may be advised for women with certain problems, up to two thirds of women are suitable for midwife-led units or home birth (DoH, 2007), and the woman has a right to choose where she gives birth.
- Women should be offered one-to-one care in labour (NICE, 2007). The presence of a caring and supportive caregiver has been proved to shorten labour, reduce intervention and improve maternal and neonatal outcomes (Green *et al.*, 2000; Hodnett *et al.*, 2011).
- Increasing numbers of women rate midwifery support as positive (CQC, 2010), although a few midwives are regarded as 'off-hand', 'bossy' or 'unhelpful' (Redshaw *et al.*, 2007).
- 5–6% of mothers develop birth-related post-traumatic stress disorder (Kitzinger and Kitzinger, 2007).
- Over two-thirds of Heads of Midwifery report they have insufficient midwife numbers to cope with their unit workload (RCM, 2009) which impacts on the quality of midwifery care women receive, reducing the chance of one-to-one care.
- The attitude of the caregiver seems to be the most powerful influence on women's satisfaction in labour (NICE, 2007).
- 89% of fathers attend the birth (Redshaw and Heikkila, 2010) but there are other relationships e.g. lesbian couples, who have been less closely studied.

Mode of delivery statistics

- The normal birth rate for England was 63% in 2010/11; in 2009/10 it was 60% in Scotland, 61% in Wales and 56% in Northern Ireland (BirthChoice UK; ESRI, 2011; ONS, 2012)

- The instrumental delivery rate was 12.5% for NHS hospitals in 2010/11; 16.7% in Northern Ireland (ESRI, 2011; ONS, 2012)
- The episiotomy rate for England is 8.3% for a normal birth; almost 20% overall (BirthChoice UK; ONS, 2012).
- The caesarean section (CS) rate for England in 2010/11 is around 25% (ONS, 2012).

The birth environment

In what kind of surroundings do people like to make love? A brightly lit bare room with a high metal bed in the centre? Lots of background noise, with a series of strangers popping in and out to see how things are going? The answers to these questions may seem obvious. If we accept that oxytocin levels for sexual intercourse are directly affected by mood and environment, why is it that women in labour receive less consideration? The intensely complex relationship between birth and sexuality is an increasing source of study and reflection by birth writers (Buckley, 2010).

Once women gave birth where and when they chose, adopting the position they wanted, using their instinctive knowledge to help themselves and each other. Recently birth has become more medicalised, and the place of birth more restricted. No-one would deny that appropriate intervention saves lives. For some women an obstetric unit is the safest choice, and for others it *feels like* the safest, so that makes them feel happier. But does it have to be the choice for everyone?

The clinical environment and increased medicalisation of many birth settings directly affects a woman's privacy and sense of control (Walsh, 2010a). Hodnett *et al.* (2010) have demonstrated that home-like birthing rooms ('alternative settings') even within an obstetric unit, lead to increased maternal satisfaction, reduced intervention and satisfactory perinatal outcomes. This may be due partly to the fact that women simply feel more relaxed at home, or in a home-like setting. However, simply changing the curtains and hiding the suction machine does not always mean a change of philosophy of care. A more telling factor may be that the type of midwives who choose to work in the community or birth centre, or who gravitate towards more home-like rooms, are those with a less interventionist approach.

Women should be able to choose where to give birth; it would be still more wonderful if women could simply decide *in labour* whether they wish to stay at home, or go to a birth centre or an obstetric unit, and indeed if they could change their mind during labour. Such choices do exist, but UK service provision is patchy, and in many countries women have little or no choice.

Whilst it has been estimated that at least two thirds of women are suitable for labour at home or a midwife-led birthing centre (DoH, 2007), for many reasons the majority of mothers and midwives in the UK will still meet in labour in an acute hospital setting. It is incumbent on all midwives to make the environment for a woman in labour, irrespective of its location, warm, welcoming and safe. Always remember that the quality of the caregiver in labour is the thing that most strongly influences a woman's satisfaction with her labour (NICE, 2007).

The *Royal College of Midwives Campaign for Normal Birth* has produced ten top tips to enhance women's birth experience: see Box 1.1.

Box 1.1 Ten top tips for normal birth (RCM, 2010).

(1) Wait and see

The single practice most likely to help a woman have a normal birth is patience. In order to be able to let natural physiology take its own time, we have to be very confident of our own knowledge and experience.

(2) Build her a nest

Mammals try to find warm, secure, dark places to give birth – and human beings are no exception.

(3) Get her off the bed

Gravity is our greatest aid in giving birth, but for historical and cultural reasons (now obsolete) in this society we make women give birth on their backs. We need to help women understand and practise alternative positions antenatally, feel free to be mobile and try different positions during labour and birth.

(4) Justify intervention

Technology is wonderful, except where it gets in the way. We need to ask ourselves 'is it really necessary?' And not to do it unless it is indicated.

(5) Listen to her

Women themselves are the best source of information about what they need. What we need to do is to get to know her, listen to her, understand her, talk to her and think about how we are contributing to her sense of achievement.

(6) Keep a diary

One of the best sources for learning are our own observations. Especially when we can look back at them and realise what we have learned and discovered since then. Write down what happened today: how you felt, what you learnt.

(7) Trust your intuition

Intuition is the knowledge that comes from the multitude of perceptions that we make which are too subtle to be noticed. With experience and reflection we can understand what these patterns are telling us – picking up and anticipating a woman's progress, needs and feelings.

(8) Be a role model

Our behaviour influences others – for better or worse. Midwifery really does need exemplars who can model the practices, behaviour and attitudes that facilitate normal birth. Start being a role model today!

(9) Give her constant reassurance – be positive

Nothing in life prepares a woman for labour. Your reassurance that contractions and emotions are all part of the normal process of giving birth is vital. Do you believe in her strength and ability to give birth normally? How equipped are you to support and encourage women through the peaks and troughs? You may be the only constant anchor during woman's labour to give her constant reassurance – be positive.

(10) From birth to abdomen – skin to skin contact

Breastfeeding gets off to a better start when mothers and their babies have time together – beginning at birth. Immediate skin to skin contact allows them to remain together and provide opportunities for babies to feed on demand for an unlimited time, stay warm and cry less. Mothers learn to recognise their baby's cues and the baby reciprocates. The relationship becomes tender and loving – a connection that lasts a lifetime begins from birth to abdomen.

www.rcmnormalbirth.org.uk/practice/ten-top-tips

Reproduced with permission (RCM, 2010).

Signs that precede labour

Women often describe feeling restless and strange prior to going into labour, sometimes experiencing energy spurts or undertaking 'nesting' activities. Physical symptoms may include:

- low backache and deep pelvic discomfort as the baby descends into the pelvis
- upset stomach/diarrhoea
- intermittent regular/irregular tightening for days/weeks before birth
- loss of operculum ('show'); usually clear or lightly bloodstained
- increased vaginal leaking or 'cervical weep'; and/or
- spontaneous rupture of membranes (SROM) – usually unmistakable; sometimes less so, particularly if the head is well engaged (see Boxes 1.2 and 1.3 for diagnosis and management of SROM). See Chapter 13 for more information on preterm SROM.

Box 1.2   Diagnosis of spontaneous ruptured membranes (SROM).

Woman's history
- This is usually conclusive in itself (Walsh, 2001a).
- Clarify the time of loss, the appearance and approximate amount of fluid.

Observe the liquor
- The pad is usually soaked: if no liquor evident ask the woman to walk around for an hour and check again.
- Liquor may be
  - Clear, straw-coloured or pink: it should smell fresh.
  - Bloodstained: if mucoid contamination this is probably a show – but perform CTG if you doubt this (NICE, 2007).
  - Offensive smelling: this may indicate infection.
  - Meconium-stained (green): a term baby may simply have passed meconium naturally, but always pay close attention to meconium. Light staining is less of a concern, but dark green or black colouring, and/or thick and tenacious meconium means it is fresh, and this could be more serious. NICE (2007) advise continuous electronic fetal monitoring (EFM) for significant meconium, and 'consider' continuous EFM for light staining, depending on the stage of labour, any other risks, volume of liquor and FHR.

Speculum examination
- If the history is unmistakable, or the woman is in labour there is no need for a routine speculum examination (NICE, 2007). However if the head is high consider it, as there is a small risk of cord prolapse.
- Avoid vaginal examination unless the woman is having regular strong contractions and there is a good reason to do so: it risks ascending infection. However there is a degree of paranoia about this: the evidence base is weak (NICE, 2007): it is not a *disaster* if VE is done, just preferable to avoid.
- To perform:
  - Suggest the woman lies down for a while to allow liquor to pool.
  - Lubricate the speculum and gently insert it: the mother may find raising her bottom (on her fists or a pillow) allows easier and more comfortable access.
  - If no liquor visible ask her to cough: liquor may then trickle through the cervix and collect in the speculum bill.
  - Amnisticks (nitraxine test) are no longer recommended due to high false positive rates.

Not all women seek advice at this stage. If they do, the midwife should act as a listener and reassure the woman that these prelabour signs are normal. Avoid negative terms such as 'false labour/alarm'.

Prelabour rupture of membranes at term

Some women experience prelabour rupture of the membranes (PROM) at term (see Box 1.3 and Chapter 19). Risks include infection, cord prolapse (see page 272) and sometimes iatrogenic consequences of intervention but most women go into labour spontaneously and have a good outcome.

Box 1.3   Management of prelabour rupture of membranes (PROM) at term.

Await labour. The woman can await the onset of labour in the comfort of her home, away from potential infection and unnecessary interventions.

Check temperature. Ask her to do this 4-hourly during waking hours (NICE, 2007).

Observe liquor and report any change in colour or smell. There is no need for vaginal swabs, or nitrazine/ferning tests (NICE, 2007).

Listen to the fetal heart. Intermittent auscultatation is fine: there is no need for a CTG unless significant meconium-stained liquor observed (NICE, 2007). Observe fetal activity.

General advice
- Suggest the woman avoids sexual intercourse or putting anything into her vagina.
- Suggest she wipes from front to back after having her bowels opened.
- Inform her that bathing or showering are not associated with any increase in infection.
- Advise her to report any reduced fetal movements, uterine tenderness, pyrexia or feverish symptoms.
- Ask her to come back after 24 hours if labour has not started.
- Tell her that 60% of women go into labour within 24 hours.

If no labour within 24 hours (NICE, 2007)
- NICE advises induction of labour after 24 hours of PROM (see IOL chapter). The woman will then be advised to remain in hospital for 12 hours afterwards so the baby can be observed.
- If a woman chooses to wait longer, continue as above and review every 24 hours.
- After birth observe asymptomatic babies (ROM >24 hours) for 12 hours: at 1 hour, 2 hours then 2 hourly for 10 hours: observe general well-being, chest movements and nasal flare, colour, tone, feeding temperature, heart rate and respiration. Ask the mother to report any concerns.

First stage of labour

There is much debate about whether it is helpful to divide labour into 'stages'. Walsh (2010b) among any others, challenges this: 'The division of the first stage of labour into latent and active is clinician-based and not necessarily resonant with the lived experience of labour'.

Midwives should always be aware of the limitations of rigid categories, but it is also true that certain broad generalisations are helpful to enable the midwife to offer the appropriate support to a woman. With some reservation, the following definitions are offered:

Latent stage

Characteristics of latent stage

NICE (2007) describes this as: 'a period of time, not necessarily continuous, when:

- there are painful contractions, and
- there is some cervical change, including cervical effacement and dilatation up to 4 cm'.

Midwifery care in latent phase

Women may be excited and/or anxious. They will need a warm response and explicit information about what is happening to them. In very early labour they may need just verbal reassurance; they may make several phone calls.

Ideally, home assessment is preferable to hospital; it reduces analgesia use, labour augmentation and CS and appears cost-effective. Women report greater feelings of control and an improved birth experience (Walsh, 2000a; Spiby *et al.*, 2008). If women do come to hospital, evidence supports an assessment unit separate from the labour ward, reducing labour ward stay, increasing perceived sense of control and reducing analgesia use (Hodnett *et al.*, 2008).

Some women experience a prolonged latent phase, which may be tiring and demoralising, requiring more support (see 'Prolonged latent phase', Chapter 9). Women may undergo repeated visits/assessments and feel something is going wrong. Most women however cope well.

The first midwife contact is important and it will establish trust:

- Greet the woman warmly and make her feel special.
- Observe, listen and acknowledge her excitement.
- Be positive but realistic: many women, especially primigravidae, can be overoptimistic about progress.
- Women whose first language is not English may need extra reassurance, careful explanations and sensitivity to personal and cultural preferences. CMACE (2011) highlights the importance of accessing translation services. A translator that the woman is comfortable with should have been arranged prior to labour, but this is sometimes not the case. Some hospitals subscribe to 'languageline' or have other local arrangements. In reality many women go through labour with little or no adequate translator.
- Physical checks include:
  - **Baseline observations.** See Table 1.1.
  - **Urinalysis.** NICE (2007) recommend testing for protein at labour onset, although this is debatable for normotensive women since vaginal secretions, e.g. liquor, commonly contaminate the sample so protein is often ignored.
  - **Abdominal palpation.** Ascertain fundal height, lie, presentation, position and engagement (see Figure 1.1). Ask about fetal movements (FMs): more/less than usual?

- ○ **Fetal heart (FH) auscultation.** See Chapter 3. Offer intermittent auscultation (IA) not a 'routine admission trace' for low-risk women (NICE, 2007) (see Chapter 3).
- **Vaginal examination** (VE) is not usually warranted if contractions are <5 min apart and lasting <60 seconds unless the woman really wants one.
- **Ruptured membranes** (see Box 1.2 for diagnosis) are usually obvious. If the woman is contracting, there is no need for a speculum examination.

Table 1.1   Maternal observations in labour.

Observation	Frequency	Significance
Blood pressure Normal range: Systolic: 100–140 mmHg Diastolic: 60–90 mmHg (NICE, 2011)	Tested at labour onset then hourly (NICE, 2007)	**Hypertension** can be caused by ○ Anxiety and pain ○ General anaesthesia ○ Essential hypertension or pre-eclampsia (See Chapter 20 for definitions of pre-eclampsia)
		Hypotension can be caused by ○ An epidural/top-up ○ Aortocaval occlusion secondary to lying supine ○ Haemorrhage and hypovolaemic shock
Pulse rate Normal range: 55–90 bpm	Tested at labour onset then hourly when checking the fetal heart (NICE, 2007)	**Tachycardia ≥100 bpm** can be caused by ○ Anxiety, pain, hyperventilation ○ Dehydration ○ Pyrexia, infection ○ Obstructed labour ○ Haemorrhage, anaemia and shock
		Bradycardia ≤55 bpm can be caused by ○ Rest and relaxation ○ Drugs, e.g. opiates, magnesium sulphate ○ Cardiac problems
Temperature Normally 36–37°C (97–98.4°F)	Tested at labour onset then 4-hourly (NICE, 2007) or hourly if in birthing pool	**Pyrexia >37.5°C** can be caused by ○ Infection ○ Epidural – usually low-grade pyrexia but rises with time ○ Dehydration ○ Overheated birth pool (see Chapter 7)

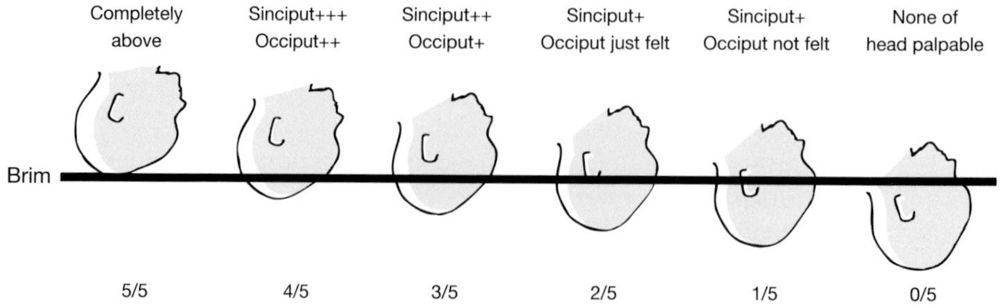

Fig. 1.1   Engagement of the fetal head: fifths palpable by abdominal palpation.

Established first stage of labour

Characteristics of established first stage

In early labour:

- The woman may eat, laugh and talk between/during contractions.
- Contractions become stronger, increasingly painful, 2–5 minutes apart lasting ≤60 seconds.
- The cervix is mid to anterior, soft, effaced (not always fully effaced in multiparous women) and <4 cm dilated.

As labour advances:

- She usually becomes quieter, behaves more instinctively, withdrawing as the primitive parts of the brain take over (Ockenden, 2001).
- During contractions she may become less mobile, holding someone/something during a contraction or stand legs astride and rock her hips. She may close her eyes and breathe heavily and rhythmically (Burvill, 2002), moaning or calling out during the most painful contractions.
- Talking may be brief, e.g. 'water' or 'back'. This is not the time for others to chat. Lemay (2000) echoes Dr Michel Odent's consistent advice: 'the most important thing is *do not disturb the birthing woman'*. Midwives are usually adept at reading cues. Others unfamiliar with labour behaviour, including her partner and students, may need guidance to avoid disturbing her, particularly during a contraction. Before FH auscultation, first speak in a quiet voice or touch the woman's arm; do not always expect an answer.

Midwifery care in established first stage

Make sure your manner is warm. Involve her partner. Clarify how they prefer to be addressed. Ideally, the woman will have already met her midwife antenatally. A good midwife, familiar or not, will quickly establish a good rapport. Kind words, a constant presence and appropriate touch are proven powerful analgesics.

- **Take a clear history:**
  - Discuss previous pregnancies, labours and births
  - Look for relevant risk factors.
  - Ask about vaginal loss, 'show' and time of onset of tightenings.
- **Review the notes:**
  - Ultrasound scan (USS) for dates and placental location
  - Blood results: group, rhesus factor, antibodies, recent haemoglobin
  - Any allergies.
- **Offer continuous support.** Cochrane review (Hodnett *et al.*, 2011) found that continuous female support in labour:
  - reduces use of pharmacological analgesia including epidural
  - makes spontaneous birth more likely (fewer instrumental/CS births)
  - shortens labour
  - increases women's satisfaction with labour.

- **Supporting male birth partner.** Some men don't cope well in hospitals, or when their partner is in pain. Encourage them to take frequent breaks, eat and drink. Some men are clumsy when offering support, annoying the woman. Men may also worry about the birth noises women make. Communicating quietly, and giving gentle guidance on anticipating his partner's needs will help both partners.

Supporting a woman and her partner in labour is an intense relationship, hour after hour, and can be physically and mentally demanding. Providing emotional support, monitoring labour and documenting care may mean that the midwife can hardly leave the woman's side. Involving the birth partner(s) or a doula can both support the midwife and enhance the quality of support the woman receives. There should be no restriction on the number of birth partners present, although be very sure that they are the people the mother really wants. Sometimes women accede to the desires of sisters or friends to be at the birth. Birth however is not a spectator sport: if they are chatting amongst themselves and not supporting the woman then the midwife may need to offer them some direction or tactfully suggest they leave the room.

- **'Listen to her' (RCM, 2010).** Talk through any birth plans early, while the woman is still able to concentrate. As labour progresses, observe her verbal and body language and tell her how well she is coping, offering simple clear information. Try not to leave her alone unless she wishes this. Many women report that they and/or their birth partner were 'left alone and worried at some time during labour' (CQC, 2010).
- **'Build her a nest' (RCM, 2010).** Make the birth environment welcoming: prepare the room before she arrives.
  - Mammals like warm dark places to nest, so keep it relaxed with low lighting.
  - Remove unnecessary monitors/equipment.
  - Noise, particularly other women giving birth, can be distressing; low music may help cut out such noise. Avoid placing a woman arriving in labour near someone who is noisy.
  - Keep interruptions to a minimum; always knock before entering a room and do not accept anyone else failing to do this.
  - If there is a bed, consider pushing it to the side so that it is not the centrepiece (NCT, 2003).
- **Eating and drinking.** Women often want to eat in early (rarely later) labour. Drinking well will prevent dehydration, and a light diet is appropriate unless the woman has recently had opioids or is at higher risk of a general anaesthetic (NICE, 2007; Singata *et al.*, 2010). Ensure her birth supporters eat too.
- **Basic observations (see Table** 1.1**).** Little evidence supports many routine labour observations (Crowther *et al.*, 2000; NICE, 2007), but NICE (2007) recommends hourly pulse (checked simultaneously with the fetal heart rate (FHR)) BP, and 4-hourly temperature. Consider hourly temperature if water birth (see Chapter 7).
- **Frequent micturition** should be encouraged, but urinalysis in labour is probably pointless.
- **Observe vaginal loss**, e.g. liquor, meconium, blood and offensive smell.
- **Do not offer a shave or enema!** Fortunately in the UK the days of routine enemas and pubic shaves have long gone, since they are at best ineffective and at worst embarrassing, painful and harmful; leading paradoxically to increased infection rates (Basevi and Lavender, 2001; Reveiz, 2007). Very occasionally a loaded rectum

can be felt, on VE or the woman may report she is constipated. A couple of glycerine suppositories may bring relief.

- **FH auscultation.** NICE (2007) recommends every 15 minutes for 1 minute following a contraction. Midwives may disagree with this guidance that is based on (largely obstetric) opinion rather than clear evidence, and does not cater for the individual. Midwives may choose to monitor less than every 15 minutes early in labour or, more frequently, at other times, e.g. following SROM or a VE. See Chapter 3.

Assessing progress in labour

'Justify intervention' (RCM, 2010).

Unless birth is imminent, most midwives undertake *abdominal palpation* when taking on a woman's care and, periodically thereafter, to ascertain the lie, position and presentation of the baby. Engagement is particularly helpful to monitor descent of the presenting part and thus labour progress (see Figure 1.1). However, some women may find this examination painful, particularly in advanced labour.

Labour progress can also be judged *observationally*: by the woman's contractions and her verbal and non-verbal response to them (Stuart, 2000; Burvill, 2002; see Table 1.2). Some midwives also observe the 'purple line', present in 76% women, which may gradually extend from the anal margin up to the nape of the buttocks by full dilatation (Hobbs, 1998; Shepherd *et al.*, 2010).

Vaginal examination, artificial rupture of the membranes and partograms

VEs in labour are an invasive, subjective intervention of unproven benefit (Crowther *et al.*, 2000) but are the 'accepted' method for assessing labour progress (see Chapter 2). It can be difficult for woman to decline a VE or for the midwife to perform one only when she/he feels it is best indicated. Even in low-risk births, midwives often feel pressured to adhere to medicalised guidelines which lack good evidence.

NICE (2007) recommends:

- Four-hourly VEs in the first stage of labour.
- Cervical dilatation of 0.5 cm/hour as reasonable progress.
- A 4-hour rather than 2-hour action line on the cervicogram/partogram. This appears to reduce intervention for primigravidae with no adverse maternal or neonatal outcomes, although Cochrane review found no benefit to the cervicogram/partogram per se, but acknowledges there would be difficulties in removing it from practice (Lavender *et al.*, 2008). For more on partograms and assessing progress see Chapter 9.
- Artificial rupture of the membranes (ARM) should not be performed routinely and may not significantly improve normal labour duration (NICE, 2007). The decision should be made in consultation with the woman, discussing evidence, with the intervention justified and not minimised (RCM, 2005). See Chapter 2 for more on ARM.
- *Document* care on partogram and in notes, including any problems, interventions or referrals (for more on record keeping see Chapter 22).

Table 1.2   Contractions and women's typical behaviour up to full dilatation.

Cervical dilatation	0–3 cm	3–4 cm	4–7 cm	7–9 cm	9–10 cm
Frequency of contractions	May be irregular and sometimes stop Gradually increasing in frequency	2:10 minutes Increasingly regular, lasting 20–40 seconds	3:10 minutes Regular, lasting ≤60 seconds	3–4:10 minutes Regular, lasting ≤60 seconds	4–5:10 minutes Sometimes almost continuous, although can 'fade away' for a while in transition
Pain of contractions	Varying from painless/ mild/stronger	Becoming more painful but usually bearable		Increasingly painful	Often almost (sometimes completely) unbearable pain although if in transitional stage may have some respite
Behaviour	Chatty, nervous, excited, able to make jokes and laugh. Often able to talk through contractions May use learned breathing techniques too early, and need reminding to pace herself		Withdrawing more Deeper 'sighing' breathing Sense of humour fading	Becoming vocal: crying out with some contractions May express irritation when touched	Appears withdrawn, in another world May not reply, or answer sharply Concentrating on breathing which slows and deepens with a contraction Throaty grunting noises, crying out with expiration: may panic and express desperate ideas: 'I *can't do* this!'
Movement and posture	Mobile during contractions		Needing to stop and concentrate during contractions	Grasps abdomen and leans forward. May rock, curl toes	Less mobile, holding on to something during a contraction; often eyes closed, but may open wide in surprise with pushing urge

N.B. This is only a broad guide, intended to stimulate awareness of external signs. There is in reality no such thing as a 'typical labour' and women's behaviour will of course vary. Most women exhibit the above to some degree.

Analgesia

Pain is a complex phenomenon and a pain-free labour will not necessarily be more satisfying. Working with women's pain rather than alleviating it underpins many midwives' practice (Downe, 2004). Indeed many would argue that some degree of pain is an essential part of labour: 'as it stimulates the brain to release a cocktail of hormones, which in turn stimulate the uterus to contract' (Walsh and Gutteridge, 2011). Leap (2010) distinguishes between midwives who 'work with pain' and those who provide 'pain relief'.

Most midwives encourage natural and non-interventionist methods first, with pharmacological methods only if these methods are deemed insufficient.

Non-pharmacological analgesia

- **Massage and touch.** These can be powerful analgesics (Figure 1.2), encouraging pain-relieving endorphin release. Never underestimate the effect of being 'with woman'. Be sensitive however. Touch can be irritating or distracting, particularly in later labour. Labour can induce flashbacks for sexual abuse victims (see Chapter 2) and some women come from cultures where *any* non-essential touching by strangers feels invasive.
- **Distraction**, e.g. breathing patterns, music, television:
  'In labour I spend a lot of time in a monotone voice quietly talking women through a contraction. *Breath in through your nose*, (pause) *blow out from your mouth . . . let your shoulders drop, arms relax, unclench your hands. . . .* Next out breath I add: *let your legs relax and sink into the chair/bed etc . . . unclench your toes!!* I don't think this is hypnobirthing but it's working with each contraction and it seems to work!' (Midwife, personal communication).
- **Position changes with aids.** Upright postures reduce the intensity of pain (Lawrence *et al.*, 2009): e.g. beanbags, wedges, stools and birthing balls (e.g. Figures 1.3 and 1.4).
- **Transcutaneous electrical nerve stimulation (TENS).** Despite conflicting opinions on its effectiveness, including possible placebo effect, many women report that it provides good analgesia, especially in the first stage of labour (Johnson, 1997): 20% of women use it (Healthcare Commission, 2008) and most say they would use it again (Dowswell *et al.*, 2009). There is no adverse effect on the mother or baby (Mainstone, 2004). However, lack of substantial non-anecdotal evidence has led NICE (2007) to conclude, controversially, that TENS should not be recommended in established labour. However, Cochrane review (Dowswell *et al.*, 2009) suggests research is insufficient and that women should have the choice of using TENS: many continue to hire TENS units, or borrow them from enlightened hospitals/birth centres.
- **Aromatherapy.** The use of essential oils may aid relaxation in labour. Oils should be diluted, preferably to half the usual dilution, in pregnancy. For a bath, adding the drops to milk prior to putting them in water helps them disperse. Some trusts have an agreed policy for use of oils in labour. Without this, a midwife who has not received any training in aromatherapy should be careful not to give uninformed advice to a woman in labour about the use of oils. Only oils known to be safe in pregnancy should be used: some are contraindicated in pregnancy (Tiran, 2000). Continuous vaporisation may impede concentration and have adverse maternal effects (Tiran, 2006).
- **Other methods, e.g. acupuncture/pressure, reflexology, shiatsu, yoga, hypnosis (including self-hypnosis), sterile water blocks, homeopathic and herbal remedies.** Normally only midwives trained in these specialist areas or qualified practitioners offer these therapies. Non-pharmacological methods are notoriously difficult to evaluate by standard research methods. Acupuncture, acupressure and hypnosis have been clinically proved to work (Smith *et al.*, 2006; NICE, 2007; Smith *et al.*, 2011a; Smith *et al.*, 2011b). A Cochrane review is underway to evaluate the effects of 0.1ml intradermal water injection (Derry *et al.*, 2011). Anecdotal accounts of interventions e.g. hypnobirthing yield extraordinary stories (http://www.hypnobirthing.co.uk).

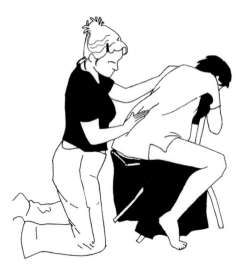

Fig. 1.2   Hands on comfort: massage and touch.

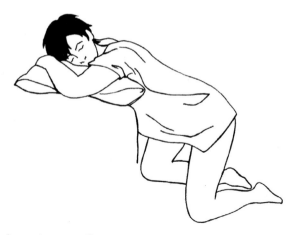

Fig. 1.3   Kneeling forwards onto a pillow.

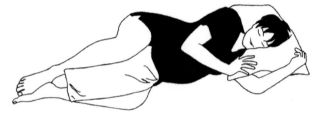

Fig. 1.4   Side lying.

- **Water.** Deep-water immersion has unique benefits. The opportunity to labour in water should be part of routine labour care. See Chapter 7.

Pharmacological analgesia

- **Entonox (nitrous oxide):** the most commonly used labour analgesic in the UK. There is little evidence on fetal/maternal effects; it appears fairly safe. Side effects are minor, e.g. dry mouth or nausea, but it is quickly excreted so effects wear off rapidly. Long-term exposure risks are well documented, including risk to pregnant staff with high labour ward workloads (Robertson, 2006).
- **Opioids, e.g. pethidine, diamorphine:** usually given intramuscularly (IM) but occasionally by patient-controlled analgesia. Antiemetics should be given prophylactically with opioids (NICE, 2007). Opioids can 'take the edge off' the pain for some women, inducing a feeling of well-being and allowing some rest. Many midwives recount stories of anxious, scared women who, on receiving pethidine, fall into a doze and wake up fully dilated. Arguably, this 'emotional dystocia' (Simkin and Ancheta, 2005) can be addressed in other ways, e.g. good caring support. There are considerable doubts about effectiveness of opioids and concern about potential maternal, fetal and neonatal side-effects. Maternal side-effects include nausea, vomiting and hypertension (Ullman *et al.*, 2010). Some women feel disorientated and out of control. Neonatal side effects include respiratory depression (which may require injection of the antagonist naloxone), subdued behaviour patterns, including a lack of responsiveness to sights and sounds, drowsiness and impaired early breastfeeding (NICE, 2007). Babies of mothers receiving opiates in labour appear more likely to become addicted to opiates/amphetamines in later life (Jacobsen *et al.*, 1988, 1990; Nyberg *et al.*, 2000).
- **Regional anaesthesia (epidural, spinal or combination)** aims to remove pain altogether from the lower half of the body, and is used by around a third of UK women for birth (NHS Maternity Statistics, 2007). Patient controlled analgesia using a pump connected via the epidural catheter gives women control and reduces breakthrough pain.
  - *Epidural anaesthesia*: administration of local anaesthetic and/or opiates into the epidural space around the spinal column
  - *Spinal anaesthesia*: an opiate, and sometimes anaesthetic drug injected through the covering of the spinal cord; faster and usually short-acting
  - *Combined epidural–spinal anaesthesia*: quicker (NICE, 2007) but gives no better pain relief than epidural alone (Simmons *et al.*, 2007).

For many women regional anaesthesia provides welcome relief from pain; if labour is complicated and/or slow, the risks may be of little consequence at the time. Women should be aware of those risks however (NICE, 2007): e.g. pyrexia, leg weakness, hypotension, poor mobility, longer labour, increased malposition, increased oxytocin augmentation and significant perineal trauma due to increased instrumental delivery (Leighton and Halpern, 2002; Lieberman and O'Donaghue, 2002; Howell, 2004, Anim-Somuah *et al.*, 2005). Cochrane review found no increase in CS, long term backache or immediate neonatal effects from epidural, although any use of opiates will result in some placental transfer, and decreased mother–baby interaction and poorer breastfeeding rates following epidural anaesthesia have been reported (Buckley, 2004b). However if a woman really wants an epidural she should be able to have one if humanly possible. Ongoing publicity about midwives denying women epidurals in the belief that all women should give birth naturally, reflects a breakdown in communication between mother and midwife (http://www.birthtraumaassociation.org.uk/).

Increasingly in the UK low-dose epidurals, often rather optimistically known as 'walking epidurals', are being offered. These are intended to increase mobility, allowing a woman to adopt upright positions, and occasionally to stand or walk. It is hoped that she may be able to push more actively, and an increase in vaginal deliveries has been recorded (COMET, 2001). More research is needed into other possible effects; a Cochrane review is underway to assess the effect of upright positions with an epidural in situ (Kibuka *et al.*, 2009).

Care for a woman with regional anaesthesia includes

- intravenous (IV) access, hourly sensory block check and continual pain assessment
- BP monitoring every 5 min for 15 min, particularly following establishment of block and following any bolus administration (top-up) (NICE, 2007)
- continuous CTG for 30 min following establishment of block and following bolus (top up) (NICE, 2007)
- regular position changes and non-supine (NICE, 2007), side lying or all fours position (if possible) (Downe, 2004) with attention to pressure areas
- bladder care: in/out or continuous catheter; and
- avoidance of aortocaval compression.

Some epidurals provide only partial pain relief or none at all (Agaram *et al.*, 2009). A woman in this situation needs particular support. She may feel panicky and out of control. A midwife may have to be a very strong advocate for her; recalling the anaesthetist, possibly a more senior one. Sometimes little can be done, and the midwife will need to give great emotional support to a disappointed distressed women.

Mobility and positions

'Get her off the bed' (RCM, 2010).

Midwives are the major influence on whether a woman is free to mobilise. Actively encouraging mobilisation during labour is a fundamental component of good midwifery practice and is a safe, cost-effective way of reducing complications caused by restricted mobility and semi-recumbent postures, as well as enriching the woman's birth experience. Cochrane review found that upright positions shorten the first stage by around an hour, and reduce epidural use (Lawrence *et al.*, 2009).

Women's expectations of how to behave in labour, unfamiliar surroundings, the labour room bed, lack of privacy and medicalised care models, all inhibit mobility in labour. Most women labouring upright say they would do the same again; those labouring supine would prefer to be upright for a subsequent labour/birth (MIDIRS, 2007). However, 20% women report they were not enabled to choose the most comfortable position in labour (Redshaw *et al.*, 2007).

'Think about how you can help the woman to adopt other positions in labour – observe what works and what doesn't, and review when and why these positions were most successful.

Your knowledge of anatomy can also help you to understand how different positions aid the physiological processes (e.g., the curve of Carus)' (RCM, 2005).

Try to witness other midwives or ask a colleague for support when the mother is giving birth in an unfamiliar non-supine position.

- Have you discussed with the woman in labour why it is important to mobilise in labour? By pointing out that labour is more likely to be shorter and less painful, you will give her 'permission' to move around freely and do what she feels is best for her.
- Women often get stuck on the bed following an examination or during electronic fetal monitoring (EFM). Suggest that she changes position or walks out to the toilet.
- Mind your back. Avoid twisting: try to be square to the woman, perhaps temporarily kneeling or squatting, depending on your preference and the mother's position.

Transition

Towards the end of the first stage contractions may become almost continuous or, conversely, space out a little. Many women may have a bearing down sensation at the peak of the contraction as the cervix approaches full dilatation. This stage may be the most painful and distressing. It can last a few contractions, but for some women it lasts much longer. Labour stress hormones peak; this has a positive effect in producing the surge of energy shortly needed to push (Odent, 1999; Buckley, 2004a).

'The diagnosis of the transitional stage . . . is a far more women-centred and subjective skill . . . essentially a midwifery observation and as such is dependent on knowing the woman . . . and recognising any changes in her behaviour. Progress can thus be diagnosed without the need to resort to a VE' (Mander, 2002).

The woman experiencing the 'extreme pain' of transition has a decreased ability to listen or concentrate on anything but giving birth. She becomes honest in vocalising her needs and dislikes, 'unfettered by politeness' (Leap, 2000)! This should not be misinterpreted by the midwife or birth partner as rejection or rudeness.

Typical behaviour may include:

- distressed/panicky statements: 'I want to go home!', 'Get me a caesarean/epidural!', 'I've changed my mind!';
- non-verbal sounds: groaning/shouting, involuntary pushing sounds;
- body language: agitated, restless, toes curling, closed eyes due to intense concentration and pain (Leap, 2000);
- withdrawing from activities/conversation of people around (Leap, 2000; Burvill, 2002).

Midwifery care in transition

Support birth partners. They can become tired, be stressed and want something done to help the woman. This common reaction sometimes leads to inappropriately timed analgesia, e.g. epidural (Mander, 2002), with subsequent discovery of a fully dilated cervix. It can be a difficult judgement call for the midwife.

Keep it calm. Change the dynamics if the women panics; e.g. suggest a walk to the toilet, a position change or focus on her breathing.

Avoid the temptation of VE. Unless the woman really wants it, VE is likely to yield disappointment: at this stage it is painful and the cervix is often 8–9 cm dilated (Lemay, 2000).

To push or not to push? Telling women that they must not push when they cannot stop themselves at the end of the first stage is unnecessary and distressing for the woman (Sleep *et al.*, 2000). The belief that pushing on an undilated cervix will cause an oedematous cervix is based on very limited evidence (Perez-Botella and Downe, 2006). 20% of women, irrespective of parity experience an early pushing urge. Downe *et al.* (2008) found that those with the urge had a better chance of a spontaneous normal birth than those who didn't.

Second stage of labour

This is traditionally defined as the stage from full cervical dilation until the baby has been born. Usually, the actual time of onset is uncertain (Walsh, 2000b) as it is technically defined by VE. Long (2006) suggests 'redefining the second stage, so that the emphasis is placed on descent and station of the presenting part instead of cervical dilation'.

Lemay (2000) describes the majority of a primigravida's pushing phase as 'shaping of the head' rather than 'descent of the head':

> *'Each expulsive sensation shapes the head of the baby to conform to the contours of the mother's pelvis. This can take time and . . . often . . . is erroneously interpreted as "lack of descent", "arrest" or "failure to progress". I tell mothers at this time, "It's normal to feel like the baby is stuck. The baby's head is elongating and getting shaped a little more with each sensation. It will suddenly feel like it has come down".'*

Characteristics of second stage

The woman may experience/exhibit the following:

- **Vomiting,** often with contractions.
- **Show** or bright red vaginal loss.
- **Spontaneous rupture of the membranes** can occur any time but often at full dilatation.
- **Urge to push.** Powerful, expulsive contractions every 2–3 minutes, often lasting ≥60 seconds. Most women make a distinctive throaty expulsive sound at the peak of a contraction. Others may groan: 'I'm *push*ing!' This urge may precede full dilatation or occur some time afterwards.
- **Rectal pressure.** The descending presenting part exerts great pressure on the bowel. The woman often feels she needs to have her bowels opened and may do so.
- **External signs,** e.g. anal dilatation, bulging perineum, gaping vagina (see Figure 1.5).

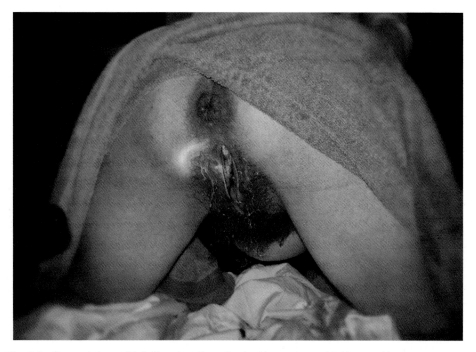

Fig. 1.5 External signs of full dilatation. *Photo by Joy Horner (www.birthjoy.co.uk).*

Midwifery care in second stage

Duration of second stage

The NICE (2007) guidelines are more flexible than previous national guidelines, although others challenge second-stage time limits if there is progress and no fetal/maternal concern, suggesting no link between time per se and poor neonatal outcome (Sleep *et al.*, 2000; Walsh, 2000b). Some evidence suggests maternal morbidity increases >3 hours second stage (Cheung *et al.*, 2004) but there is also known maternal morbidity with the alternative: i.e. instrumental delivery (Sleep *et al.*, 2000; Dupuis *et al.*, 2004).

NICE (2007) suggests:

- Delay pushing for women with epidurals for at least one hour after full dilatation unless the head is visible or the woman has an urge to push: birth should take place within 4 hours.
- Perform a VE after an hour of 'active second stage' for nulliparous women, then offer ARM if membranes intact, and consider further analgesia.
- If no birth after 2 active hours (or 1 hour for multigravidae), then obstetric review every 15 min if no fetal well-being concerns: do not start oxytocin.
- Instrumental delivery after 3 hours of active pushing for a nulliparous woman and 2 hours for a multiparous woman.

Walsh (2000a) suggests that only allowing an extra hour before pushing if women have epidurals is illogical, since many women without epidurals may need to rest semi-recumbent for a while before pushing, and many writers including Odent (2000) suggest that it is not full dilatation that makes women want to push: it is the descent of the head to the pelvic floor. Odent believes the true role of the midwife in the second stage is to protect the woman, to allow the fetus ejection reflex to be triggered.

Rightly or wrongly, midwives have been known to 'fudge' VE results in the face of restrictive policies, claiming that a woman has an anterior lip, to allow her more time without intervention.

Vaginal examination. It has become the norm for full dilatation to be confirmed by VE. It should not be automatic, particularly for multigravidae or if external signs are evident.

Monitoring the fetal heat rate. NICE (2007) recommends auscultation every 5 minutes in the second stage following a contraction. As the baby descends the FH can be difficult to locate and monitoring may feel invasive/uncomfortable. Early decelerations are more common in the second stage due to head compression, sometimes becoming variable, late or leading to bradycardia due to cord compression (see Chapter 3).

Pushing

Bergstrom *et al.* (1997) ask, 'Why does the clinician's definition of second stage take precedent, regardless of what the woman's body is instinctively doing?'

Bergstrom *et al.* describe how midwives expend great energy discouraging a woman from pushing prior to confirmation of full dilatation, and then coerce her into exaggerated active pushing once full dilatation is confirmed. As stated earlier, there is no evidence that cervical swelling occurs with premature pushing (Walsh, 2000b) and active pushing is known to do more harm than good (see also Chapter 2, 'Anterior lip', page 45).

Enable spontaneous involuntary pushing. Women simply push as they wish; most take a short breath, hold their breath for up to 6 seconds as they bear down and then give an expiratory grunt (Thomson, 1995). They may give multiple short pushes with a contraction.

Push only when ready. Women naturally push as the contraction builds up and the urge is present. The earliest part of the contraction pulls the vagina taut, preventing it from being pushed down in front of the descending presenting part (Gee and Glynn, 1997).

Forced pushing (valsalva). Directed, prolonged breath-holding/bearing down (Sleep *et al.*, 2000), particularly if held for ten seconds or more, can result in FH abnormalities, lower Apgars, perineal trauma, episiotomy, instrumental birth (Thomson, 1995; Sleep *et al.*, 2000; Lemos *et al.*, 2011), pelvic dysfunction and urinary incontinence (Schaffer *et al.*, 2005).

Try stopping pushing or even trying to 'suck the baby back in' for a few contractions if pushing feels ineffective: paradoxically (perhaps it is psychological) some women find that this increases their pushing urge (Lemay, 2000).

Pushing with an epidural. Many women do not experience a pushing urge and may need more direction. Delaying pushing for 1-2 hours (Roberts *et al.*, 2004) and allowing a 3–4-hour second stage (NICE, 2007), may help achieve a normal delivery and avoid complications (Simpson and James, 2005). Discontinuing the epidural can be distressing for the woman and does not increase the spontaneous birth rate (Torvaldsen *et al.*, 2004).

Slow progress may be normal for that woman or problematic (see Chapter 9).

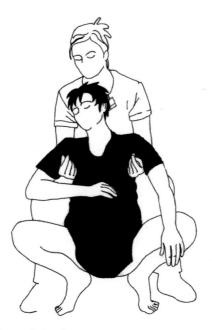

Fig. 1.6   Supported squat (second stage).

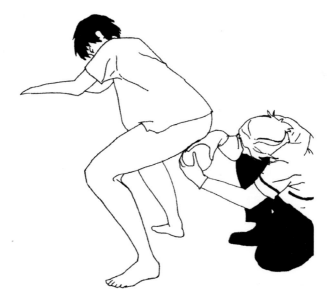

Fig. 1.7   Standing/hanging from a bed (second stage).

Verbal support. Speak soothingly, give simple explanations and praise the woman for doing so well. Insincere, over-effusive praise sounds false. Most midwives instinctively know the right thing to say and when to say it.

Birthing positions. Squatting, kneeling or side-lying, as opposed to lying semi-recumbent, increases the maximum pelvic outlet significantly. Gravity-enhancing up-right positions (Figures 1.1, 1.3, 1.5, 1.6 and 1.7) appear less painful and may shorten the second stage compared with supine or lithotomy positions which increase fetal heart anomalies, dystocia, episiotomy and instrumental delivery (Gupta *et al.*, 2012; RCM, 2005). Side-lying appears to reduce perineal trauma the most, while squatting may increase it (Shorten *et al.*, 2002; Bedwell, 2006). Blood loss appears higher following upright birth (Gupta *et al.*, 2012), but this may be due to the ease of measuring blood loss when upright. Upright positions may also benefit the perineum in making episiotomies difficult to perform (Albers *et al.*, 2005): as a result there are more second-degree tears instead (Gupta *et al.*, 2012). Many women instinctively take up the position that feels right for them if encouraged to do so.

Amazingly a survey of 25 000 mothers in England found that only 13% gave birth in an active position, i.e. standing, squatting or kneeling (CQC, 2010). Over half the women experiencing normal deliveries gave birth lying down (54%), while 16% of 'normal' births occurred in stirrups, something which shocked the NCT: ... 'it seems we have gone back in time to the 'production line' approach where ... active birth is not promoted despite all the known benefits' (Phipps, quoted by Duff, 2011). Most midwives will admit that occasionally trying a semi-recumbent position – even stirrups – will sometimes shift a baby that is stuck, and there is no position that is per se undesirable. We have all also seen women who labour in an upright position then suddenly turn on their back to give birth. However it would be straining good sense to suggest a 13% upright birth rate reflects good practice.

The birth

As the birth approaches the perineum bulges, the vagina gapes and the anus flattens. Often the woman opens her bowels when pushing. The presenting part becomes visible, advancing with contractions. The 'fetal ejection reflex', a surge of birth hormones, including oxytocin and catecholamines, increases the energy needed to expel the baby (Odent, 2000). The woman may cry out as she feels the stretching, burning sensation of the stretching perineum. She may be immensely focused or, conversely, may panic, and writhe around, maybe even resisting pushing because of the pain.

Low lighting and privacy. There is no justification for putting on bright fluorescent lights. They are harsh and likely to cause a stress reaction, inhibiting natural oxytocin production. Birthing mammals tend to prefer darker environments and need nests where they feel safe (Johnston, 2004). A light source near the perineum may reassure some midwives who wish to view the perineum, but continual staring and focusing on the perineum and/or the woman's face may put her under pressure and make her feel exposed. This can feel particularly voyeuristic for sexual abuse victims (Kitzinger, 1992). Also consider the baby: the transition from womb to outside world is likely to be quite a shock as it is, without a bright light shining into its eyes.

Reassurance. This can be a key moment where trust between midwife and woman staves off panic. A calm voice telling her she is nearly there, that she can do it, can help get her through this most challenging of episodes. Try to minimise noise: the mother may sob, grunt, moan or even scream at the point of birth, but there is a big difference between a woman's need to cry out and the cacophony of shouting and exhorting that birth supporters sometimes create. While there is occasionally a place for an energy injection from onlookers, midwives need to be very skilled to avoid the woman feeling shrieked at by tense carers. Imagine the difference for the baby if it is born into a peaceful room, perhaps with its mother's or father's voice the first that it hears.

Warm moist compresses may be soothing and have been found to reduce perineal pain and the incidence of severe trauma (Aasheim, 2011). Some women may prefer a cool compress.

Perineal massage in labour is invasive and appears ineffective; NICE (2007) recommends avoiding it in the second stage. This is again for the woman to decide: some find any perineal touch excruciating now.

Episiotomy is performed much less often these days: around 20% of UK births (ONS, 2012). Some clinicians do none at all. It is justified only for suspected fetal compromise (Sleep *et al.*, 2000) or some instrumental deliveries (NICE, 2007). It should not be routinely offered for a previous third/fourth-degree tear as it confers no protection (NICE, 2007). Avoid in your impatience classifying an uncomplicated slow delivery as a 'rigid perineum' – this is rare. Even if you think the perineum is about to tear, there is more chance of an intact perineum if you wait and see. Cochrane review suggests restrictive episiotomy reduces perineal trauma, suturing and complications, doesn't affect pain measures or severe vaginal/perineal trauma, but increases risk of anterior perineal trauma. The benefits of midline versus mediolateral episiotomy are unclear (Carroli and Mignini, 2009), although NICE (2007) recommends mediolateral (with tested effective analgesia – unless in an emergency).

Head awareness. The woman may wish to touch her baby's head or watch in a mirror as she pushes. Some women find this encouraging, while others absolutely do not want to touch or watch.

Slow birth. Controlled pushing of the crowning head between contractions appears to reduce perineal trauma (Albers *et al.*, 2005): also a calm relaxed atmosphere may help (Jackson, 2000). At the point of crowning some midwives encourage gentle shallow breaths and slow small pushes.

Hands on or poised? Whether midwives put hands on (flexing the head and touching the perineum with the other hand) or off (both hands off but poised to prevent the baby emerging rapidly) does not appear to significantly affect perineal trauma (McCandlish *et al.*, 1998; Caroci and Riesco, 2006; NICE, 2007). Neither appears to do harm so this is an individual decision.

Await restitution. While some babies deliver quickly, most await the next contraction for the shoulders to rotate into the anteroposterior diameter, as the baby's head appears to turn. With the next contraction (or earlier) the shoulders should gently emerge. This final contraction may take ≥ 2 min to arrive. Beware of overdiagnosing shoulder dystocia (see Chapter 17). Two minutes can seem like a long wait. Resist the urge to apply traction before the next contraction.

Checking for cord. This is often painful, usually unnecessary and may cause posterior wall tearing (MacLellan and Lang, 2011). Unless the baby seems slow to deliver, untangle any nuchal cord after the birth (ARM, 2000). If the cord (not an impacted shoulder) genuinely seems to be preventing delivery then clamp and cut, but remember you have now removed the baby's oxygen supply; birth should be imminent to prevent neonatal compromise.

The moment of birth (Figures 1.8 and 1.9). Do not rush to deliver the body; perineal damage can occur with a shoulder or a hand. A gentle unhurried birth of the body is just as important as the head. The mother or father may wish to put their hands down as well and feel the baby birthing. The midwife should already have checked that the

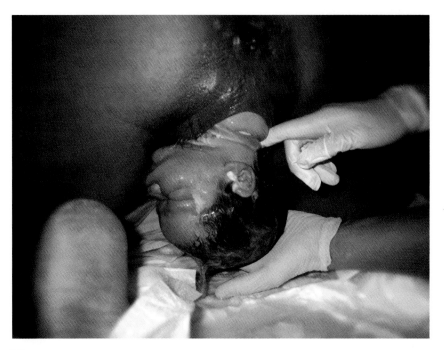

Fig. 1.8

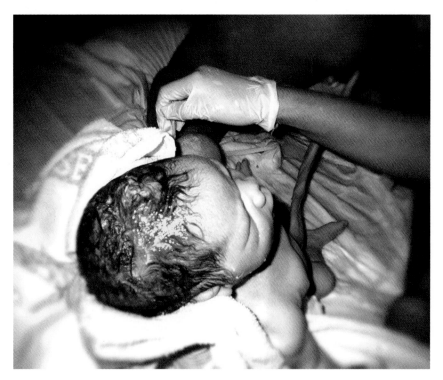

Fig. 1.9

Box 1.4   The benefits of skin-to-skin contact.

Immediate skin-to-skin (SSC) contact between mother and baby appears to
- Improve mother and baby interaction at birth
- Keep babies warmer
- Decrease infant crying
- Improve neonatal heartrate and respiratory stability
- Make breastfeeding more likely, and improves duration of breastfeeding
- Probably improve the early relationship between mothers and babies
- There appear to be no short-term or long-term negative effects.

(Moore *et al.*, 2012)

It also appears to help maintain neonatal blood sugar: failure to offer SSC or early breastfeeding may be one reason why too many babies of diabetic mothers are admitted to NICU (CEMACH, 2007).

Benefits of fathers offering SSC
- Fathers offering SSC to preterm babies felt earlier positive feelings towards them (Sullivan, 1999)
- Babies given SSC with their fathers following CS cry less and appear calmer (Erlandsson *et al.*, 2007)

Preterm babies appear to benefit too! See Chapter 13.

mother is happy to have her baby put straight into her arms for immediate skin-to-skin contact (see Box 1.4). Occasionally, parents are squeamish in advance about wet bloodstained babies, but the reality is usually quite different. Most women will reach out instinctively to their baby.

Third stage of labour

There are two options for assisting the third stage of labour: (a) physiological (expectant) management or (b) active management. There are various controversies around both methods.

- NICE (2007) recommends **active management** with **early cord clamping**, but states that women requesting physiological management should be supported. The World Health Organization recommends **active management** with **delayed cord clamping** (DCC) of 1–3 minutes (Begley *et al.*, 2010).
- The RCM (2012) recommends DCC of 3–5 minutes if active management is practised, while the RCOG (2009) state "the cord should not be clamped earlier than necessary, based on a clinical assessment of the situation".
- Physiological management is suitable if the woman has had a physiologically normal labour and birth (no epidural, no IV oxytocin).

Pros and cons of physiological versus active management

- Active management is usually quicker: typically 5–20 minutes versus 20–60 minutes for expectant waiting. Some women want the whole thing over with quickly so they opt for an oxytocic.

- Some women simply want a natural delivery of the placenta and dislike the idea of receiving drugs.
- Active management reduces blood loss immediately following birth, so it is advisable for anyone at significant risk of immediate postpartum haemorrhage (PPH) (Prendiville *et al.*, 2004).
- Overall blood loss by 36 hours is similar with active or physiological management (Wickham, 1999) so long-term effects appear similar for both methods. No-one really knows what is an optimal blood loss immediately following birth.
- Cochrane review found active management increases the risk of later readmission with bleeding, and increases oxytocin side-effects, i.e. headache, nausea, vomiting and severe afterpains (Liabsuetrakul *et al.*, 2007; Begley *et al.*, 2010).
- Neither method appears to have any significant ill effects on the baby (Prendiville and Elbourne, 2000; Begley *et al.*, 2010).

All midwives should be knowledgeable about both methods of third stage management. Some lack experience/confidence in physiological management, having assisted few physiological third stages and have never really learned what to do – and what, more importantly, not to do.

Physiological third stage (expectant management)

If the woman has had a positive birth followed by unhurried, quality contact with her newborn, this will facilitate oxytocin release (Odent, 1999), which stimulates uterine muscle contraction. Breastfeeding and/or nipple stimulation will also increase natural oxytocin. The woman may use her contractions, upright postures and maternal pushing efforts to aid placenta delivery, or it may just suddenly emerge.

Midwifery care for a physiological third stage

The key to good support is 'watchful waiting'. If all appears well then resist the urge to intervene! An anxious clock-watching midwife is likely to unsettle the woman and interfere with oxytocin release.

Do not

- Administer an oxytocic (unless there is heavy bleeding: if so, proceed to active management).
- Repeatedly palpate the uterus ('fundal fiddling'!). This is painful, causes poor contractility and increases PPH risk.
- Apply cord traction.
- Clamp the maternal end of the cord. If mother and baby need to be separated (e.g. the mother wishes to move from a pool to deliver the placenta and/or the cord is short) Levy (1990) suggests clamping the baby's end of the cord and then cutting, leaving the maternal end of the cord free to bleed into a bowl. Indeed recent Cochrane review (Soltani *et al.*, 2011) suggests that there may be benefits to *routinely* cutting the cord and allowing the maternal end to drain, but this is by no means accepted practice at present. It seems wise to recommend cord cutting only if essential during physiological management , in view of the possible benefits to the

baby of delayed cord clamping. If planning to cut the cord, wait until it has stopped pulsating so that the baby receives plenty of maternal blood, unless the situation is urgent. If the cord has to be cut quickly for whatever reason, there may be a benefit in milking the cord (two or three times along the whole length of the cord towards the baby) before clamping to increase neonatal blood volume expansion and haematocrit and haemoglobin levels (Mercer and Erikson-Owens, 2010).

Do

- Encourage skin-to-skin contact.
- Encourage breastfeeding to increase oxytocin levels (consider nipple self-stimulation if not).
- Keep the mother warm and comfortable; avoid loud noise and bright lights.

Watch blood loss and observe for signs of separation, e.g.:

- Cord lengthening
- Trickle of blood/small clots
- The woman may groan, feel a contraction or (sometimes slight) pushing urge
- Visible placenta at vagina.

Assist her to an upright posture, e.g. kneeling, squatting or sitting: gravity will help her birth the placenta.

Push with a contraction; expulsive efforts are usually more effective then.

If the placenta does not emerge after several attempts, relax and wait before trying again. Try changing position:

'Sure enough, the moment I moved, out it came – masterfully caught by a midwife with a kidney dish and reflexes a rattlesnake would be proud of' (Brenda (mother) http://www.homebirth.org.uk/thirdstage.htm 2012).

A quiet darkened room may reduce stress hormones and increase oxytocin production. Some midwives, especially at home, encourage the mother to sit on the toilet with the lights dimmed; perhaps the one place where a woman feels truly private and undisturbed. If the woman has tried pushing, utilising gravity, changing position, breastfeeding and passing urine, you may wish to check that the placenta has actually separated: a gentle VE may reveal the partially/totally separated placenta in the os or vagina.

If the placenta is slow, but there is no heavy bleeding, then encourage the baby to nuzzle and feed at the breast. Encourage the woman to relax . . . and try to do the same.

Most women (95%) deliver the placenta within one hour of physiological third stage (NICE, 2007); multiparous women average 20 minutes (Begley, 1990). There is little good evidence to guide midwives in the safe time to wait for the placenta, as most PPH studies look only at active management. NICE (2007) recommends proceeding to active management (oxytocic + cord traction) after one hour, citing one study suggesting PPH risk rises after 30 minutes, peaking at 75 minutes with both active and physiological management (Combs and Laros, 1991), but this old US data (i.e. 1976–1985) may not be applicable to current UK physiological management.

Active management of the third stage of labour

Active management usually achieves placenta delivery within 10–15 minutes of birth. Initial blood loss is reduced (Prendiville and Elbourne, 2000; Begley *et al.*, 2010).

- **Give a prophylactic oxytocic** after delivery of the anterior shoulder or following birth. Syntometrine (ergometrine-oxytocin) is commonly used: Cochrane review suggests it reduces blood loss of 500–1000 ml (but not >1000 ml) more effectively than oxytocin alone (McDonald *et al.*, 2004) but has side-effects of hypotension, nausea and vomiting. NICE (2007) recommends oxytocin (Syntocinon) 10 IU IM, stating it appears as effective as syntometrine at preventing haemorrhage and re-duces the likelihood of retained placenta.

Box 1.5   Benefits of delayed cord clamping (DCC).

Some prefer the expression 'physiological cord clamping' as 'delay' implies that immediate cord clamping is normal, and a 'delay' a deviation from the norm (Main, 2012). We use 'DCC' – with reservations – here, as most research uses it.

- DCC expands neonatal blood volume by 20–50%, increasing neonatal haemoglobin and haematocrit (Prendiville & Elbourne, 2000; Mercer & Erikson-Owens, 2010). Iron deficiency at 4 months of age is significantly reduced by DCC of three minutes or more with no increased risk of jaundice (Andersson et al., 2011).
- DCC may reduce fetomaternal transfusion, benefiting rhesus negative mothers delivering rhesus positive babies (Prendiville & Elbourne, 2000).
- DCC particularly benefits babies in developing countries, reducing anaemia, which is more common there (NICE, 2007) but Andersson (2011) suggests that the benefit to babies born even in countries with low anaemia prevalence means that DCC should be universal.
- Current UK Resuscitation Council (UKRC) guidelines recommend DCC for *at least* 1 minute, or until the cord stops pulsating; also for vigorous preterm babies who benefit more, so should have a longer DCC period than term babies (Richmond & Wiley, 2010).
- Possible small increase in jaundice (Hutton & Hassan, 2007; McDonald & Middleton, 2008) although increased need for phototherapy outweighed by other benefits. Other meta-analyses suggest no increase in symptomatic polycythaemia/jaundice (Vento *et al.*, 2009).
- DCC can be performed after CS with the baby on the mother's legs or chest (Cernadas *et al.*, 2006).
- DCC may benefit a baby requiring resuscitation (NLS, 2010). Why cut off a major source of oxygen to an already compromised baby? Consider leaving the cord uncut initially, bringing the ambubag to the mother and baby; give the recommended first 90 seconds of inflation in air on the bed/floor in front of the mother. Paradoxically the compromised baby is usually the quickest to be whisked away from its mother to a resuscitaire: arguably these babies benefit most from DCC.
- Milking the cord towards the baby before clamping may help if early separation is necessary, e.g. for continued resuscitation (Mercer & Erikson-Owens, 2010).
- Some believe that placing the baby lower than the mother significantly increases mother–baby blood flow (for good or ill) but little evidence supports/refutes this (Airey *et al.*, 2010).

- **Clamp and cut the cord.** Some mistakenly believe the cord should be clamped immediately, even prior to giving an oxytocic, to avoid neonatal overtransfusion, leading to jaundice. It is sad to see inexperienced staff frantically trying to close a cord clamp in the quickest possible time, with shaking hands, as if something terrible is about to happen if that cord is not clamped! This is a misconception. Firstly, if Syntocinon has been given IM as NICE suggests, which may take more than 2 minutes to take effect through an intramuscular route (Crafter, 2002), then clamping the cord before two minutes is mixing physiological and active management, and, at the very least, unnecessary. Secondly, there is ample evidence that delayed cord clamping (DCC), even after early oxytocic administration, is beneficial: see Box 1.5. Main (2012) points out that the baby has received continual maternal-fetal transfusion with labour contractions, up to 500 ml every 2–3 minutes (Ndala, 2007) so an additional transfusion following birth is unlikely to be excessive.

- Once the decision has been taken to finally cut the cord, Cochrane review suggests **unclamping the maternal end** and allowing it to drain into a bowl reduces the length of the third stage, and slightly reduces blood loss (Soltani *et al.*, 2011).
- **Deliver the placenta by controlled cord traction.** while guarding the uterus with the other hand, typically several minutes after the administration of the oxytocic. Many midwives wait for placental separation first, i.e. a small gush of blood indicating that the placenta has sheared off the uterine wall, as traction prior to separation is believed to cause pain and risk haemorrhage.
- **Retained placenta.** NICE (2007) defines a 'prolonged third stage' as an undelivered placenta after 30 minutes active management since PPH risk increases after this time. It may be necessary to proceed to manual removal of placenta (MROP) under regional or general anaesthesia, although there is some interesting evidence that oral tocolytics e.g. nitroglycerin tablets may reduce the need for MROP (Abdel-Aleem *et al.*, 2011). (See Chapter 16 for PPH management/MROP.)

Possible third-stage problems (physiological or active management)

The placenta is delivered, but the membranes remain stuck:

- Suggest that the mother gives a few good coughs: this usually releases the membranes and they slide out.
- It is also possible to gently twist the placenta round and move it up and down, to coax the membranes out (Davis, 1997).

Bleeding is heavy, gushing or continuous:

- Rub up a contraction.
- Administer oxytocic: local policy may apply. Syntocinon may be preferable to Syntometrine/ergometrine if the placenta is still in situ as the latter cause the cervical os to close (Crafter, 2002) but ergometrine is faster acting; consider IV administration if giving Syntocinon.
- Refer to Chapter 16 for full PPH management.

Following delivery of the placenta

Check the uterus is well contracted and blood loss normal. Examine the placenta: some women are fascinated by their placenta and wish to watch.

After the birth

Immediately after the birth. Women's reactions vary enormously. Some may enjoy being congratulated: others are in their own new world at this point and simply do not know the midwife exists. Stand back: let her or her birth partner explore the baby to discover the sex; resist the urge to talk loudly or take control unless it is clear that guidance is wanted. Feel free to smile a huge smile!

The baby. Babies are individuals too and may have had a hard birth. Some gaze calmly around: others cry pitifully and need lots of comfort. Mothers instinctively use a unique high soothing voice to their newborn.

Babies are vulnerable to heat loss. Keep the baby snuggled up with its mother and/or birth partner for skin-to-skin contact for as long as they want. A warm hat and blanket over the outside of the mother and baby will keep them both warm. For babies needing **resuscitation** see Chapter 18.

For **examination of the newborn** see Chapter 5.

Breastfeeding. As with labour, it is important for midwives to 'sit on their hands' at this point: try to minimise interruption, giving the mother and baby space to explore each other. Most babies are very alert immediately after a natural birth. They will readily root towards the breast, nuzzle, lick and suckle when they are ready. The first hour after birth is a special time. Some animals are known not to attach to their young unless they are able to lick and smell them immediately after birth (Buckley, 2004b).

Examine the perineum (see Chapter 4) for trauma when the woman is ready. Many will want this to be over as soon as possible so that they can relax and enjoy their baby.

Offer analgesia. Multigravid women, in particular, can experience strong afterpains, and all women are vulnerable to perineal and rectal pain, even with an intact perineum. Excessive perineal pain may indicate a haematoma (see Chapter 16).

Records. Carefully record the birth. Computer details are usually also required. This gives the opportunity for a physical and psychological break for the midwife who may have been under intense pressure for some hours. Most parents relish being left on their own to explore and enjoy their baby. Others may prefer to have a midwife hovering. Most of the paperwork can be done in the room so be flexible.

Think about the birth partner. They can feel exhausted, overwhelmed and even traumatised by experiencing birth. Congratulate them on their support; show that you realise their needs are important. Remember they, like their partner, may need time later to recount their story.

Offer food and drink. There is nothing like the smell of tea and toast in the middle of the night to remind you a baby has been born.

Get her settled. The mother should not be hurried to have a bath or move to a fresh bed: some will feel the need to freshen up earlier than others. If the birth is at home, she can have all the time in the world. The 'routine' postbirth bath has become almost a ritual after birth for many midwives: many mothers (and babies) may enjoy the experience but some mothers may be too tired to want to move. It has been suggested that some shivery women may value being warmly wrapped and left for some time (Simkin and Ancheta, 2005): the cooling by evaporation that occurs following a bath may chill them further. Bathing should be optional, not routine practice.

Post-birth check. Check pulse, temperature, blood pressure, fundus and lochia. Encourage her to pass urine, within six hours of birth if possible, and measure the first void. On a busy labour ward there is often pressure to transfer the woman quickly to the postnatal area. Sometimes this is just habit, and midwives are pressured to rush even if the labour ward is quiet. Resist this coercion. Sometimes, however, it is necessary for the safety of other mothers who may need a birth room and the midwife's attention imminently. If this is necessary, consider continuing skin-to-skin contact by suggesting that the baby bathes with the mother if she wants a bath, or goes to the father for skin-to-skin contact, and/or tucks inside the mother's or father's clothes for further contact during transfer to the postnatal area.

Summary

Latent phase

- Ideally spent at home
- Women may need lots of support if prolonged

Established first stage

- Continuous midwifery support is effective analgesia
- Encourage:
  - Mobilisation and position changes
  - Regular bladder emptying, eating and drinking
  - Natural coping methods
- Observe/monitor:
  - Basic vital signs, contractions and woman's response
  - Progress/descent by palpation and VE (if required)
  - FHR intermittently unless concerns
- Avoid:
  - Unnecessary VE/ARM/other interventions
  - Arbitrary time limits

Second stage

- Monitor descent by external signs, palpation and/or VE
- Auscultate FHR intermittently unless concerns
- Encourage:
  - Upright posture, non-directed pushing
  - Low lighting, privacy
  - Slow, gentle birth, immediate SSC
- Avoid:
  - Non-indicated episiotomy
  - Arbitrary time limits

Third stage

- Physiological management:
  - Leave cord unclamped (or cut and leave maternal end unclamped).
  - Encourage SSC and breastfeeding.
  - Deliver by maternal effort. Hands off!

- Active management:
  - ○ Give oxytocic: NICE recommends syntocinon 10 IU IM.
  - ○ Consider DCC for at least 3–5 minutes or until cord stops pulsating.
  - ○ Controlled cord traction with fundal guarding.

Useful contacts and information

An amazing video on life from conception to birth using scanning technology that won its inventors the Nobel Peace Prize. http://www.youtube.com/watch_popup?v=fKyljukBE70

Association for Improvements in the Maternity Services (AIMS). www.aims.org.uk

Doulas UK. www.doula.org.uk

Maternity Care Working Party (2007) Making Normal Birth a Reality. Consensus statement from the Maternity Care Working Party. *NCT, RCM, RCOG.* www.appg-maternity.org.uk

National Childbirth Trust (NCT). www.nct-online.org

Nursing and Midwifery Council (NMC). www.nmc-uk.org

Royal College of Midwives (RCM). www.rcm.org.uk

RCM position paper on normal birth (2010): www.rcm.org.uk/college/policy-practice/guidelines/rcm-position-statements/position-statements/

References

Aasheim, V., Nilsen, A. B. V., Lukasse, M., Reinar, L. M. (2011) Perineal techniques during the second stage of labour for reducing perineal trauma. *Cochrane Database of Systematic Reviews* Issue 12.

Abdel-Aleem, H., Abdel-Aleem, M. A., Shaaban, O. M. (2001) Tocolysis for management of retained placenta. *Cochrane Database of Systematic Reviews*, Issue 1.

Agaram, R., McTaggart, R. A., Gunka, V. (2009) Inadequate pain relief with labour epidurals: a multivariate analysis of associated factors. *Journal of Obstetric Anaesthesia* 18(1), 10–4.

Airey, R., Farrar, D., Duley, L. (2010) Alternative positions for the baby at birth before clamping the umbilical cord. *Cochrane Database of Systematic Reviews*, Issue 10.

Albers, L., Sedler, K., Bedrick, E., Teaf, D. Peralta, P. (2005) Midwifery care measures in the second stage of labour and reduction of genital tract trauma at birth: a randomised trial. *Journal of Midwifery and Women's Health* 50, 563–72.

Andersson, O., Hellström-Westas, L., Andersson, D., Domellöf, M. (2011) Effect of delayed versus early umbilical cord clamping on neonatal outcomes and iron status at 4 months: a randomised controlled trial. *BMJ* 343, d7157.

Anim-Somuah, M., Smyth, R., Howell, C. (2005) Epidural versus non-epidural or no analgesia in labour. *Cochrane Database of Systematic Reviews*, Issue 4.

Association of Radical Midwives (ARM) (2000) Association of Radical Midwives Nettalk: checking for cord. *Midwifery Matters* 87, 28–30.

Basevi, V., Lavender, T. (2001) Routine perineal shaving on admission in labour. *Cochrane Database of Systematic Reviews*, Issue 1.

Baston, H. (2001) Blood pressure measurement: midwifery basics. *The Practising Midwife* 4(9), 10–14.

Bedwell, C. (2006) Are third degree tears unavoidable? The role of the midwife. *British Journal of Midwifery* 14(9), 212.

Begley, C. (1990) A comparison of 'active' and 'physiological' management of the third stage of labour. *Midwifery* 63, 3–17.

Begley, C., Gyte, G., Murphy, D., Devane, D., McDonald, S., McGuire, W. (2010) Active versus expectant management for women in the third stage of labour. *Cochrane Database of Systematic Reviews*, Issue 7.

Bergstrom, L., Seedily, J., Schulman-Hull, L. *et al.* (1997) 'I gotta push. Please let me push!' Social interactions during the change from first stage to second stage of labour. *Birth* 24(3), 173–80.

BirthChoice UK *website www.birthchoiceuk.com*

Buckley, S. (2004a) Undisturbed birth – nature's hormonal blueprint for safety, ease and ecstasy. *MIDIRS Midwifery Digest* 14(2), 203–9.

Buckley, S. (2004b) What disturbs birth? *MIDIRS Midwifery Digest* 14(3), 353–7.

Buckley, S. (2010) Sexuality in labour and birth: an intimate perspective. In: Downe, S., Walsh, D. (eds) *Intrapartum Care*. Wiley-Blackwell: Oxford.

Burvill, S. (2002) Midwifery diagnosis of labour onset. *British Journal of Midwifery* 10(10), 600–5.

Care Quality Commission (CQC) (2010) *Maternity Services 2010*. www.cqc.org.uk

Caroci, A., Riesco, M. (2006) A comparison of 'hands off' vs 'hands on' for decreasing perineal lacerations during birth. *Journal of Midwifery Women's Health* 51, 106–11.

Carroli, G., Mignini, L. (2009) Episiotomy for vaginal birth. *Cochrane Database of Systematic Reviews*, Issue 1.

CMACE (Centre for Maternal and Child Enquiries) (2011) Saving Mothers' Lives: Reviewing maternal deaths to make motherhood safer: 2006–2008. The Eighth Report of the Confidential Enquiries into Maternal Deaths in the United Kingdom BJOG 118, supplement 1, 1-203. http://onlinelibrary.wiley.com/doi/10.1111/j.1471-0528.2010.02847.x/pdf

CEMACH (Confidential Enquiry into Maternal and Child Health) (2007) *Diabetes in Pregnancy: Caring for the Baby After Birth. Findings of a National Enquiry. England, Wales and Northern Ireland*. CEMACH, London. www.cemach.org.uk

Cheung, Y., Hopkins, I., Caughey, A. (2004) How long is too long: does a prolonged second stage of labour in nulliparous women affect maternal and neonatal morbidity? *American Journal of Obstetrics and Gynaecology* 191, 933–8.

Combs, C., Laros, R., Jr (1991) Prolonged third stage of labor: morbidity and risk factors. *Obstetrics and Gynecology* 77(6), 863–7.

COMET (Comparative Obstetric Mobile Epidural) Study Group UK (2001) Effect of low-dose mobile versus traditional epidural techniques on mode of delivery: a randomised controlled trial. *Lancet* 358, 19-23.

Crafter, H. (2002) Intrapartum and primary postpartum haemorrhage. In *Emergencies Around Childbirth – A Handbook for Midwives* (Boyle, M., ed.), pp. 113–26. Radcliffe Medical Press, Oxford.

Crowther, C., Enkin, M., Keirse, M., Brown, I. (2000) Monitoring progress in labor. In *A Guide to Effective Care in Pregnancy and Childbirth*, 3rd edn (Enkin, M., Keirse, M. J. N. C., Neilson, J., Crowther, C., Duley, L., Hodnett, E. and Hofmeyr, J., eds), pp. 210–18. Oxford University Press, Oxford.

Davis, E. (1997) *Hearts and Hands: A Midwife's Guide to Pregnancy and Birth*, 3rd edn. Berkeley, California, Celestial Arts.

Department of Health (DoH) (2004) *National Service Framework for Children, Young People and Maternity Services*, pp. 27–9. DoH, London.

Department of Health (DoH) (2007) *Maternity Matters: choice, access and continuity of care in a safe service*. London, DoH. www.dhgov.uk

Derry, S., Straube, S., Moore, R. A., Hancock, H., Collins, S. (2011) Intracutaneous or subcutaneous sterile water injection for relieving pain in labour (Protocol). *Cochrane Database of Systematic Reviews*.

Downe, S. (ed.) (2004) *Normal Childbirth: Evidence and Debate*. Oxford, Churchill Livingstone.

Downe, S., Young, C., Hall-Moran, S., Trent Midwifery Research Group (2008). Multiple midwifery discourses: the case of the early pushing urge. In: Downe, S. (ed.) *Normal Birth, Evidence and Debate*, 2nd edn. Oxford, Elsevier.

Dowswell, T., Bedwell, C., Lavender, T., Neilson, J. P. (2009) Transcutaneous electrical nerve stimulation (TENS) for pain management in labour. *Cochrane Database of Systematic Reviews*, Issue 2.

Duff, E. (2011) Too few women offered choice in maternity care. *Perspective (NCT journal)* June, 11.

Dupuis, O., Madelenat, P., Rudigoz, R. (2004) Faecal and unrinary incontinence and delivery: risk factors and prevention. *Gynaecology, Obstetrics and Fertility* 32, 540–48.

Erlandsson, K., Dsilna, A., Fagerberg, I., Christensson, K. (2007) Skin-to-skin care with the father after caesarean birth and its effect on newborn crying and prefeeding behaviour. *Birth* 34(2), 105–13.

ESRI (The Economic and Social Research Institute) (2011) *Perinatal Statistics Report 2009*. Health Research and Information Division, ESRI. http://www.esri.ie

Gee, H., Glynn, M. (1997) The physiology and clinical management of labour. In *Essential Midwifery*, Henderson, C., Jones, K. (eds), pp. 171–202. London, Mosby.

Green, J., Renfrew, M., Curtis, P. (2000) Continuity of carer: what matters to women? A review of the evidence. *Midwifery* 16(3), 187–96.

Gupta, J., Hofmeyr, G., Shehmar, M. (2012) Position in the second stage of labour for women without epidural anaesthesia. *Cochrane Database of Systematic Reviews*, Issue 5.

Hatem, M., Sandall, J., Devane, D., Soltani, H., Gates, S. (2008) Midwife-led vs other models of care for childbearing women. *Cochrane Database of Systematic Reviews*, Issue 4.

Healthcare Commission (2008) *Towards Better Births: a review of maternity services in England*. London: Commission of Healthcare Audit and Inspection, 35.

Hobbs, L. (1998) Assessing cervical dilatation without VEs. *The Practising Midwife* 1(11), 34–5.

Hodnett, E. D., Stremler, R., Willan, A. R., Weson, J. A., Lowe, N. K., Simpson, K. R., Fraser, D., Gafni, A. (2008) Effect on birth outcomes of a formalised approach to care in hospital labour assessment units: international, randomised controlled trial. *BMJ* 28, 337.

Hodnett, E. D., Downe, S., Walsh, D., *et al.* (2010) Alternative versus conventional institutional settings for birth. *Cochrane Database of Systematic Reviews*, Issue 9.

Hodnett, E. D., Hofmeyr, G. J., Sakala, C., Weston, J. (2011) Continuous support for women during childbirth. *Cochrane Database of Systematic Reviews*, Issue 2.

Howell, C. (2004) Epidural versus non-epidural analgesia for pain relief in labour (Cochrane Review). *Cochrane Database of Systematic Reviews*, Issue 1.

Hutton, E. K., Hassan, E. S. (2007) Late vs early clamping of the umbilical cord in full-term neonates: systematic review and meta-analysis of controlled trials. *JAMA* 297, 1241–52.

Jackson, K. (2000) The bottom line: care of the perineum must be improved. *British Journal of Midwifery* 8(10), 609–14.

Jacobsen, B., Nyberg, K., Eklund, G., Bygdeman, M., Rydberg, U. (1988) Obstetric pain medication and eventual adult amphetamine addiction in offspring. *Acta Obstetrica et Gynecologica* 67, 677–82.

Jacobsen, B., Nyberg, K., Gronbladh, L., Eklund, G., Bygdeman, M., Rydberg, U. (1990) Opiate addiction in adult offspring through possible imprinting after obstetric treatment. *BMJ* 301(6760), 1067–70.

Johnson, C., Keirse, M. J. N. C., Enkin, M., Chalmers, I. (2000) Hospital practices – nutrition and hydration in labor. In Enkin, M., Keirse, M. J. N. C., Neilson, J., Crowther, C., Duley, L., Hodnett, E., Hofmeyr, J. (eds) *A Guide to Effective Care in Pregnancy and Childbirth*, 3rd edn, pp. 255–66. Oxford, Oxford University Press.

Johnson, M. (1997) TENS in pain management. *British Journal of Midwifery* 5(7), 400–5.

Johnston, J. (2004) The nesting instinct. *Birth Matters Journal* 8, 21–2.

Lemos, A., Amorim, M. M. R., Dornelas de Andrade, A., de Souza, A. I., Cabral Filho, J. E., Correia, J. B. (2011) Pushing/bearing down methods for the second stage of labour (Protocol). *Cochrane Database of Systematic Reviews*, Issue 5.

Kibuka, M., Thornton, J., Kingswood, C. (2009) Position in the second stage of labour for women with epidural anaesthesia (Protocol). *Cochrane Database of Systematic Reviews*.

Kitzinger, C., Kitzinger, S. (2007) Birth trauma: talking to women and the value of conversation analysis. *British Journal of Midwifery* 15(5), 256–64.

Kitzinger, J. V. (1992) Counteracting, not re-enacting, the violation of women's bodies: the challenge for perinatal caregivers. *Birth* 19(4), 219–22.

Lauzon, L., Hodnett, E. (2001) Labour assessment programs to delay admission to labour wards *Cochrane Database of Systematic Reviews*, Issue 3.

Lavender, T., Hart, A., Smyth, R. M. D. (2008) Effect of partogram use on outcomes for women in spontaneous labour at term. *Cochrane Database of Systematic Reviews*, Issue 4.

Lawrence, A., Lewis, L., Hofmeyr, G., Dowswell, T., Styles, C. (2009) Maternal positions and mobility during first stage labour. *Cochrane Database of Systematic Reviews*, Issue 2.

Leap, N. (2000) Pain in labour. *MIDIRS Midwifery Digest* 10(1), 49–53.

Leap, N., Dodwell, M., Newburn, M. (2010) Working with pain in labour: an overview of evidence. *New Digest* 49, 22–6.

Leighton, B., Halpern, S. (2002) The effects of epidural analgesia on labor, maternal and neonatal outcomes: a systematic review. *American Journal of Obstetrics and Gynaecology* 186, 69–77.

Lemay, G. (2000) Pushing for first time moms. *Midwifery Today* 55, 9–12.

Levy, V. (1990) The midwife's management of the third stage of labour. In Alexander, J., Levy, V. and Roch, S. (eds) *Intrapartum Care 1–1 A Research Based Approach*, pp. 139–43. Basingstoke, Macmillan.

Liabsuetrakul, T., Choobun, T., Peeyananjarassri, K., Islam, Q. M. (2007) Prophylactic use of ergot alkaloids in the third stage of labour. *Cochrane Database of Systematic Reviews*, Issue 2.

Lieberman, E., O'Donaghue, C. (2002) Unintended effects of epidural analgesia in labour: a systematic review. *American Journal of Obstetrics and Gynaecology* 186, 531–68.

Long, L. (2006) Redefining the second stage of labour could help to promote normal birth. *British Journal of Midwifery* 14, 104–6.

MacLellan, J., Lang, I. (2011) Supporting the perineum: a technique from practice. *MIDIRS* Sept 21(3), 354–7.

Main, C. (2012) Changing practice: physiological cord clamping. *The Practising Midwife* Jan, 30–33.

Mainstone, A. (2004) TENS. *British Journal of Midwifery* 12(9), 578–81.

Mander, R. (2002) The transitional stage – pain and control. *The Practising Midwife* 5(1), 10–12.

McCandlish, R., Bower, U., van Asten, H., Berridge, G., Winter, C., Sames, L., Garcia, J., Renfrew, M., Elbourne, D. (1998) A randomised controlled trial of care of the perineum during the second stage of normal labour (HOOP trial). *British Journal of Obstetrics and Gynaecology* 105, 1262–72.

McDonald, S. J., Abbott, J. M., Higgins, S. P. (2004) Prophylactic ergometrine-oxytocin versus oxytocin for the third stage of labour. *Cochrane Database of Systematic Reviews,* Issue 1.

McDonald, S. J., Middleton, P. (2008) Effect of timing of umbilical cord clamping of term infants on maternal and neonatal outcomes. *Cochrane Database of Systematic Reviews,* Issue 2.

McNiven, P., Williams, J., Hodnett, E., Kaufman, H. M. (1998) An early labour assessment program: a randomised controlled trial. *Birth* 25(1), 5–10.

Mercer, J., Erikson-Owens, D. (2010) Evidence for neonatal transition and the first hour of life. In Walsh, D., Downe, S. (eds) *Intrapartum Care.* Oxford, Wiley-Blackwell.

MIDIRS (2007) *Positions in Labour and Delivery.* Informed Choice Leaflet. Bristol, MIDIRS.

Moore, E. R., Anderson, G. C., Bergman, N., Dowswell, T. (2012) Early skin-to-skin contact for mothers and their healthy newborn infants. *Cochrane Database of Systematic Reviews,* Issue 5.

NCT (National Childbirth Trust) (2003) *Creating a Better Birth Environment: An Audit Toolkit.* London, NCT.

National Institute for Health and Clinical Excellence (NICE) (2007) *Clinical Guideline 55: Intrapartum Care.* London, NICE.

NICE (2011) *Clinical Guildeline 107: Hypertensive disorders of pregnancy.* London, NICE.

Ndala, R. (2007) The third stage of labour. In Stables, D., Rankin, J. (eds) *Physiology in Childbearing,* 2nd edn. London, Elsevier.

NHS Maternity Statistics 2005–2006 (2007) *The Information Centre.* www.ic.nhs.uk

Nyberg, K., Buka, S., Lipsitt, L. (2000) Perinatal medication as a potential risk factor for adult drug abuse in a North American cohort. *Epidemiology* 11(6), 715–16.

Ockenden, J. (2001) The hormonal dance of labour. *The Practising Midwife* 4(6), 16–17.

Odent, M. (1999) *The Scientification of Love.* London, Free Association Books.

Odent, M. (2000) Insights into pushing: the second stage as a disruption of the fetus ejection reflex. *Midwifery Today International Midwife* 55, 12.

ONS (Office for National Statistics) (2012) HES online NHS Maternity Statistics 2010–2011. ONS. http://www.hesonline.nhs.uk

Perez-Botella, M., Downe, S. (2006) Stories as evidence: the premature urge to push. *British Journal of Midwifery* 14(11), 636–42.

Prendiville, W., Elbourne, D. (2000) The third stage of labor. In Enkin, M., Keirse, M. J. N. C., Neilson, J., Crowther, C., Duley, L., Hodnett, E. and Hofmeyr, J. (eds) *A Guide to Effective Care in Pregnancy and Childbirth,* 3rd edn. Oxford, Oxford University Press.

Prendiville, W. J., Elbourne, D., McDonald, S. (2004) Active versus expectant management in the third stage of labour. *Cochrane Database of Systematic Reviews,* Issue 1.

Redshaw, M., Heikkila, K. (2010) *Delivered with Care: a national survey of women's experience of maternity care 2010.* National Perinatal Epidemiology Unit, University of Oxford https://www.npeu.ox.ac.uk/files/downloads/reports/Maternity-Survey-Report-2010.pdf

Redshaw, M., Rowe, R., Hockley, C., Brocklehurst, P. (2007) *Recorded Delivery: The findings from a national survey of women's experience of maternity care.* National Perinatal Epidemiology Unit, Oxford. Available at: www.npeu.ox.ac.uk (accessed March 2008).

Reveiz, L., Gaitán, H. G., Cuervo, L. G. (2007) Enemas during labour. *Cochrane Database of Systematic Reviews*, Issue 4.

Richmond, S., Wyllie, J. (2010) Newborn Life Support Resuscitation Council (UK). http://www.resus.org.uk/pages/nls.pdf

Roberts, C. L., Torvaldsen, S., Cameron, C. A., Olive, E. (2004) Delayed versus early pushing in women with epidural analgesia: a systematic review and met-analysis. *British Journal of Obstetrics and Gynaecology* 111(12), 1333–40.

Robertson, A. (2006) Nitrous oxide – no laughing matter. *MIDIRS Midwifery Digest* 16(1), 123–8.

Royal College of Obstetricians and Gynaecologists (RCOG) (2009) Clamping of the umbilical cord and placental transfusion (SAC Opinion Paper 14) www.rcog.org.uk

Royal College of Midwives (RCM) (2005) *Campaign for Normal Birth*. London, RCM. www.rcmnormalbirth.org.uk

RCM (2009) *Results of the RCM Survey of Heads of Midwifery*. London, RCM, www.rcm.org.uk

RCM (2010) Ten top tips for a normal birth www.rcmnormalbirth.org.uk/practice/ten-top-tips

RCM (2012) Clamping update to be delivered. Midwives 5, 15. www.rcm.org.uk

Schaffer, J., Bloom, S., Casey, B., McIntire, D., Nihira, M., Leveno, K. (2005) A randomised trial of the effects of coached vs uncoached pushing during the second stage of labour on postpartum pelvic floor structure and function. *American Journal of Obstetrics and Gynecology* 192, 1692–6.

Shepherd, A., Cheyne, H., Kennedy, S., McIntosh, C., Styles, M., Niven, C. (2010) The purple line as a measure of labour progress: a longitudinal study. *BMC Pregnancy Childbirth* 10, 54.

Singata, M., Tranmer, J., Gyte, G. (2010) Restricting oral fluid and food during labour. *Cochrane Database of Systematic Reviews*, Issue 1.

Shorten, A., Donsante, J., Shorten, B. (2002) Birth position, accoucheur, and perineal outcomes: informing women about choices for vaginal birth. *Birth* 29(1), 18–27.

Simkin, P., Ancheta, R. (2005) *The Labor Progress Handbook*. Oxford, Blackwell Science.

Simmons, S. W., Cyna, A. M., Dennis, A. T., Hughes, D. (2007) Combined spinal-epidural versus epidural analgesia in labour. *Cochrane Database of Systematic Reviews*, Issue 3.

Simpson, K., James, D. (2005) Effects of immediate vs delayed pushing during second stage on fetal well-being: a randomised controlled trial. *Nursing Research* 54, 149–57.

Sleep, J., Roberts, J., Chalmers, I. (2000) The second stage of labor. In Enkin, M., Keirse, M. J. N. C., Neilson, J., Crowther, C., Duley, L., Hodnett, E., Hofmeyr, J. (eds) *A Guide to Effective Care in Pregnancy and Childbirth*, 3rd edn, pp. 289–99. Oxford, Oxford University Press.

Smith, C. A., Collins, C. T., Cyna, A. M., Crowther, C. A. (2006) Complementary and alternative therapies for pain management in labour. *Cochrane Database of Systematic Reviews*, Issue 4.

Smith, C. A., Collins, C. T., Crowther, C. A., Levett, K. M. (2011a) Acupuncture or acupressure for pain management in labour. *Cochrane Database of Systematic Reviews*, Issue 7.

Smith, C. A., Collins, C. T., Crowthern, C. A. (2011b) Aromatherapy for pain management in labour. *Cochrane Database of Systematic Reviews*, Issue 7.

Soltani, H., Poulose, T. A., Hutchon, D. R. (2011) Placental cord drainage after vaginal delivery as part of the management of the third stage of labour. *Cochrane Database of Systematic Reviews*, Issue 9.

Spiby, H., Green, J., Renfrew, M. *et al.* (2008) Improving care at the primary/secondary interface: a trial of community-based support in early labour. *The ELSA trial.* York: Mother and Infant Research Unit, Department of Health Sciences, University of York. www.york.ac.uk/

Stuart, C. (2000) Invasive actions in labour. Where have all the 'old tricks' gone? *The Practising Midwife* 3(8), 30–33.

Sullivan, J. R. (1999) Development of father-infant attachment in fathers of preterm infants. *Neonatal Network* 18(7), 33–9.

Thomson, A. (1995) Maternal behaviour during spontaneous and directed pushing in the second stage of labour. *Journal of Advanced Nursing* 22(6), 1027–34.

Tiran, D. (2000) *Clinical Aromatherapy for Pregnancy and Childbirth*, 2nd edn. Edinburgh, Churchill Livingstone.

Tiran, D. (2006) Midwives responsibilities when caring for women using complementary therapies during labour. *MIDIRS* 16(1), 77–8.

Torvaldsen, S., Roberts, C. L., Bell, J. C., Raynes-Greenow, C. H. (2004) Discontinuation of epidural in labour for reducing the adverse delivery outcomes associated with epidural analgesia. *Cochrane Database of Systematic Reviews*, Issue 4.

Ullman, R., Smith, L. A., Burns, E., Mori, R., Dowswell, T. (2010) Parenteral opioids for maternal pain relief in labour. *Cochrane Database of Systematic Reviews*, Issue 9.

Walsh, D. (2000a) Evidence-based care. Part 3: assessing women's progress in labour. *British Journal of Midwifery* 8(7), 449–57.

Walsh, D. (2000b) Evidence-based care. Part 6: limits on pushing and time in the second stage. *British Journal of Midwifery* 8(10), 604–8.

Walsh, D. (2010a) Evolution of intrapartum care. In Downe, S., Walsh, D. (eds) *Intrapartum Care.* Oxford, Wiley Blackwell.

Walsh, D. (2010b) Labour rhythms. In Downe, S., Walsh, D. (eds) *Intrapartum Care.* Oxford, Wiley Blackwell.

Walsh, D., Gutteridge, K. (2011) Using the birth environment to increase women's potential in labour. *MIDIRS* 21(2), 143–7.

Wickham, S. (1999) Further thoughts on the third stage. *The Practising Midwife* 2(10), 14–15.

World Health Organization (WHO) (1997) *Safe Motherhood: Thermal Protection of the Newborn: A Practical Guide.* WHO, Geneva.

2 Vaginal examinations and artificial rupture of the membranes

Vicky Chapman

Vaginal examinations

'Practitioners should be continuously aware of the need to show respect and consideration for the dignity of a woman undergoing vaginal examination in labour. Although this seems an obvious statement to make it is reiterated because some practitioners display insensitivity in this regard. Each woman should be treated with courtesy and respect, and her modesty protected by minimal exposure and examiners/examinations' (Lai and Levy, 2002).

Digital vaginal examination (VE) assesses cervical dilatation, descent of the presenting part, presentation and position, and determines intact/ruptured membranes. Most midwives agree there is a place for selective VEs in labour care, but many question the prescriptive and inflexible way that regular labour VEs are carried out, challenging their usefulness, frequency and necessity. Walsh (2000a) suggests VEs have become so routine that they are no longer seen as an intervention. They are part of biomedical model of care that subscribes to surveillance and early intervention in labours deemed 'too slow'. There have been few clinical studies on use of VEs (Warren, 1999; Crowther

The Midwife's Labour and Birth Handbook, Third Edition. Edited by Vicky Chapman and Cathy Charles.
© 2013 John Wiley & Sons, Ltd. Published 2013 by John Wiley & Sons, Ltd.

et al., 2000; Walsh, 2000a; Enkin 2000, cited by RCM, 2005) and studies on VE accuracy are often limited, using a simulated cervix.

Most women regard a VE as something to be endured. Some, especially abuse victims, find it intolerable and/or withhold consent. They may meet staunch resistance from staff, and pressured to comply. Midwives too may feel pressure to perform the ubiquitous 4-hourly labour VE, regardless of their clinical judgement.

Midwives have long relied on other methods to assess labour progress, e.g. frequency and strength of contractions; maternal behaviour and vocalisation. The 'purple line' presents in 76% of labours (Shepherd *et al.*, 2010) (see Chapter 1, page 12). Ultrasound scan (USS) appears more accurate than digital VE in determining cervical dilatation, station and fetal position (Chou *et al.*, 2004; Souka *et al.*, 2003; Kabawata *et al.*, 2010), although studies are small and further research is needed. Some might argue however that USS is technologically more invasive than a low-tech VE which can be performed in any setting (e.g. home) at any time. VE remains a core labour skill: its over-use in labour surveillance should not be a prerequisite for mass condemnation, but midwives should always be aware of its limitations and the woman's right to decline it. It is only a tool among many others used to assess labour progress.

Incidence and facts

- While women feel that the examiner's attitude and approach is generally more important than their gender, some say they feel embarrassed when examined by a male doctor (Lai and Levy, 2002).
- Women find VEs intrusive, embarrassing and unpleasant (Shepherd *et al.*, 2010). They can trigger feelings of sexual intimacy, invasion of privacy and vulnerability and can be especially difficult for women who have been sexually abused (Nolan, 2001). Women with a history of fetal loss or previous gynaecological surgery have reported feeling distressed during a VE (Menage, 1993).
- VEs risk ascending infection which increases with frequency of examinations, and therefore are contraindicated in preterm prelabour rupture of the membranes (RCOG, 2010).
- Latex gloves can cause skin sensitivity or allergic reactions in either clinician or patient. Sensitivity is more prevalent among healthcare workers (7–10%). Severe reactions such as anaphylaxis/death are rare (0.125%) but clinicians should be aware of this risk (Sussman and Beezhold, 1995).
- In multigravidae, cervical dilatation does not always reliably indicate progress, which is sometimes more accurately reflected in women's labour behaviour and vocalisation.

Accuracy and timing of VEs

'Repeated VEs are an invasive intervention, of, as yet, unproven value. Those who advocate their use thus have the responsibility to test their belief in an appropriately controlled trial' (RCM, 2005 citing Enkin, 2000).

Some recommend that the timing of labour VEs should be individualised in order to permit adequate assessment of a woman's progress; not performed too frequently or for the sake of 'routine' (Crowther *et al.*, 2000). Conversely, NICE (2007) advocates VEs at routine, fixed 4-hourly time intervals in the first stage of labour.

Definitions of progress vary (Crowther *et al.*, 2000) but a cervical dilatation of 0.5 cm/ hour is advised in the NICE (2007) intrapartum guidelines. Labour progress issues are discussed further in Chapter 9.

Studies suggest:

- VEs can be imprecise and subjective, particularly when performed by different examiners (Crowther *et al.*, 2000). Ideally the same clinician should perform serial VEs (RCM, 2005).
- Comparing USS and VE: determining fetal head position by VE was incorrect in one third of cases in the first stage of labour, particularly <7 cm. VE was incorrect in two thirds of cases in the second stage (Souka *et al.*, 2003; Kabawata *et al.*, 2010) and less accurate in diagnosing non-OA positions (Souka *et al.*, 2003; Chou *et al.*, 2004; Kabawata *et al.*, 2010).
- Simkin and Ancheta (2011) describe the importance of additional measures of progress including cervical consistency, thinning and effacement, movement from posterior to anterior and the importance of good cervical application to the presenting part.

Consent or compliance?

'Women accept the necessity for vaginal examinations, but expressed the need to be able to trust that the examiner would respect them as individuals and try to maintain their dignity, perform the examination skilfully and communicate the findings to them' (Lai and Levy, 2002).

A study of women's experiences of labour VE found that two thirds of midwives provided good or very good information, 60% of women said their permission was sought prior to a VE, 40% felt they could refuse, but 42% felt they couldn't refuse (Lewin *et al.*, 2005).

Performing a VE without *express consent* could constitute assault and has medicolegal implications (RCM, 2005). To be valid, consent must be given voluntarily and freely, without pressure or undue influence being exerted on the person to accept or refuse (DoH, 2009). *Implied consent* may not be sufficient evidence that someone has given *express consent*.

If consent is withheld it is important to remain sensitive, open and accept the woman's decision. Document this in the notes and use alternative methods of assessing labour progress (see Chapter 1). The GMC states that clinicians must respect a patient's decision to refuse an investigation, examination or treatment even if they think that decision is wrong or irrational. While they should explain their concerns they must not put pressure on a patient to accept their advice (GMC, 2008).

Informed consent:

- Discuss the indication for the examination.
- Explain what it may feel like and how long it may last.
- The guidelines issued by the GMC Standards Committee recommend that, wherever possible, patients undergoing an intimate examination should be offered a chaperone, irrespective of the clinician's gender.
- In non-English speaking women, ensure an interpreter/advocate is available (RCOG, 1997).

Performing a VE

Despite VEs being undertaken frequently, the procedure lacks good evidence to guide best practice. In the absence of clinical evidence, it seems prudent to wear *sterile* gloves if the membranes are ruptured, labour is preterm, prolonged or if infection is a possibility.

Stewart (2006) found that midwives sanitise their terminology, using abbreviations (a 'VE') and euphemisms (an 'internal') to distance themselves from intimacy and embarrassment. Stewart describes how some midwives ceremonially prepare a trolley, opening sterile packs with the ritualised wash down of the woman's genitalia demonstrating power and an affirmation that women's body fluids are in some way 'dirty' (Stewart, 2006). Such practices expose women to a protracted examination and embarrassing levels of genital touching. Evidence suggests a douche or wash down, using water or chlorhexidine is of no benefit in reducing ascending infection (Lumbiganon *et al.*, 2004). Alternatively use an informal, speedier approach: omit the genital wash down, squeeze lubricant inside the opened packet of sterile gloves, put on the gloves, then apply the lubricant to gloved fingers.

Before a VE

- Ensure the woman's bladder is empty.
- Perform abdominal palpation.
- Ask any unnecessary people to leave the room. Never underestimate someone's potential embarrassment or vulnerability even if attending a home birth. To ensure privacy, make sure doors are closed, blinds/curtains drawn and in hospital display a 'please knock and wait' sign on the door.
- Cover up the woman's lower half with a sheet/dressing gown.

VE procedure

- Tell the woman that if she wants you to stop at any point or the VE 'hurts' she can trust that you will respond appropriately.
- Wash your hands and put on gloves.
- Sit next to the woman and encourage her to relax her thighs and bottom before commencing the VE. Use plenty of lubricant and gently advance two fingers inside the vagina.

- Never start a VE during a contraction: it is unnecessary and painful. If the woman has a contraction during the VE (commonly triggered by touching the os), reassure her calmly that you won't move your fingers. If she becomes distressed then stop the VE. During a VE it can be reassuring if you explain what you are doing, particularly when moving your fingers anteriorly (usually the most uncomfortable and sensitive area) and be aware of the woman's body language; ask her directly if she is okay.
- Avoid looking worried, disappointed or disconnected from what is happening.

Following the examination

- Always smile and congratulate the woman on how well she coped and discuss the findings.
- Offer the woman a sanitary towel and assist her into a comfortable position, ideally upright, or help her off the bed.
- Remove the gloves; wash your hands.
- Listen to the fetal heart rate (FHR).
- Document your findings – see Box 2.1, Figures 2.1 and 2.2.

Box 2.1   Information obtained from a vaginal examination.

Remember to perform abdominal palpation first!

Vulva and vagina
- Healthy or identify problems e.g. female genital mutilation/circumcision, genital warts, offensive discharge

Cervix
- Location (posterior, mid, central, anterior or lateral)
- Consistency (soft/firm, thick/thin, rigid/stretchy)
- Application (loosely, moderately or well applied)
- Effacement (uneffaced, partially/fully effaced)
- Dilatation (os closed, 1–9 cm, anterior lip, 10 cm or fully dilated)

Presenting part
- Presentation (cephalic, breech, other)
- Position (see Fig. 2.1 for various vertex positions)
- Station (ballotable, −3, −2, −1, at spines, +1, +2)
- Caput/moulding (absent/present, amount of caput, degree of overlap of skull bones)

Membranes
- Intact or absent. If ARM performed, give indication
- Liquor absent/present; approximate quantity: +, ++, +++; colour (if meconium present: light/dark green or black, thin or thick/tenacious, any lumps present)

Document
- Findings
- FH

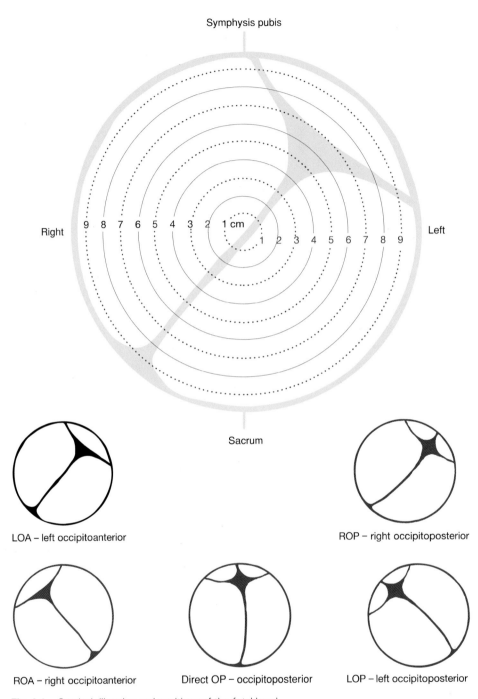

Fig. 2.1   Cervical dilatation and positions of the fetal head.

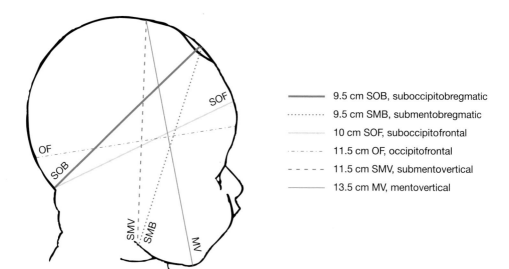

Fig. 2.2 Diameters of the fetal skull.

Some common problems

Poor progress

Poor progress can be hard to accept. It can be very demoralising for the woman, creating self-doubt about her ability to labour and birth. It is important to sound optimistic and say something encouraging if possible, e.g. 'the cervix is so much thinner' or 'the baby is moving down really well'. Chapter 9 considers slow progress in depth.

Misleading results

Stewart describes how midwives may perceive VE as a form of surveillance bordering on the punitive. Midwives may modify and monitor their behaviour in response, by fudging or obscuring findings (Stewart, 2010). Some deliberately record different cervical measurements to their clinical findings; e.g. a cervix of 3–4 cm may be recorded as 2 cm to ensure the woman has longer to establish and progress before the formal surveillance of active labour commences.

This practice illustrates the powerlessness of midwives and how they subvert information to work within the limitations of medicalised care.

Anterior lip

This is a small anterior portion of undilated cervix that precedes full dilatation. Multiparous women usually push this away with ease, but in some nulliparae the cervix may take sometime to dilate.

If the cervix is not too resistant some midwives gently slip it over the presenting part during a contraction. This can be painful and the woman will need to understand and want to cooperate. It may slip back down so may need to be held back for several contractions, then when the woman pushes the presenting part advances and the cervix can no longer move back.

Sometimes when a cervix is fully dilated, the midwife will deliberately record an 'anterior lip', to allow the woman a longer second stage and therefore increased chance of achieving a normal vaginal birth. This knowledge is something midwives keep among themselves and pass on to their students. Stewart (2010) suggests that because midwives fail to challenge obstetric definitions regarding the 'normal' duration of second stage, these definitions will never stand corrected, and the dominant view remains unchallenged.

Oedematous cervix

This is when the cervix swells anteriorly, feeling tense and enlarged. It has been a long held belief that women who push prior to full dilatation have the greatest risk of a swollen cervix. However, Walsh (2000b) and Downe and Schmid (2010) suggest that there is no evidence to support this. Downe *et al.* (2008) found that at least 20% of women irrespective of parity experience an early pushing urge, and in fact they seem to have a better chance of normal birth than those who don't. Walmsley (2000) suggests that a premature pushing urge, common in occipito-posterior (OP) babies, may be physiologically desirable to rotate the baby into an optimum position prior to full dilatation and descent.

Downe and Schmid (2010) note how some midwives vary the methods, initially 'going with the flow' (letting the woman push if her body wants to), but if unsuccessful switching to the contrasting method of encouraging the woman to resist the pushing urge and adopt a position to reduce it, e.g. side lying, all fours or knee-chest positions.

Be patient and give loads of encouraging support. With time an oedematous cervix usually dilates, with or without midwifery intervention. If it really will not budge further intervention is likely; an epidural may bring welcome relief. Anecdotally, midwives who discover a swollen cervix *midway* through labour suggest it rarely resolves and a caesarean section (CS) usually becomes necessary (ARM, 2000).

'Shrinking' cervix

Some midwives argued that a shrinking cervix is not always a misdiagnosis. Possibly the presenting part, or even the bag of membranes, may initially press hard on the cervix, causing it to dilate. If then the membranes rupture, or if the presenting part increases/decreases its degree of flexion during labour, this may alter the pressure on the cervix causing it to appear less dilated at the next VE. A shrinking cervix has been recognised between delivery of twins sometimes born weeks apart; however, anecdotal evidence suggests that it is more common in OP positions and can be a sign of dystocia (ARM, 2000).

Invasive examinations and sexual abuse

Many women may not disclose if they have been sexually abused/raped as a child or adult. Symptoms associated with sexual abuse survivors are often misinterpreted and women can be labelled as 'difficult' patients. This lack of awareness by health professionals can result in inappropriate treatment, resulting in further trauma (Aldcroft, 2001). Sociologists have observed how carers can act in a paternalistic manner, with the woman feeling powerless and childlike, regressed back to her former role as a victim (Kitzinger, 1992).

Women experiencing any intervention have to comply and let someone do something to their body, which may feel invasive, unpleasant and possibly painful. 'Submitting' to the midwife or doctor can be reminiscent of past abuse. They may be left feeling vulnerable, powerless, violated and dirty (Kitzinger, 1992).

Women who have suffered previous sexual abuse are more likely to have a difficult birth experience which results in a higher level of obstetric intervention (Gutteridge, 2001).

Phobias and behaviours linked to past abuse

- Fear or obvious dislike of VEs, invasive procedures, needles or going to the dentist.
- History of depression, poor self-esteem and emotional problems (Riley, 1995).
- There is a correlation between women who have been sexually abused as children and psychiatric/emotional dysfunction and postnatal depression (Riley, 1995).
- Disclosure of previous abuse.
- Behaviour during intimate procedures may include:
  - 'Shutting off' during the procedure.
  - Crying or becoming distressed.
  - Regressive or infantile behaviour including talking in a childish voice (Gutteridge, 2001).
  - Tensing up or refusing to proceed with the examination.

What can the midwife do to help?

Try not to replicate abuse:

- **Give the woman control.** Let her know you will stop if she wants you to. Squeezing your free hand as a sign to stop may avoid her having to speak (Aldcroft, 2001).
- **Avoid voyeurism.** The presence of others may replicate abusive situations. Send others out of the room, particularly male midwives/doctors (Kitzinger, 1992).
- **Language.** Avoid patronising or disempowering terms. Even well-intended words can regress women back to their former victim status, with the midwife now as the perpetrator (Mayer, 1995), e.g. 'That's a good girl', 'Open your legs a bit wider', 'Lie still, this won't hurt', 'shhh . . .' (Gutteridge, 2001).
- **Reality check.** Ground the woman in the 'here and now' explaining what is happening as it happens. Keep the situation focused on the cervix, the labour, and the baby, rather than let her return to her former victim state (Aldcroft, 2001).

Artificial rupture of the membranes

For the vast majority of women experiencing normal labour, their membranes tend to remain intact throughout the first stage, often rupturing spontaneously around the time of full dilatation, heralding the onset of the second stage. This is physiologically normal and works perfectly well.

The RCM (2005) and NICE (2007) conclude that artificial rupture of the membranes (ARM) is an intervention which should not be considered a routine part of normal labour care. Performing ARM carries risks (see below) including increased FHR abnormalities, increased uterine contractions and is linked to a small increase in CS. Following ARM, many women feel their contractions worsen and describe feelings of loss of control and self-doubt.

A large Cochrane review suggests that ARM has a smaller effect on labour duration and other outcomes than some might think. Routine ARM does not appear to affect first stage of labour duration, maternal satisfaction, analgesia use, infection, maternal morbidity or fetal morbidity. It appears to have little effect on multiparous women, although it shortens the second stage for some primigravidae. For nulliparae with slow progress however ARM did seem to have a positive effect on subsequent labour progress and duration, although even then it did not reduce the need for oxytocin augmentation (Smyth *et al.*, 2007).

Many midwives may doubt this quantitative evidence, believing ARM enables rapid progress and speedy birth in multigravid women, and will recount numerous episodes where an ARM is quickly followed by strong contractions and an urge to push.

Occasionally a woman – often a multigravida – will request ARM to speed up her labour even if she is progressing normally. Some women believe that they have uniquely tough membranes(!): 'They had to break my waters last time'. Often mutual discussion dispels this misconception. However some women retain a deeply held belief that ARM is necessary or desirable. This is a tricky issue and one of those ethical dilemmas where midwives face a conflict between published evidence and a woman's right to choice.

The RCM (2005) recommends that the decision to ARM should only be taken in direct consultation with the woman, when the evidence is discussed and the intervention justified and not minimised (RCM, 2005). This discussion should not take place just before or during a VE. 'I'm just going to break your waters' is in no way seeking consent.

Indications for ARM

- If progress is slow ARM appears to improve subsequent labour progress and duration in nulliparous women (Smyth *et al.*, 2007).
- ARM can be used as a method of inducing labour. It may be used alone, or in conjunction with prostaglandins and/or oxytocics.

Contraindications to ARM

- Maternal choice.
- Placenta praevia (have you checked placental location on the USS report?).
- Cord presentation: CS is usually undertaken immediately.
- High or mobile presenting part. ARM is neither life-saving nor essential. ARM with a high/mobile presenting part resulting in a cord prolapse could be deemed

negligent. In over 50% of cases of cord prolapse, ARM is a direct cause; cord prolapse is associated with poor perinatal outcomes (Prabulos and Philipson, 1998).

- Preterm, growth-restricted or breech babies, oligohydramnios: again risk of cord compression/prolapse.
- Women with a sexually transmitted disease, genital tract infection or carrying Group B Streptococcus (or only if the latter is receiving appropriate antibiotic treatment).
- Undiagnosed/untreated HIV positive women have a risk of mother-to-child transmission (MTCT) if their membranes rupture. Studies conducted before the advent of highly active retroviral therapy (HAART) found that rupture of membranes >4 hours doubles the HIV transmission risk (International Perinatal HIV Group, 2001). Known HIV positive women treated with HAART are *not* at increased risk of MTCT even if the membranes have ruptured (Mark *et al.*, 2012). However, ARM is an invasive procedure, best avoided if possible in HIV positive women; furthermore not all women know their HIV status.

Summary

- VEs have become routine practice but have not been well researched.
- NICE recommends 4-hourly labour VE; others challenge routine VE.
- Cervical dilatation can be inaccurate and may not reflect labour progress, especially in multigravidae.
- Women in general find VEs uncomfortable, invasive and unpleasant.
- For some women VEs can be a very distressing experience.
  Do
  - Ensure privacy and gain clear informed consent.
  - Tell her you will stop if she asks; be aware of your body language.
  - Be caring and gentle.
  - Say something positive and always explain/discuss the findings.
  Don't
  - Start or continue a VE during a contraction.
  - ARM unless there is slow progress and no contraindications: it involves risk.

References

Aldcroft, D. (2001) A guide to providing care for survivors of child sex abuse. *British Journal of Midwifery* 9(2), 81–5.

ARM (Association of Radical Midwives) (2000) ARM nettalk: incredible shrinking cervices. *Midwifery Matters* 87, 30.

Chou, M. R., Kresier, D., Taslimi, M., Druzin, M. L., El-Sayed, Y. Y. (2004) Vaginal versus ultrasound examination of the fetal head position during the second stage of labor. *American Journal of Obstetrics and Gynecology* 191, 521–4.

Crowther, C., Enkin, M., Keirse, M. J. N. C., Brown, I. (2000) Monitoring progress in labour. In Enkin, M., Keirse, M. J. N. C., Neilson, J. (eds) *A Guide to Effective Care in Pregnancy and Childbirth*, 3rd edn, pp. 281–8. Oxford, Oxford University Press.

DoH (2009) *Reference Guide to Consent for Examination or Treatment*, 2nd edn. DoH. www.dh.gov.uk/consent

Downe, S., Schmid, V. (2010) Midwifery skills for normalising unusual labours. In Walsh, D., Downe, S. (eds) *Essential Midwifery Practice: Intrapartum Care*, pp. 178–179. Oxford, Wiley-Blackwell.

Downe, S., Young, C., Hall-Moran, S. (Trent Midwifery Research Group) (2008). Multiple Midwifery Discourses: the case of the early pushing urge. In Downe, S. (ed.) *Normal Birth, Evidence and Debate*, 2nd edn. Oxford, Elsevier.

Enkin, M. (2000) Infection in pregnancy. In Enkin, M., Keirse, M. J. N. C., Neilson, J. *et al.* (eds) *Guide to Effective Care in Pregnancy and Childbirth*, 3rd edn, pp. 154–68. Oxford, Oxford University Press.

GMC (General Medical Council) (2008) *Consent: patients and doctors making decisions together*. www.gmc-uk.org/guidance/current/library/consent.asp#forms

Gutteridge, K. (2001) Failing women: the impact of sexual abuse on childbirth. *British Journal of Midwifery* 9(5), 312–15.

International Perinatal HIV Group (2001) Duration of ruptured membranes and vertical transmission of HIV-1: a meta-analysis from 15 prospective cohort studies. *AIDS* 15, pp. 357–68.

Kawabata, I., Nagase, A., Oya, A., Hayashi, M., Miyake, H., Nakai, A., Takeshita, T. (2010) Factors influencing the accuracy of digital examination for determining fetal head position during the first stage of labor. *J Nippon Med School* 77 (6). www.jstage .jst.go.jp/article/jnms/77/6/290/_pdf.

Kitzinger, J. V. (1992) Counteracting, not re-enacting, the violation of women's bodies: the challenge for perinatal caregivers. *Birth* 19(4), 219–22.

Lai, C. Y., Levy, V. (2002) Hong Kong Chinese women's experiences of vaginal examinations in labour. *Midwifery* 18(4), 296–303.

Lewin, D., Fearon, B., Hemmings, V., Johnson, G. (2005) Informing women during VEs. *British Journal of Midwifery* 13(1), 26–9.

Lumbiganon, P., Thinkhamrop, J., Thinkhamrop, B., Tolosa, J. E. (2004) Vaginal chlorhexidine during labour for preventing maternal and neonatal infections (excluding Group B Streptococcal and HIV). *Cochrane Database of Systematic Reviews*, Issue 4.

Mark, S., Murphy, K. E., Read, S., Bitnun, A., Yudin, M. H. (2012) HIV mother-to-child transmission, mode of delivery, and duration of rupture of membranes: experience in the current era. *Infectious Diseases in Obstetrics and Gynecology* 2012, Article ID 267969, 5 pages. doi:10.1155/2012/267969

Mayer, L. (1995) The severely abused woman in obstetric and gynaecological care. Guidelines for recognition and management. *Journal of Reproductive Medicine* 40(1), 13–18.

Menage, J. (1993) Post-traumatic stress disorder in women who have undergone obstetric and/or gynaecological procedures. *Journal of Reproductive and Infant Psychology* 11, 221–8.

NICE (National Institute for Health and Clinical Excellence) (2007) *Clinical Guideline 55: Intrapartum Care*. London, NICE.

Nolan, M. (2001) VEs in labour (Expert View). *The Practising Midwife* 4(6), 22.

Prabulos, A. M., Philipson, E. H. (1998) Umbilical cord prolapse. Is time from diagnosis to delivery critical? *Journal of Reproductive Medicine* 43(2), 129–32.

Riley, D. (1995) *Perinatal Mental Health*. Oxford, Radcliffe Medical Press.

RCM (Royal College of Midwives) (2005) *Midwifery Practice Guidelines. Evidence Based Guidelines for Midwifery-Led Care in Labour*. RCM Press. www.rcm.org.uk

RCOG (Royal College of Obstetricians and Gynaecologists) (1997) *Guidelines on Intimate Examinations*. RCOG, London.

RCOG (2010) *Preterm Prelabour Rupture of Membranes. RCOG Green-top Guideline No 44*. RCOG, London.

Shepherd, A., Cheyne, H., Kennedy, S., McIntosh, C., Styles, M., Niven, C. (2010) The purple line as a measure of labour progress: a longitudinal study. *BMC Pregnancy Childbirth* 10, 54.

Simkin, P., Ancheta, R. (2011) *The Labour Progress Handbook*, 3rd edn. Oxford, Wiley-Blackwell.

Smyth, R. M. D., Allderd, S. K., Markham, C. (2007) Amniotomy for shortening spontaneous labour. *Cochrane Database of Systematic Reviews*, Issue 4.

Souka, A. P., Haritos, T., Basayiannis, K., Noikokyri, N., Antsaklis, A. (2003) Intrapartum ultrasound for the examination of the fetal head position in normal and obstructed labor. *Journal of Maternal and Fetal Neonatal Medicine*, 13, 5963.

Stewart, M. (2006) 'I'm just going to wash you down' sanitizing the VE. *MIDIRS Midwifery Digest* 16(1), 30–6.

Stewart, M. (2007) Midwives' and women's discourse about vaginal examination in labour. PhD thesis. University of the West of England, Bristol.

Stewart, M. (2010) Feminism and intrapartum care. In Walsh, D., Downe, S. (eds). *Essential Midwifery Practice: Intrapartum Care*, pp. 273–88. Oxford, Wiley-Blackwell.

Sussman, G. L., Beezhold, D. H. (1995) Allergy to latex rubber. *Annals of Internal Medicine* 122(1), 43–6.

Walmsley, K. (2000) Managing the OP labour. *MIDIRS Midwifery Digest* 10(1), 61–2.

Walsh, D. (2000a) Evidence-based care. Part 3: assessing women's progress in labour. *British Journal of Midwifery* 8(7), 449–57.

Walsh, D. (2000b) Evidence-based care. Part 6: limits on pushing and time in the second stage. *British Journal of Midwifery* 8(10), 604–8.

Warren, C. (1999) Why should I do VEs? *The Practising Midwife* 2(6), 12–13.

3 Fetal heart rate monitoring in labour

Bryony Read

Introduction

Fetal heart monitoring, whether intermittent or continuous, is performed with the intent of assessing the well-being of the fetus and detecting the few who are hypoxic. Continuous electronic fetal monitoring (EFM) became widely popular in the 1970s, often used routinely without evidence of benefit. Iatrogenic intervention frequently resulted. More recently, EFM has been targeted at higher-risk pregnancies, even though its efficacy even in this area remains unproved. Women may find themselves caught in the centre of this debate, and become anxious, often unnecessarily, about the well-being of their unborn baby.

Intermittent auscultation

Intermittent auscultation (IA) is the auscultation of the fetal heart rate (FHR) at intermittent intervals, using a pinards stethoscope or a hand-held doppler device. Midwives have traditionally monitored according to the stage of labour, increasing IA frequency when the woman is in established, advanced labour. In the absence of any substantive evidence, NICE (2007) has made IA recommendations based only on

The Midwife's Labour and Birth Handbook, Third Edition. Edited by Vicky Chapman and Cathy Charles.
© 2013 John Wiley & Sons, Ltd. Published 2013 by John Wiley & Sons, Ltd.

medical expert committee opinion, recommending auscultation after a contraction for 1 minute:

- Every 15 minutes in the first stage of labour
- Every 5 minutes in the second stage of labour.

Beech Lawrence (2001) and Spiby (2001) suggest that frequent IA may be as restrictive as continuous EFM, and Martis *et al.* (2010) propose to review the safety and effectiveness of methods and timings used in IA.

Using a pinards/hand-held doppler

One benefit of the pinards is that it will only pick up the fetal, rather than the maternal, heart rate. It can be used throughout labour. Women may find the pressure required for good pinards auscultation uncomfortable. A hand-held doppler device (Figure 3.1) can be placed more lightly on the abdomen and also allows others to hear the fetal heart. A water-resistant device can be used in baths/birthing pools. Some midwives/women may prefer the simplicity of the pinards and are aware that while the use of doppler ultrasound appears to be safe, it has never been proved unequivocally to be so.

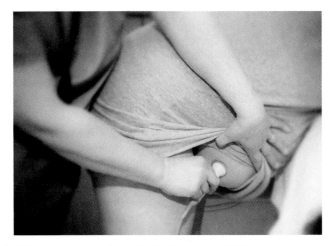

Fig. 3.1 Hand held doppler device. *Photo by Debbie Gagliano-Withers.*

Effective use of a pinards requires a precise awareness of the baby's position, and indeed it can be used to confirm position. Following palpation, place the bell end over the baby's torso (Figure 3.2). Press your ear to the flat end to secure it and let go of the pinards; carefully listen for a muffled thudding, the same sound as putting an ear directly over someone's chest to hear their heart. Midwives can purchase their own wooden or plastic pinards from various online suppliers including the National Childbirth Trust (NCT).

If there are any FHR concerns the assessment of variability becomes important. The FHR should vary at least five beats from the baseline rate over a period of 1 minute. However, it is particularly difficult to assess by audibility alone. A hand-held doppler that displays the FHR is useful, as it shows heart rate variations.

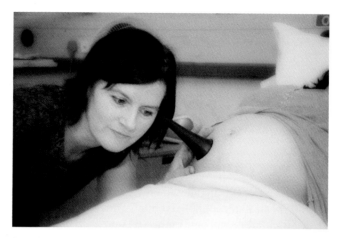

Fig. 3.2   Listening with a pinards. *Photo by Debbie Gagliano-Withers.*

If there is any deviation from the norm, e.g. decelerations, bradycardia or tachycardia, then a cardiotocograph (CTG) should be commenced or, if at home, consider transfer to hospital for EFM. However, FH decelerations often occur in the second stage, and if delivery is imminent a CTG may be impractical and pointless. Midwives may find it difficult to implement IA due to pressure to conform to their individual unit's policies, which may not always adhere to NICE guidelines.

Electronic fetal monitoring

'EFM was introduced with the aim of reducing perinatal mortality and cerebral palsy. This reduction has not been demonstrated in the systematic reviews of randomised controlled trials. However an increase in maternal intervention rates has been shown' (NICE, 2007).

When EFM is used on low risk women as a predictor of cerebral palsy it has a 99.8% false positive rate (Nelson *et al.*, 1996). It is difficult to imagine another area of medicine where such a false positive would be tolerated, particularly when the intervention is as major as a caesarean section (CS) (Pateman *et al.*, 2008). Despite the lack of evidence to support EFM, even for women deemed 'high-risk', NICE (2007) continues to recommend its routine use for any woman with a 'risk' factor. For a variety of complex reasons, EFM technology has become part of the hospital birth culture (Walsh, 2001). Consequently obstetricians and hospital midwives rely heavily on EFM as part of their skill base, even if evidence suggests their confidence is misplaced. It may be difficult for many clinicians to re-skill themselves physically and psychologically and to therefore avoid coercing women into accepting EFM. Although midwives may state that it is theoretically preferable to use IA, many continue to rely on EFM for fear of missing a pathological FH feature (Hindley *et al.*, 2006). EFM also continues to be used on busy shifts when one-to-one care is unavailable.

Units using EFM should have fetal blood sampling (FBS) available before a CS is performed (see Appendix and 'fetal blood tests', page 376). FBS can, in theory, (a) confirm the need for a CS or (b) reassure and avoid an unnecessary CS which otherwise would have been carried out based on CTG evidence alone. However, Cochrane review found no evidence of higher CS rates when FBS was unavailable (Alfirevic *et al.*, 2006) and NICE (2007) reports increased instrumental delivery but no difference in outcomes. NICE (2007) recommends:

- No 'admission trace' for low-risk women. Cochrane review also found no evidence to support the admission CTG for low-risk woman, suggesting it increases CS risk by 20% (Devane *et al.*, 2012).
- EFM should be *offered* to 'high-risk' cases (see appendix) e.g. fresh bleeding in labour, oxytocin augmentation, VBAC.
- Meconium-stained liquor
  - Light staining: *consider* EFM based on assessment of other risks, e.g. stage/progress of labour
  - Significant staining, e.g. thick/tenacious dark green/black, or lumps of meconium: advise continuous EFM.

To perform a CTG

- Explain to the mother why it is being offered. Obtain consent.
- Record the indication in the notes and on CTG.
- Label CTG with date, mother's name, hospital/NHS number and maternal pulse (to differentiate it from FHR).
- Set date and time correctly; paper speed 1 cm/min (in UK).
- Palpate for position and presentation.
- Auscultate using pinards prior to positioning FH monitor, as the ultrasound transducer can 'double up' maternal pulse and show a false FHR.
- Attach toco (pressure-sensitive) contraction monitor around top of the uterus and FH monitor over fetal heart area. Secure with belts.
- Explain simply to the parents the FH range and contraction line. Explain that 'loss of contact' does not mean the baby's heartbeat has stopped.
- Undo monitor belts and encourage periodic mobilisation, if possible, to reduce discomfort and complications caused by restricted mobility.
- Consider any external factors that may cause a FHR change, e.g. lying flat for an examination, vomiting or pethidine; note them on the CTG. A position change to left lateral or sitting more upright may resolve anomalies (Figure 3.3). Lying flat can cause aortocaval compression, when the inferior vena cava and aorta are compressed by the gravid uterus, producing maternal hypotension and fetal hypoxia.
- Consider a 'fresh eyes' approach, where another midwife reviews the trace. Local policies may vary on frequency; NICE (2007) suggests hourly.
- Anyone asked to review should note their findings on the trace and/or in more detail in the maternal notes, with date, time and signature.

Following the birth, sign the CTG and write the time of birth. File it securely in the notes: CNST (2012) recommend resealable hole-punched envelopes. If the outcome is poor, photocopy CTG(s) as the original may deteriorate over time. Ensure the machine is cleaned and checked.

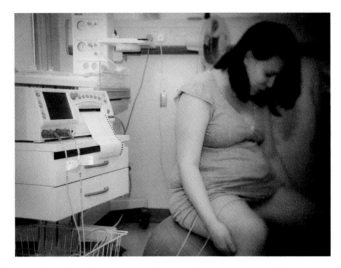

Fig. 3.3   CTG monitoring: There is no reason why most women cannot sit in a chair or on a ball unless their legs are numb from an epidural. *Photo by Debbie Gagliano-Withers.*

Fetal scalp electrode

A fetal scalp electrode (FSE) is an accurate but invasive form of FHR monitoring. Once frequently used, it is now generally only used where there is significant FHR concern with poor contact from the external CTG. It can occasionally cause scarring and/or neonatal infection.

Do not apply FSE if:

- The woman's consent is not obtained (most women dislike the idea of a clip piercing their baby's skin).
- The baby is <34 weeks gestation or has a bleeding disorder, e.g. haemophilia.
- There is a non-cephalic or non-vertex presentation.
- The woman has an infection, pyrexia, human immunodeficiency virus, hepatitis, sexually transmitted disease, or is at high risk for these conditions (e.g. intravenous drug user).

ST analysis

A more recent method for FHR interpretation has been developed, requiring the use of an FSE, called ST wave analysis, or STAN. This combines CTG interpretation with automatic analysis of the ST interval in the electrocardiogram complex of the fetus (Heintz *et al.*, 2008). STAN rates the significance of abnormalities shown by the CTG. Modest evidence supports STAN in labours where CTG would be used (Neilson, 2006) as it is associated with a reduction in FBS and operative vaginal deliveries, although there was no difference in the CS rate or neonatal outcomes at birth.

Classification of fetal heart rate features

The CTG is classified as normal (Figure 3.4), suspicious or pathological. The classification is obtained by examining the features of the CTG (see Table 3.1 and 3.2).

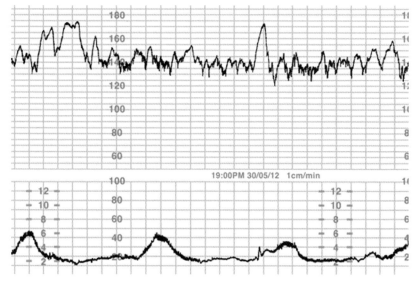

19:00PM 30/05/12 1cm/min

Fig. 3.4 Normal CTG.

Table 3.1 Classification of FHR trace features (NICE, 2007).

Feature	Baseline (bpm)	Variability (bpm)	Decelerations	Accelerations
Reassuring	110–160	≥5	None	Present
Non-reassuring	100–109 161–180	<5 for 40–90 min	Typical variable decelerations with over 50% of contractions, for over 90 min Single prolonged deceleration for up to 3 min	The absence of accelerations with otherwise normal trace is of uncertain significance
Abnormal	<100 >180 Sinusoidal pattern ≥10 min	<5 for 90 min	Either atypical variable decelerations with over 50% of contractions or late decelerations, both for over 30 min Single prolonged deceleration for more than 3 min	

NICE (2007) Reproduced with permission.

Table 3.2 Definition of normal, suspicious and pathological FHR traces (NICE, 2007).

Category	Definition
Normal	All four features are classified as reassuring
Suspicious	One feature classified as non-reassuring and the remaining features classified as reassuring
Pathological	Two or more features classified as non-reassuring or one or more classified as abnormal

NICE (2007) Reproduced with permission.

Baseline: mean level of FHR when stable, determined over 5–10 mins: normally 110–160 bpm: *baseline bradycardia*: 100–110 bpm, *baseline tachycardia*: >160 bpm.

Baseline variability: Variation of baseline within a bandwidth, excluding accelerations and decelerations. Normal variability: >5 bpm.

Acceleration: transient FHR increase of ≥15 bpm above the baseline, lasting for ≥15 seconds.

Deceleration: transient FHR decrease of ≥15 bpm below the baseline, lasting for ≥15 seconds.

Decelerations are early, late or variable:

- True *early decelerations* are rare and benign (NICE, 2007); these are synchronous with the contraction, usually associated with fetal head compression.
- *Late decelerations* occur after a contraction and are usually, but not exclusively, pathological.
- *Variable decelerations* vary in shape and timing and can be *typical or atypical*:
  - *Typical variable decelerations* (*often simply called 'variable decelerations'*): a variable intermittent slowing of FHR with rapid onset and recovery (see Figure 3.5). Typified by 'shouldering' (intermittent increase in FHR before and after deceleration). Attributed to cord compression which the fetus is tolerating.
  - *Atypical variable decelerations* are considered more serious, as they suggest cord compression that that the fetus is less able to cope with. These are variable decelerations with any of the following components
    - loss of, or exaggerated, shouldering
    - delayed recovery to baseline after deceleration
    - prolonged rise in baseline after deceleration
    - loss of variability during deceleration

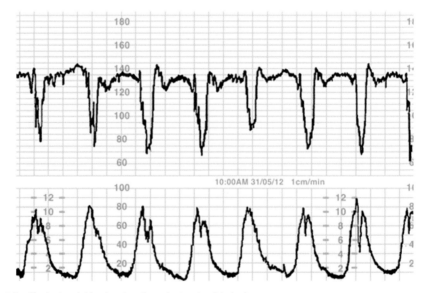

Fig. 3.5 Typical variable decelerations (note shouldering).

- biphasic deceleration
- persistence of secondary deceleration (overshoot) (NICE, 2007; Gibb and Arulkumaran, 2008); Draycott *et al.*, 2008).

CTGs can also be documented using the acronym DR C BRAVADO (see Box 3.1).

Box 3.1   DR C BRAVADO CTG documentation.

Determine **R**isk
Contractions (frequency and strength)
Baseline **RA**te
Variability
Accelerations
Decelerations
Overall assessment

AAFP (2012).

Positive and negative aspects of EFM

Positive aspects

- The belief underpinning EFM is that it may identify a hypoxic fetus and enable early intervention and delivery.
- Some women/partners feel reassured hearing the baby's heartbeat, as it shows their baby is alive (Grant, 2000; Sinclair, 2001), especially if they can see the monitor (Grant, 2000).
- Clinicians often feel reassured they are doing something physical, measurable and observable when recording a CTG.
- A CTG trace may protect against litigation (although it may equally be used appropriately or inappropriately as 'evidence' to condemn practitioners).
- Although not best practice, there are times on a busy delivery suite where EFM is used to 'keep an eye' on the FH when the midwife is busy elsewhere.

Negative aspects

- Lack of evidence to demonstrate benefit even for 'high-risk' women. Perhaps this is why NICE (2007) uses the term 'offer' or 'advise' as opposed to 'recommend' when discussing EFM with women.
- EFM is associated with a reduction in neonatal seizures, but it does not reduce cerebral palsy, infant mortality or other standard measures of neonatal well-being (Alfirevic *et al.*, 2006; Graham *et al.*, 2006).
- EFM increases interventions, e.g. FBS, episiotomy, instrumental delivery and CS resulting in iatrogenesis (pathology caused by medical intervention). This is unacceptable because it is entirely preventable (Walsh, 2001). Iatrogenic risks of EFM are rarely discussed with women. 'Is this because clinicians are unaware of these complications?' questions Wagner (2000), who challenges clinicians, asking 'Is ignorance misconduct?' Interventions can be unpleasant and stressful; particularly unjustifiable when the delivery is expedited and the baby delivered without evidence of hypoxia. Wagner (2000) poignantly suggests doctors are rarely sued or criticised for unnecessary interventions.

- Beech Lawrence (2001) argues that not all risk is 'high risk' and that some conditions are notoriously misdiagnosed, e.g. oligohydramnios and growth-restriction, and meconium-stained liquor can be irrelevant or ominous. Preterm infants have different heart rates from term infants due to the baby's immature autonomic nervous system and evidence that EFM offers any advantage over IA in preterm labours is not forthcoming (Alfirevic *et al.*, 2006).
- Women undergoing EFM experience discomfort and restricted movement, which is likely to prolong labour, increase the need for analgesia and increase FHR abnormalities (Gupta *et al.*, 2012). NICE (2007) recommends that women are informed that EFM will restrict mobility. Some women feel EFM interferes with their relationship with their partner/caregivers. Women undergoing IA tend to report a more positive labour experience (Grant, 2000).
- The monitor, rather than the mother, can become the focus of attention and interest, and both staff and parents may become overly anxious (Walsh, 2000, 2001).
- The NHS Litigation Authority (2009) states that 'CTG misinterpretation' accounts for 34% of stillbirth cases, the most frequent example of alleged negligence encountered in the study.

The skill of interpreting EFM is of key importance. However, CTG interpretation is subject to human error and is not an exact science. Several studies have highlighted CTG interpretation inconsistencies both between different practitioners and for the same practitioner on different days (Devane and Lalor, 2005). Even STAN requires accurate CTG interpretation underpinning it (Jomeen *et al.*, 2010). Altaf *et al.* (2006) report that many midwives feel ambivalent about EFM. They may react to traces, consciously or subconsciously, differently from obstetricians, as identifying a problem may create a shift from midwifery to medical control. Education and training are vital. Midwives and obstetric staff should have regular updates; CNST recommends 6-monthly CTG analysis updates (CNST, 2012). Training may help reduce, but will not eliminate, differences in interpretation.

Summary

- Most babies go through labour with no problems. FH monitoring aims to detect the few who become hypoxic.
- Women/partners may find FH monitoring reassuring or distracting/disturbing.
- Express consent must always be obtained for any form of FH monitoring.
- IA is the method of choice for low-risk women in labour.
- Do not perform a 'routine' CTG admission trace.
- Continuous EFM is offered to women with increased risk factors, although there is no evidence of its efficacy.
  - Encourage movement and frequent mobilisation during EFM.
  - Always consider the CTG context: i.e. what else might be causing FHR changes.
  - If EFM is used then FBS facilities should be available before a CS is performed.
  - Label CTG traces clearly and store safely.
- Midwives must interpret CTGs knowledgeably and undertake regular CTG updates.

References

AAFP (American Academy of Family Physicians) (2012) Advanced Life Support in Obstetrics (ALSO) Provider Manual.

Alfirevic, Z., Devane, D., Gyte, G. M. L. (2006) Continuous cardiotocography as a form of electronic fetal monitoring for fetal assessment in labour. *Cochrane database of Systemic Reviews*, Issue 3. www.thecochranelibrary.com

Altaf, S., Oppenheimer, C., Shaw, R., Waugh, J., Dixon-Woods, N. (2006) Practices and views on fetal heart monitoring: a structured observation and interview study. *British Journal of Obstetrics and Gynaecology* 113(4), 409–18.

Atalla, R., Kean, L., McParland, P. (2000) Preterm labour and predator rupture of the membranes. In Kean, L.H., Baker, P., Edelstone, D.I. (eds) *Best Practice in Labour Ward Management*, pp. 111–39. Edinburgh, WB Saunders.

Beech Lawrence, B. (2001) Electronic fetal monitoring: do NICE's new guidelines owe too much to the medical model of childbirth? *The Practising Midwife* 4(7), 31–3.

Clinical Negligence Scheme for Trusts (2012) *Maternity Clinical Risk Management Standards*. NHS Litigation Authority. www.nhsla.com

Devane, D., Lalor, J. (2005) Midwives' visual interpretation of intrapartum cardiotocographs: intra- and inter-observer agreement. *Journal of Advanced Nursing* 52(2), 133–41.

Devane, D., Lalor, J. G., Daly, S., McGuire, W., Smith, V. (2012) Cardiotocography versus intermittent auscultation of fetal heart on admission to labour ward for assessment of fetal wellbeing. *Cochrane Database of Systematic Reviews*, Issue 2.

Draycott, T., Winter, C., Crofts, J., Barnfield, S. (eds) (2008) *PROMPT PRactical Obstetric MultiProfessional Training*. London, RCOG Press.

Jomeen, J., Cross, D., Cairns, J. (2010) Cardiotocography and ST analysis (STAN): a retrospective review. *British Journal of Midwifery* 18(9), 568–74.

Gibb, D., Arulkumaran, S. (2008) *Fetal Monitoring in Practice*, 3rd edn. London, Elsevier.

Graham, E. M., Petersen, S. M., Christo, D. K., Fox, H. (2006) Intrapartum electronic fetal heart rate monitoring and the prevention of perinatal brain injury. *Obstetrics and Gynaecology* 108 (3, part 1), 656–66.

Grant, A. (2000) Care of the fetus during labour. In Enkin, M., Keirse, M. J. N. C., Neilson, J., Crowther, C., Duley, L., Hodnett, E., Hofmeyr, J. (eds) *A Guide to Effective Care in Pregnancy and Childbirth*, 3rd edn, pp. 267–80. Oxford, Oxford University Press.

Gupta, J., Hofmeyr, G., Shehmar, M. (2012) Position in the second stage of labour for women without epidural anaesthesia. *Cochrane Database of Systematic Reviews*, Issue 5. www.thecochranelibrary.com

Heintz, E., Brodtkorb, T. H., Nelson, N., Levin, L. A. (2008) The long term cost-effectiveness of fetal monitoring during labour: a comparison of cardiotocography complemented with ST analysis versus cardiotocography alone. *British Journal of Obstetrics and Gynaecology* 115, 1676–87.

Hindley, C., Wren Hinsliff, S., Thomson, A. M. (2006) English midwives' views and experiences of intrapartum fetal heart rate monitoring in women at low obstetric risk: conflicts and compromises. *Journal of Midwifery and Women's Health* 51(5), 354–60.

Martis, R., Emilia, O., Nurdiati, D. S. (2010) Intermittent auscultation (IA) of fetal heart rate in labour for fetal well-being (Protocol). *Cochrane Database of Systematic Reviews*, Issue 9.

National Childbirth Trust (NCT) www.nct-online.org

National Health Service Litigation Authority (NHSLA) (2009) Study of Stillbirth Claims http://www.nhsla.com/NR/rdonlyres/3DCA11D2-49E9-4E4F-97B0-260B0BDD0E6C/0/NHSLitigationAuthorityStudyofStillbirthClaims.pdf

NICE (National Institute for Health and Clinical Excellence) (2007) *Clinical Guideline 55: Intrapartum Care*. London, NICE.

Neilson, J. P. (2006) Fetal electrocardiogram (ECG) for fetal monitoring during labour. *Cochrane Database of Systematic Reviews*, Issue 3. www.thecochranelibrary.com

Nelson, K. B., Dambrosia, J. M., Ting, T. Y., Grether, J. K. (1996) Uncertain value of electronic fetal monitoring in predicting cerebral palsy. *New England Journal of Medicine* 334(10), 613–8.

Pateman, K., Khalil, A., O'Brien, P. (2008) Electronic fetal heart rate monitoring: help or hindrance? *British Journal of Midwifery* 16(7), 454–7.

Sinclair, M. (2001) Birth technology. *RCM Midwives Journal* 4(6), 168.

Spiby, H. (2001) The NICE guidelines on electronic fetal monitoring. *British Journal of Midwifery* 9(8), 489.

Wagner, M. (2000) Choosing caesarean section. *The Lancet* 356, 1677–80.

Walsh, D. (2000) Evidence-based care. Part 4: Fetal monitoring should be controlled. *British Journal of Midwifery* 8(8), 511–16.

Walsh, D. (2001) Midwives and birth technology: a debate that's overdue. *MIDIRS Midwifery Digest* 11 (Suppl. 2), 53–6.

Appendix: Continuous EFM algorithm (NICE, 2007)

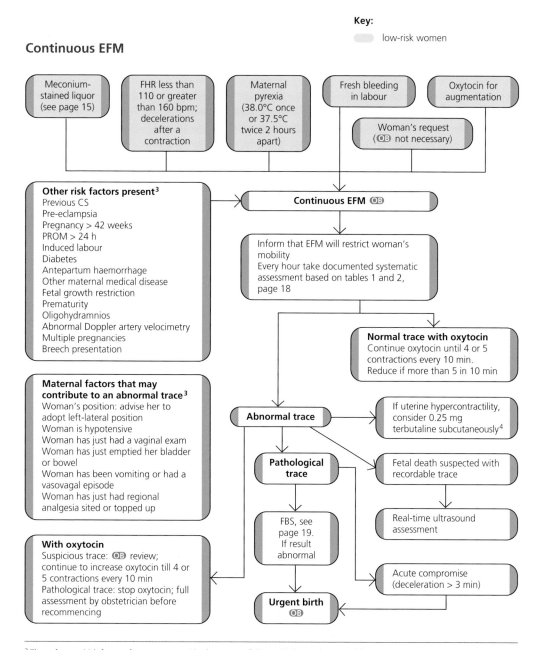

[3] These factors (risk factors for women outside the scope of this guideline and maternal factors that may contribute to an abnormal trace) are from 'Electronic fetal monitoring' (NICE inherited guideline C) which this guideline updates and replaces.
[4] At the time of publication (September 2007), terbutaline did not have UK marketing authorisation for this indication. Informed consent should be obtained and documented.

National Institute for Health and Clinical Excellence (2007) CG 55 Intrapartum care: care of healthy women and their babies during childbirth. London: NICE. Available from www.nice.org.uk/guidance/CG55. Reproduced with permission.

4 Perineal trauma and suturing

Vicky Chapman

Introduction

Many women sustain perineal trauma when giving birth. Some will heal without intervention, while some require suturing. The midwife is in a key position to offer advice and support, suturing if necessary or referring to a more specialist professional if required.

Incidence

- Perineal trauma rate for vaginal births in England 2010–2011 (ONS, 2012):
  - perineal tears 52–53%
  - episiotomy 19.5%
  - combined episiotomy and tears 72% for vaginal births in England
- The Aarhus Birth Cohort (2008) over 30 000 Danish births found:
  - labial trauma in primiparas 40%
  - second degree tears primiparas 34%, multiparas 20.5%
- 0.5–2.5% of women sustain a third/fourth degree tear, with a small risk of recurrence in a subsequent vaginal birth of 4.5% (Byrd *et al.*, 2005).

The Midwife's Labour and Birth Handbook, Third Edition. Edited by Vicky Chapman and Cathy Charles.
© 2013 John Wiley & Sons, Ltd. Published 2013 by John Wiley & Sons, Ltd.

Facts

- Studies on suturing versus non-suturing second degree tears have found no significant statistical differences between the two groups (Metcalfe *et al.*, 2006; Elharmeel *et al.*, 2011).
- Women report the experience of being sutured as highly unpleasant and those receiving local anaesthetic, as opposed to regional, report high levels of pain throughout the procedure (Saunders *et al.*, 2002).
- Using the correct repair material and suture technique reduces postnatal pain (Kettle *et al.*, 2010; Kettle *et al.*, 2007).
- Long-term physical, psychological and social problems may result from incorrect wound approximation and unrecognised trauma to the external anal sphincter (RCOG, 2007).
- Postpartum faecal and flatus incontinence are commonly (although not exclusively) associated with third- and fourth-degree tears.
- Episiotomy increases the incidence of more serious tearing, including third/fourth degree tears, faecal incontinence, perineal pain and dyspareunia (Carroli and Belizan, 2007).
- Performing a rectal inspection and examination *prior* to suturing improves the detection of third/fourth degree tears (Andrews *et al.*, 2005; NICE, 2007).
- Appropriate training increases practitioner confidence, improves evidence-based practice and knowledge of anal sphincter injuries (Andrews *et al.*, 2005), so should help reduce morbidity and associated litigation.
- Regular pelvic floor exercises are effective in maintaining or re-establishing urinary continence (Chiarelli and Cockburn, 2002).
- Women prefer their own midwife to conduct the perineal repair (Jackson, 2000).
- Most long-term morbidity is not reported to health professionals (Bedwell, 2006).

Reducing perineal trauma

There are few studies on midwifery techniques to protect the perineum during spontaneous delivery (Eason *et al.*, 2000). Factors such as primiparity, episiotomy, instrumental birth (especially forceps) and heavier babies are associated with greater trauma (Dahlen *et al.*, 2006).

There is little good evidence to inform midwifery practice on how to improve perineal outcomes. Evidence suggests that perineal trauma (including third/fourth degree tears) can be reduced by applying a warm, moist compress during the second stage (Dahlen *et al.*, 2009; Aasheim *et al.*, 2011), antenatal perineal massage in primigravidas (Labrecque *et al.*, 1999; Beckmann and Garrett, 2006), home birth (Aikins Murphy and Feinland, 1998; NICE, 2007) and continuous support in labour (Hodnett *et al.*, 2011). There is some evidence of benefit in non-active pushing and a gentle, unhurried birth (Jackson, 2000; Albers *et al.*, 2006). Birth position may affect perineal outcome (Shorten *et al.*, 2002); the lateral birth position has the highest intact perineum rate and upright/squatting postures the lowest (Shorten *et al.*, 2002; Bedwell, 2006). However, upright and hand and knees position (though not squatting) seemed to reduce trauma in one study (Soong and Barnes, 2005). Flexing the head does not reduce trauma (Bedwell, 2006). See Chapter 1, p. 22–23, for more on preventing perineal trauma.

Assessment of perineal trauma

Prior to deciding whether suturing is required (see also Table 4.1), examine the genitalia using a good light source. It is thought best practice to perform a *digital* and *visual* inspection of the anus to ascertain any anal involvement (NICE, 2007).

- Explain what you are about to do, and obtain consent for this intimate, often uncomfortable, examination; offer Entonox.
- Be gentle and careful, using wet gauze to part and inspect the labia.
- Gently insert two fingers in the vagina and move slowly outwards towards the perineum; remove any clots as you go, checking for trauma.

Table 4.1   Classification of perineal trauma.

Anterior perineal trauma
- Injury to the labia varying from painful grazes to deeper – sometimes bilateral – labial lacerations which may require sutures
- Less commonly involves the anterior vagina, urethra or clitoris

Posterior perineal trauma
- **First degree:** Injury to just the skin
- **Second degree:** Injury to the skin, vaginal tissue and perineal muscle. The trauma may be small, medium or large, long and deep; sometimes a branch tear (extending up both sides of the vagina)
- **Third degree:** Injury to skin, perineal muscle and involves the anal sphincter. Sultan (2002) suggests this can be subdivided into:
  - **3a** Partial tear of the anal sphincter
  - **3b** Complete tear of the anal sphincter
  - **3c** Internal sphincter also torn
- **Fourth degree:** Injury to the skin, perineal muscle and extending into the anal sphincter and rectal mucosa

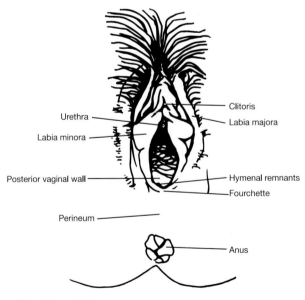

Fig. 4.1   Anatomy of female genitalia.

- Part the perineum where it meets the anus: an absence of 'puckering' around the anterior aspect of the anal sphincter suggests possible trauma (NHS QIS, 2008).
- Gently insert a lubricated finger into the rectum: if you suspect trauma ask the woman to squeeze her sphincter. If the external anal sphincter is damaged the separated ends may be seen to retract backwards (NHS QIS, 2008).
- Slowly withdraw the finger to feel for injury to the surface of the normally smooth rectal mucosa and anus. Finally, with the fingertip just inside the anal sphincter, use your thumb to 'pill roll' i.e. palpate the top of the anal sphincter between your finger and thumb. This may mean your thumb is palapating through a perineal tear to feel if the anal sphincter is damaged or very thin.

Labial tears

Labial trauma may consist of a graze or laceration; unilateral, bilateral or even multiple. Most labial trauma is minor and heals well. Assessment, classification and repair of this type of injury is poorly researched. Jenkins (2011) found that labial trauma comprised:

- 55% grazes
- 36% lacerations
- 6.3% both trauma types.

   Labial tears were sutured in 67% of cases and grazes in 26%. Doctors were more likely to suture labial trauma than midwives, possibly because midwives tend to leave minor lacerations alone and/or or refer more deep/complex cases.

   Bilateral tears or grazes are particularly painful during urination. Commonly midwives advise women to part the labia daily postnatally, to minimise the danger of labial fusion, although the literature suggests this is phenomenom is rare (Jenkins, 2011). Arkin and Chern-Hughes (2002) note that spontaneous approximation of minor labial lacerations (labial fusing) can result in distorted anatomical healing, with resultant dyspareunia and other distressing morbidity.

Urethral tears

Rare in the developed world, trauma involving the urethra should be referred immediately to a urologist, as serious urinary tract/bladder injury is possible, particularly if labour has been prolonged and/or ending in forceps or ventouse delivery. Trauma of the urethral meatus should *not* be sutured, since this risks urethral damage. A catheter is *contraindicated* as this risks extending any internal urethral injury. Urinary tract injuries usually present with a triad of symptoms: pain, problems passing urine and haematuria (Rackley *et al.*, 2009).

First and second degree tears: to suture or not to suture?

Women dislike being sutured, but endure it because they believe it to be beneficial (NICE, 2007). The trend towards not suturing first/second degree tears has evolved on the strength of limited evidence, and Yiannouzis (2002) suggests several reasons, including increased maternal choice, increased midwifery autonomy and staffing pressures. Non-suturing avoids the pain and unpleaseant experience of being sutured

(Lundquist *et al.*, 2000) and for this reason many women – and staff – find it attractive. Underconfident suturers may also readily avoid suturing.

There have been various small studies involving non-suturing of first/second degree tears (Head, 1993; Lundquist *et al.*, 2000; Fleming *et al.*, 2003) and several larger studies (Langley *et al.*, 2006; Metcalfe *et al.*, 2006; Leeman *et al.*, 2007). Midwives and women may have strong views on which option they prefer, often resulting in difficulties in recruiting participants and staff compliance in randomised studies.

NICE (2007) recommends suturing for the following:

- First degree tears if the skin is not well opposed
- All second degree tears.

However, this advice is based on limited evidence from one small randomised controlled trial (Fleming *et al.*, 2003). Larger studies suggest (Langley *et al.*, 2006; Metcalfe *et al.*, 2006; Leeman *et al.*, 2007):

- Slower initial healing in non-sutured groups with poorer wound approximation in the immediate postnatal period
- Similar outcomes at six weeks of (subjectively assessed) 'gaping', asymmetrical or open perineal wounds in some studies (Langley *et al.*, 2006; Leeman *et al.*, 2007)
- Conversely, poorer wound approximation at six weeks in some unsutured women in other studies (Fleming *et al.*, 2003; Metcalfe *et al.*, 2006)
- No difference in *reported* postnatal pain, but increased analgesia use following suturing (Langley *et al.*, 2006; Leeman *et al.*, 2007)
- Overall, few differences in secondary measures of pain, longer-term healing times, incontinence, dyspareunia, pelvic floor strength, infection rates and resumption of sexual intercourse.

To date there have been no randomised controlled trials of the quality and size to reach statistical power and draw clear evidence-based conclusions on the non-suturing of second degree tears. Langley *et al.* (2006) suggest that while the balance of evidence tends towards suturing, it is based on limited evidence and weak trials.

A Cochrane review of suturing versus non-suturing concluded. '*At present there is insufficient evidence to suggest that one method is superior to the other with regard to healing and recovery in the early or late postnatal periods. Until further evidence becomes available, clinicians' decisions whether to suture or not can be based on their clinical judgement and the women's preference after informing them about the lack of long-term outcomes and the possible chance of a slower wound healing process, but possible better overall feeling of well-being if left unsutured*' (Elharmeel *et al.*, 2011).

Women should be aware that *suturing remains strongly advisable for* extensive perineal trauma, a large second degree tear, a third/fourth degree tear, if bleeding continues, if the wound is very misaligned/complicated or the result of an unnatural straight-edged cut from an episiotomy. While midwives will no doubt hold a preference for a particular choice, it must be the woman who ultimately makes her feelings and preferences known.

Third and fourth degree tears

Many third/fourth degree tears are unpreventable, although there are associated risk factors:

- Large baby
- Malposition, malpresentation
  - Persistent occipitoposterior position (3%)
- Forceps delivery (7%)
- Shoulder dystocia (4%)
- Prolonged second stage (4%)
- Midline episiotomy (3%)
- Epidural (2%) (RCOG, 2007).

Evidence review demonstrates that third/fourth degree tears are not associated with delivery technique *nor are they preventable* (Bedwell, 2006). Midwives often feel guilty and personally responsible, but they should be reassured that such tears remain the unavoidable outcome for a tiny percentage of births.

Failure to diagnose third/fourth degree tears however *may* be considered substandard care; this contributes to most perineal trauma litigation. A third/fourth degree tear should be referred, and properly assessed and repaired by an experienced doctor in theatre, usually under regional anaesthesia. Care following repair includes indwelling catheter for 24 hours, stool softeners and bulk agents as well as antibiotic cover for seven days (RCOG, 2007). Follow-up reviews by six weeks postpartum in the UK now commonly include a course of obstetric physiotherapy.

Providing care for survivors of childhood sexual abuse

Women may not disclose that they have been sexually assaulted as a child or adult. Symptoms exhibited by abuse survivors can be misinterpreted and result in women being labelled as 'difficult patients'. This lack of awareness can result in inappropriate treatment, causing further psychological trauma (Aldcroft, 2001).

For some women the restriction of the lithotomy position makes them feel they are at the mercy of an authoritative figure and are submitting to a painful, invasive and sexually threatening procedure. This can leave them feeling violated and powerless (Kitzinger, 1992) and can have far-reaching psychological consequences. It may affect the relationship with the baby who may inadvertently be blamed for 'putting them through this' (Aldcroft, 2001). (For more information see Chapter 2.)

Suturing procedure

Pain relief

> *'The doctor who sewed me up was the most cruel person I ever experienced . . . he didn't speak to me once, throughout the whole fifty minutes, except to say 'stop jiggling about'. . . . I cried and cried with pain the whole time and I am not the sort of person who cries publicly . . . I was extremely conscious that if I complained he would sew me up more tightly'* (Salmon, 2000).

Studies on the experience of women undergoing perineal repair make for uncomfortable reading: many experience high levels of pain during suturing (Green *et al.*, 1998; Salmon, 1999; Saunders *et al.*, 2002) and current approaches to pain relief for suturing are inadequate. Saunders *et al.* (2002) found 17% of women reported 'distressing', 'horrible' or 'excruciating' pain. Several studies suggest that local anaesthetic is *inadequate* for >50% of women undergoing perineal repair (Kindberg, 2008).

Secondary to poor pain management is the issue of substandard communication; frequently the woman's distress is treated as inconsequential (Kindberg, 2008).

Salmon (1999) identified three elements that were particularly important in shaping women's experience of perineal repair:

- **Gender of the practitioner**: women continue to raise the issue of gender in studies on perineal issues. Suturing involves the private, sexual parts of a woman's body; it is sexually invasive and potentially threatening.
- **Good quality pain relief throughout suturing**
  - Current local anaesthetic dosages and route of administration may be inadequate (Kindberg, 2008).
  - Epidural (if in situ) should be adequate or 'topped-up' as this offers superior pain relief during suturing compared to local anaesthetic (Saunders *et al.*, 2002).
  - Topical, local anaesthetic cream (EMLA) applied an hour before injectable local anesthetic results in lower pain scores in women compared to injectable anaesthetic: 83.8% versus 53.3% in one small study (Franchi *et al.*, 2009). These interesting results combining topical and injectable local anaesthetic raise issues around maximum dosage as lidocaine has the potential for toxcitiy.
- **Practitioner's attitude**: pain control and the relationship between the woman and the suturer are intertwined. *Communication* and *sensitivity* are important components of effective analgesia.

Optimising the effect of local anaesthetic

Local anaesthetic's duration of action is related to the time it is in contact with nervous tissue. Anything that prolongs contact time increases its effectiveness. The golden rule if giving local anaesthetic is: ***really wait for it to work!*** So why not get into the habit of giving it first, then going to grab a coffee?

Local anaesthetic is absorbed readily into the systemic circulation after administration, affecting peripheral nerves. It can therefore have side effects. See Table 4.2.

Suturing materials

The suture material of choice is rapid-absorption polyglactin 910 (Vicryl™); a good second choice is polyglycolic acid. These synthetic sutures are associated with less perineal pain, analgesic use, dehiscence and resuturing (but increased suture removal) when compared with catgut (Kettle *et al.*, 2010). Catgut has been withdrawn in the UK since 2002.

Table 4.2   Lidocaine (lignocaine®).

Action:	Local anaesthetic
Dosage:	5–20 ml, depending on concentration and effectiveness **Maximum dose 200 mg** 0.5% (5 mg/ml) 1% (10 mg/ml) 2% (20 mg/ml)
Route:	Tissue infiltration by injection.
Contraindications:	Cardiac problems including bradycardia, sinoatrial disorders and complete heart block.
Side effects:	Dizziness, paraesthesia, drowsiness, hypovolaemia, hypotension, bradycardia, rarely anaphylaxis, respiratory depression, convulsions; may lead to cardiac arrest (JFC, 2012).
Cautions:	Epilepsy, hepatic or respiratory or cardiac impairment, bradycardia.
Reducing pain when injecting local anaesthetics	• Ideally apply *topical* anaesthetic an hour before suturing (e.g. EMLA cream). • **Warm** the lignocaine: then injection is less painful. You can use your pocket or hand. • **Location.** Drizzle a little over the wound before actually injecting: this is less painful than piercing the tough, nerve-rich skin. • **Inject *slowly:*** this is less painful (Palmon *et al.*, 1998, Taylor & Bayat, 2007) • **Aspirate** – pulling back the plunger of the syringe before injecting allows you to check that you are not in a blood vessel and is standard practice. • Always aspirate every time you move/relocate the needle.

Local anesthetic toxicity
Talk to the woman and ask her how she feels while you are injecting: look out for **confusion, dizziness**, and **abnormal taste. The most common cause of local anaesthetic toxicity is inadvertent intravenous injection** (Taylor & Bayat, 2007). Also a very vascular site can cause rapid absorption and maternal collapse.
In toxicity get help and think **ABCD** (airway, breathing, circulation, drugs).

Suturing techniques

Suturing is an aseptic technique. The tear may involve different layers (see also Table 4.1) so will influence the suturing technique:

- **Muscle layer.** Current evidence supports a loose, continuous non-locking technique for vaginal tissue and perineal muscle. Subsequent stitch tightness and tension from reactionary oedema are transferred more evenly throughout the whole length of the single knotless suture, which appears to reduce short-term pain and subsequent suture removal for tightness and discomfort (Kettle *et al.*, 2007). See also 'Perineal suturing procedure'.
- **Skin layer.** Subcuticular continuous suturing is superior to interrupted sutures for the perineal skin (Kettle *et al.*, 2007). All midwives should learn and use this simple technique as it reduces postnatal pain and constitutes best practice.

- **Skin layer unsutured.** Studies have evaluated suturing only the vaginal and perineal muscle layers but leaving the skin unsutured. NICE (2007) suggests if the edges are apposed, the perineal skin can remain unsutured. This is also preferable to interrupted sutures to the skin, resulting in a significant reduction in adverse outcomes, but was associated with a slight increase in wound gaping up to ten days following birth. Petrou *et al.* (2001) suggest it is also cost-effective in using fewer healthcare resources.

Figure 4.2 shows the basic sequence of inserting a stitch and tying a knot for right-handed individuals.

Left-handed suturing

Twelve per cent of the population are left-handed. Left-handed surgeons report difficulties in handling and using instruments designed for right-handed use: one third felt more prone to needlestick injury among other hazards (Adusumilli *et al.*, 2004). The needlestick injury risk is 1.6 times greater for left-handed than right-handed health care workers (Naghavi and Sanati, 2009). It is wise to **double glove** to protect against needle stick injury when training (especially if having to learn using right-handed instruments).

Needlestick injuries may be more likely because of the difficulties of operating and releasing right-handed ratcheted instruments when working within the awkward and somewhat restricted space of the vagina. Needle-holders are designed to be secured and released easily by the action of the thumb and forefinger of the right hand. However, this action is reversed when used by a left-hander so the ratchet actually locks tighter rather than releasing; some force is required to open the teeth. This makes releasing needle-holders very clumsy and uncomfortable, risking inadvertent needlestick injury.

Left-handers who have learned to suture the 'right-handed way' may have become accustomed to this and be content to continue. However, for those who struggle, or the novice suturer, being taught by another left-hander and practising left-handed suturing techniques is likely to improve their technique, improve speed and reduce injury risk. Practitioners should not struggle to use right-handed techniques, just as they would not attempt skills requiring fine motor control, like writing, with a weaker non-dominant hand (Chapman, 2009). See Figure 4.3 for suturing the left-handed way.

Raise the issue of the availability of appropriate left-handed instruments for suturing under risk management and health and safety protocols.

Suturing at home

Midwives must be resourceful! A good fixed light source is essential. Ensure the woman can lie comfortably with her bottom on the edge of a firm bed with the midwife positioned on the floor or low stool. The woman may find it most comfortable to rest her legs on separate chairs or she can abduct them herself but this is only usually comfortable for a short time. If both woman and midwife are on the floor it is very hard on the midwife's back and visualising/accessing the perineum can be awkward. Serious/complex tears may require transfer to hospital.

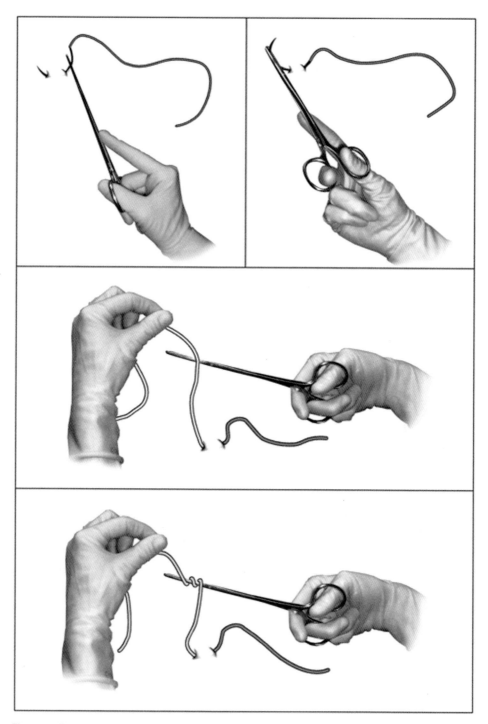

Fig. 4.2   Right-handed suturing. Knots can be hand-tied if preferred. *Artwork by Vicky Chapman.*

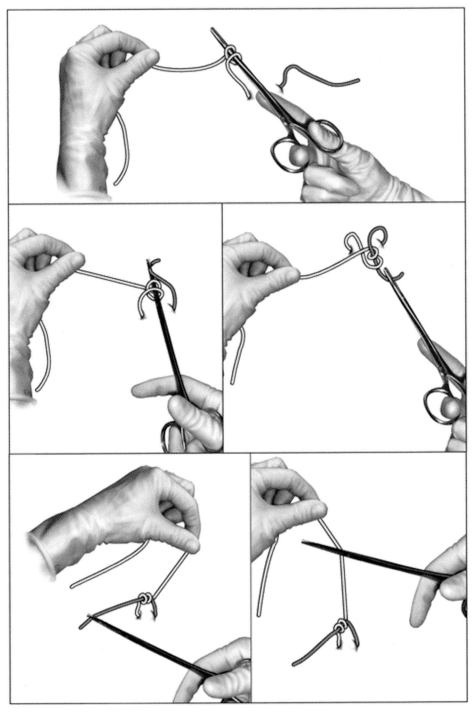

Fig. 4.2 continued   Right-handed suturing. Knots can be hand-tied if preferred. *Artwork by Vicky Chapman.*

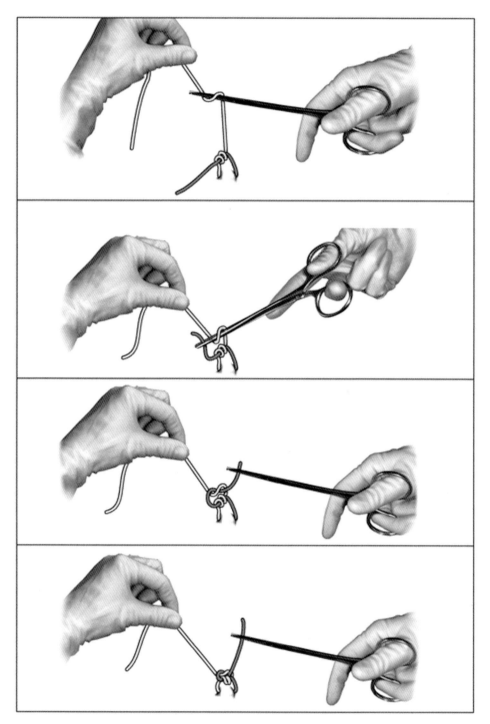

Fig. 4.2 continued   Right-handed suturing. Knots can be hand-tied if preferred. *Artwork by Vicky Chapman.*

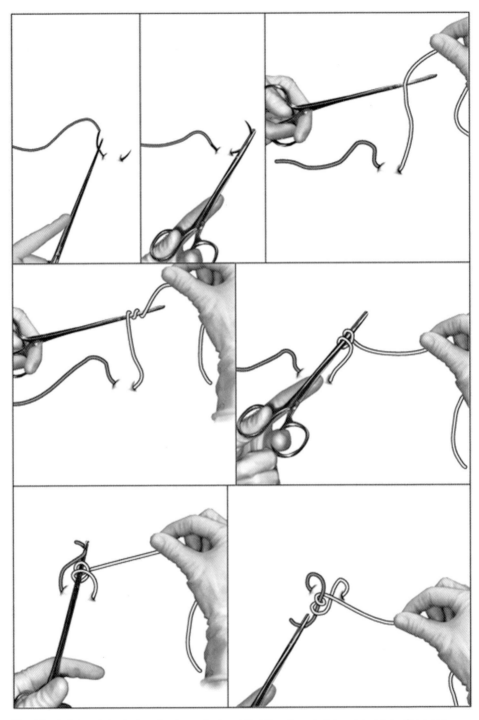

Fig. 4.3   Left-handed suturing. Knots can be hand-tied if preferred. *Artwork by Vicky Chapman.*

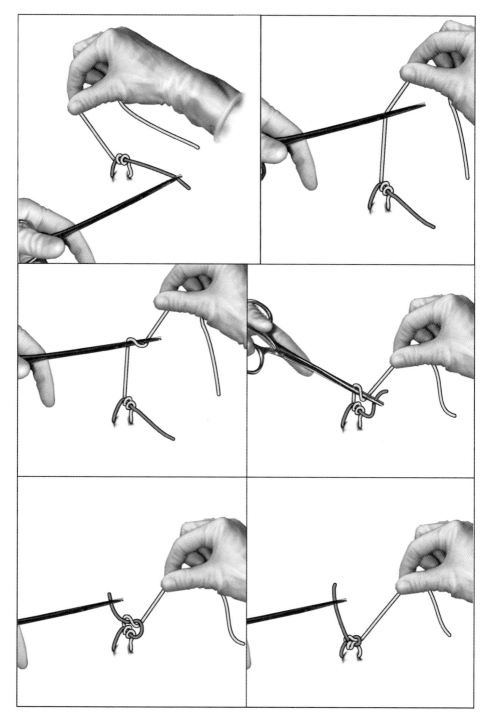

Fig. 4.3 continued Left-handed suturing. Knots can be hand-tied if preferred. *Artwork by Vicky Chapman.*

Perineal suturing procedure

'When was the last time a woman thanked you for stitching with Vicryl Rapide or for using a subcuticular method instead of another repair technique?' Walsh, 2007.

Research around perineal care and repair reflects medical priorities. As Walsh highlights, most clinical trials have concentrated on outcomes that are important to professionals and have, on the whole, ignored women's experiences. Women are more interested in the sensitivity of staff, receiving adequate pain relief and whether suturing is an intervention than can be avoided if necessary.

Following discussion, explanations, reassurance and informed consent, prepare everything ready for suturing, including a fixed light source and post-suturing analgesia.

Before starting the repair address the following questions:

- Is the woman as comfortable as possible?
- Does she understand what has to be done and how long it will take?
- Can I see what has to be done?
- Can I do it?

An overview of the perineum is shown in Figure 4.1.

Placing the woman's legs in lithotomy is no longer routine practice in many hospitals with some women resting their knees against obsolete lithotomy poles. However, the midwife must feel confident that s/he can see and access properly. A particularly nervous woman may feel more in control with her legs resting apart and, while she may need to close them if something hurts or distresses her; the midwife's patience and sensitivity will help her through this ordeal.

Ensure the woman is comfortable and skin-to-skin with her baby. Many women are unsure of this, fearing the pain may make them jump. In reality, their baby is a positive distraction from pain.

Even optimum analgesia will not eradicate all sensations. Women often find the sensations of pressure, tugging, wiping and tampon insertion unpleasant, uncomfortable and sometimes distressing: something many clinicians fail to recognise. Prepare the woman verbally prior to each occurrence and also offer *adequate* Entonox (at least 6 breaths).

- Extend the sterile field by placing a sterile sheet under the woman's buttocks.
- Warn the woman before touching, wiping or injecting anything. As you earn her confidence, she will begin to trust you, relax and stop anticipating pain.
- Infiltration of local anaesthetic more than 15 minutes before suturing will give a better block. Initially clean only enough of the perineum to inject the local anaesthetic, otherwise this will burn and sting: not a good start . . .
- Infiltrate local anaesthetic (offer Entonox): drizzle over wound first, avoid injecting through the sensitive skin, instead go through the wound.
- Prepare instruments and count swabs.
- Clean area more thoroughly if required.
- Insert a tampon. This keeps the area blood-free and visually clear. Warn the woman this is very uncomfortable; she may wish to use Entonox again. Secure tampon string to drapes (if used) or the sheet covering the woman (the end of the string does not need to be sterile).

- Move the tear 'back together' to realign and visualise significant meeting points; ensure no anal involvement.
- Locate apex in vagina; secure the first stitch just above it.
- Using a continuous suture technique, bring the muscle layers together (see Figures 4.4a–c).
- Avoid placing sutures in the fourchette skin as it can result in an unyielding scar, which forms an 'introtial bridge' at the fourchette. This stretches during intercourse causing pain; a Fentons perineorrhaphy is sometimes required to cure it.
- If a stitch appears misplaced then unfortunately the needle needs to be cut free to allow unpicking, then a knot tied. Recommence a new set of continuous sutures from the point left off.
- **For the skin:** if the edges are apposed after suturing the muscle layer, skin can be left unsutured (NICE, 2007). If sutures are required, use a subcuticular continuous suturing technique (Figures 4.4d–h). Do not insert interrupted stitches.
- Visually inspect the stitches and alignment.
- Inform the woman and gain consent before checking her rectum. Gently insert a lubricated finger, fleshy side up and slowly withdraw it, checking the anus visually as well as feeling for any stitches that may have gone through, for 'buttonholes' or a tear.
- Prepare the woman for the uncomfortable removal of the tampon.
- If the woman wishes (providing no contraindications), administer diclofenac 100 mg rectally post-suturing. This reduces additional analgesia use and perineal pain for around 24 hours, even up to 48 hours (Parsons and Crowther, 2007).
- Place a sanitary pad over the perineum and assist her back into a comfortable position.
- Count up and account for all needles, swabs and instruments.

Document findings accurately and comprehensively in black ink, including a diagram to illustrate the trauma, anaesthetic used, suture material and repair technique (e.g. 'continuous, loose non-locking sutures in vagina and perineal muscle; subcuticular to skin'). Document anything unusual, e.g. difficulty controlling bleeding, tying off a bleeding vessel (see page 264), a branch tear, graze, skin flap or awkwardly shaped tear.

Some general information can be shared with the woman during suturing:

- Suggest to the woman she tries to pass urine following suturing; it may be less painful as the local anaesthetic may still be effective. The timing and volume of the first void should be monitored and documented (NICE, 2006).
- Discuss pain control, sitting and different breastfeeding positions for comfort. Oral analgesia, cool packs and bathing offer the best evidence-based pain relief (Steen, 2011).
- Warn her of the possibility of knot migration to the perineal surface with long-acting or non-absorbable suture materials (RCOG, 2007). Interrupted skin stitches can separate under the skin; the knot suddenly appears on her pad, or as she wipes herself, sometimes many months later. A word of warning can pre-empt anxiety!
- Most women do not have their bowels opened until day three postpartum; discuss this and explain she will not 'come undone'. Advise about hygiene and washing, wiping gently from front to back, supporting the perineum with a pad when having bowels open.

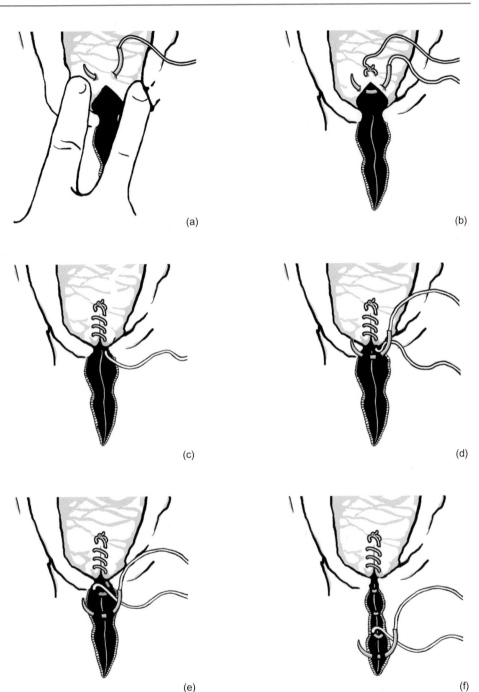

(a)

(b)

(c)

(d)

(e)

(f)

Fig. 4.4 Suturing a second degree tear. Place the first stitch above the apex of the vaginal trauma, in order to secure any deeper bleeding points (a, b). Place the loose, continuous sutures from the apex along the tear. Do not use a locking or blanket stitch, or pull sutures too tight (c). The perineum stitches are placed loosely and deeply in the subcuticular tissue (d–g). Place subcuticular, continuous sutures just under the skin (avoid placing any sutures in the fourchette) (h–k). Finish with the thread in the vagina, where a knot is tied (l).

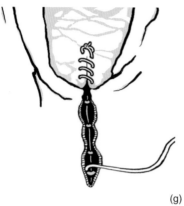

(g)

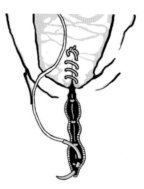

(h)

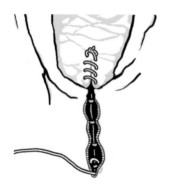

(i)

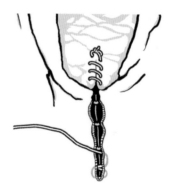

(j)

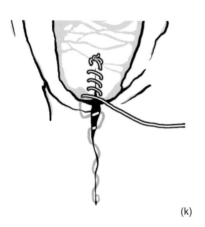

(k)

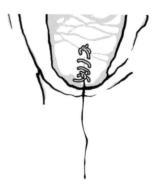

(l)

Fig. 4.4 continued   Suturing a second degree tear.

- Around 20% of childbearing women suffer from urinary incontinence. Layton (2004) suggests that midwives may give women insufficient information about this unpleasant and socially embarrassing problem. Suturing can be an opportunity for midwives to communicate to women the importance of regular pelvic floor exercises, explaining that these have been proved to be effective in maintaining continence to a significant degree (Chiarelli and Cockburn, 2002).
- It may be appropriate to discuss first sexual intercourse after the baby. Suggest the couple both feel relaxed and aroused enough before having full intercourse and consider using lubricating jelly.

Summary

- There are few studies on midwifery techniques to protect the perineum during birth.
- A rectal examination prior to suturing may improve the diagnosis of third/fourth-degree tears, which should be sutured only by an experienced doctor.
- Studies suggest little difference in non-suturing or suturing for second degree tears.
- It is *the woman's choice* whether to accept or decline suturing.
- Clinicians must be sensitive and responsive to any pain or anxiety expressed during the procedure.
- Women who have experienced sexual abuse may be especially vulnerable.

Suturing

- Use an aseptic technique with *effective* analgesia.
- Rapidly absorbed polyglactin 910 (Vicryl) is the suture material of choice.
- The muscle layer should be sutured with a loose, non-locking, continuous suture.
- The perineal skin can be left unsutured or repaired with continuous (not interrupted) suture technique.

Recommended reading

Salmon, D. (1999) A feminist analysis of women's experiences of perineal trauma in the immediate post-delivery period. *Midwifery*; 15(4), 247–56. A humbling, insightful and essential read.

References

Aasheim, V., Nilsen, A. B. V., Lukasse, M., Reinar, L. M. (2011) Perineal techniques during the second stage of labour for reducing perineal trauma. *Cochrane Database of Systematic Reviews*, Issue 12.

Adusumilli, P., Kell, C., Chang, J., Tuorto, S., Leitman, I. (2004) Left-handed surgeons: Are they left out? *Current Surgery* 61(6), 587–91.

Aikins Murphy, P., Feinland, J. B. (1998) Perineal outcomes in a home birth setting. *Birth* 25(4), 226–34.

Albers, L. L., Sedler, K. D., Bedrick, E. J. (2006) Factors related to genital tract trauma normal spontaneous vaginal births. *Birth* 33(2), 94–100.

Aldcroft, D. (2001) A guide to providing care for survivors of child sex abuse. *British Journal of Midwifery* 9(2), 81–5.

Andrews, V., Thakar, R., Sultan, A. H., Kettle, K. (2005) Can hands-on perineal repair courses affect clinical practice? *British Journal of Midwifery* 13(9), 562–6.

Arkin, A. E., Chern-Hughes, B. (2002) Case Report: labial fusion postpartum and clinical management of labial lacerations. *Midwifery Women's Health* 47(4), 290–2.

Beckmann, M. M., Garrett, A. J. (2006) Antenatal perineal massage for reducing perineal trauma. *Cochrane Database of Systematic Reviews*, Issue 1.

Bedwell, C. (2006) Are third degree tears unavoidable? The role of the midwife. *British Journal of Midwifery* 14(9), 212.

Byrd, L. M., Hobbiss, J., Tasker, M. (2005) Is it possible to predict or prevent third degree tears? *Colorectal Disease* 7, 311–18.

Carroli, G., Belizan, J. (2007) Episiotomy for vaginal birth. *Cochrane Database of Systematic Reviews*, Issue 1. Update Software, Oxford.

Chapman, V. (2009) Clinical skills: issues affecting the left-handed midwife. *British Journal of Midwifery* 17(9), 588–92.

Chiarelli, P., Cockburn, J. (2002) Promoting urinary continence in women after delivery: a randomised controlled trial. *British Medical Journal* 324(7348), 1241–4.

Dahlen, H. G., Ryan, M., Homer, C. S., Cooke, M. (2006) An Australian prospective co-hort study of risk factors for severe perineal trauma during childbirth. *Midwifery* 23(2), 196–203.

Dahlen, H. G., Homer, C. S., Cooke, M., Upton, A. M., Nunn, R. A., Brodrick, B. S. (2009) 'Soothing the ring of fire': Australian women's and midwives' experiences of using per-ineal warm packs in the second stage of labour. *Midwifery* 25(2), e39–48.

Eason, E., Labrecque, M., Wells, G., Feldman, P. (2000) Preventing perineal trauma during childbirth: a systematic review. *Obstetrics and Gynecology* 95(3), 464–71.

Elharmeel, S. M. A., Chaudhary, Y., Tan, S., Scheermeyer, E., Hanafy, A., van Driel, M. L. (2011) Surgical repair of spontaneous perineal tears that occur during childbirth versus no intervention. *Cochrane Database of Systematic Reviews*, Issue 8.

Fleming, V. E. M., Hagen, S., Niven, C. (2003) Does perineal suturing make a difference? SUNS trial. *British Journal of Obstetrics and Gynaecology* 110(7), 684–9.

Franchi, M., Cromi, A., Scarperi, S., Gaudino, R. M., Siesto, G., Ghezzi, F. (2009) Comparison between lidocaine-prilocaine cream (EMLA) and mepivacaine infiltration for pain relief during perineal repair after childbirth: a randomized trial. *American Journal of Obstetrics and Gynecology* 201(2), 186.e1-5 E-pub.

Green, J., Coupland, V., Kitzinger, J. (1998) *Great Expectations A Prospective Study of Women's Expectations and Experiences of Childbirth*. Cheshire: Books for Midwives Press.

Head, M. (1993) Dropping stitches. Do unsutured tears to the perineum heal better than sutured ones? *Nursing Times* 89(33), 64–5.

Hodnett, E. D., Hofmeyr, G. J., Sakala, C., Weston, J. (2011) Continuous support for women during childbirth. *Cochrane Database of Systematic Reviews*, Issue 2.

Jackson, K. (2000) The bottom line: care of the perineum must be improved. *British Journal of Midwifery* 8(10), 609–14.

Jenkins, E. (2011) Suturing of labial trauma: An audit of current practice. *British Journal of Midwifery* 19(11), 699–705.

JFC (Joint Formulary Committee) (2012) *British National Formulary*, 63rd edn. London, BMJ and Pharmaceutical Press.

Kettle, C. (2002) Materials and methods for perineal repair. Are you sitting comfortably? Issues around perineal trauma. *RCM Midwives Journal* 5(9), 298–301.

Kettle, C., Hills, R. K., Jones, P., Darby, L., Gray, R., Johanson, R. (2002) Continuous versus interrupted perineal repair with standard or rapidly absorbed sutures after spontaneous vaginal birth: a randomised controlled trial. *The Lancet* 359, 2217–22.

Kettle, C., Hills, R. K., Ismail, K. M. K. (2007) Continuous versus interrupted sutures for repair of episiotomy or second degree tears. *Cochrane Database of Systematic Reviews*, Issue 4.

Kettle, C., Dowswell, T., Ismail, K. M. K. (2010) Absorbable suture materials for primary repair of episiotomy and second degree tears. *Cochrane Database of Systematic Reviews*. Issue 6.

Kindberg, S. F. (2008) Perineal Lacerations after Childbirth. Studies within midwifery practice on suturing and pain relief. PhD thesis. Faculty of Health Sciences, University of Aarhus, Denmark.

Kitzinger, J. V. (1992) Counteracting, not re-enacting, the violation of women's bodies: the challenge for perinatal caregivers. *Birth* 1(4), 219–22.

Labrecque, M., Eason, E., Marcoux, S., Lemieux, F., Pinault, J.-J., Feldman, P., Laperriere L. (1999) Randomised controlled trial of prevention of perineal trauma by massage during pregnancy. *American Journal of Obstetrics and Gynecology* 10(3), 593–600.

Langley, V., Thoburn, A., Shaw, S., Barton, A., (2006) Second degree tears: to suture or not? A randomized controlled trial. *British Journal of Midwifery* 14(9), 550–4.

Layton, S. (2004) The effect of perineal trauma on women's health. *British Journal of Midwifery* 12(4), 231–6.

Leeman, L. M., Rogers, R. G., Greulich, B., Albers, L. L. (2007) Do unsutured second-degree perineal lacerations affect postpartum functional outcomes? *Journal of the American Board of Family Medicine* 20(5), 451–7.

Lundquist, M., Olisson, A., Nissen, E., Normal, M. (2000) Is it necessary to suture all lacerations after a vaginal delivery? *Birth* 27(2), 79–85.

McCandlish, R. (2001) Routine perineal suturing: is it time to stop? *MIDIRS Midwifery Digest* 11(3), 296–300.

Metcalfe, A., Bick, D., Tohill, S., Williams, A., Haldon, V. (2006) A prospective cohort study of repair and non-repair of second degree perineal trauma: results and issues for future research. *Evidence Based Midwifery* 4(2), 60–4.

Naghavi, S. H., Sanati, K. A. (2009) Needle stick injuries: does left-handedness matter? *American Journal of Infection Control* 37(4), 341.

National Institute for Health and Clinical Excellence (NICE) (2007) *Intrapartum Care: Care of Healthy Women and Their Babies During Childbirth. Clinical Guideline 55.* London, NICE.

National Institute for Health and Clinical Excellence (NICE) (2006) *Postnatal care: Routine postnatal care for women and their babies. Clinical Guideline 37.* London, NICE.

NHS QIS (NHS Quality Improvement Scotland) (2008) Perineal repair after childbirth. A Procedure and Standards tool to support Practice Development. *NHS Quality Improvement Scotland.* p. 6. www.nhshealthquality.org

ONS (Office for National Statistics) (2012) HES online NHS Maternity Statistics 2010–2011. ONS. http://www.hesonline.nhs.uk

Palmon, S. C., Lloyd, A. T., Kirsch, J. R. (1998) The effect of needle gauge and lidocaine pH on pain during intradermal injection. *Anesthesia and Analgesia.* 86(2), 379–81.

Parsons, J., Crowther, C. A. (2007) Rectal analgesia for pain from perineal trauma following childbirth. *Cochrane Database for Systematic Review*, Issue 1.

Petrou, S., Gordon, B., Mackrodt, C., Fern, E., Ayers, S., Grant, A., Truesdale, A., McCandlish R. (2001) How cost-effective is it to leave the skin unsutured? *British Journal of Midwifery* 9(4), 209–14.

Rackley, R., Vasavada, S. P., Battino, B. (2009) Bladder trauma. *Medscape.* http://emedicine.medscape.com/article/441124-overview

Royal College of Obstetricians and Gynaecologists (RCOG) (2007) The management of third and forth degree preineal tears. *Clinical Green Top Guideline 28.* http//www.rcog.org.uk/guidelines

Salmon, D. (1999) A feminist analysis of women's experiences of perineal trauma in the immediate post-delivery period. *Midwifery* 15(4), 247–56.

Saunders, J., Campbell, R. and Peters, T. J. (2002) Effectiveness of pain relief during suturing. *BJOG: An International Journal of Obstetrics and Gynaecology* 109, 1066–8.

Shorten, A., Donsante, J., Shorten, B. (2002) Birth position, accoucheur, and perineal outcomes: informing women about choices for vaginal birth. *Birth* 29(1), 18–27.

Soong, B., Barnes, M. (2005) Maternal position at midwife-attended birth and perineal trauma: is there an association? *Birth* 32, 164–9.

Stamp, G., Kruzins, G., Crowther, C. (2001) Perineal massage in labour and prevention of perineal trauma: randomised controlled trial. *BMJ* 322, 1277–80.

Steen, M. (2011) Care and consequences of perineal trauma. *British Journal of Midwifery* 18(11), 710–15.

Sultan, A. (2002) 'Have I missed a third degree tear?' The identification, treatment and follow-up of women who experience perineal trauma. Are you sitting comfortably? Issues around perineal trauma. *RCM Midwives Journal* 5(9), 298.

Sultan, J. (2007) BestBets: the effect of warming local anaesthetics on pain of infiltration. Lancashire Teaching Hospitals NHS Trust. http://www.bestbets.org/bets/bet.php?id=1480

Taylor B., Bayat, A. (2007) Basic plastic surgery techniques and principles: Using local anaesthetics. *Student BMJ archive.* http://archive.student.bmj.com/issues/03/07/education/227.php

The Aarhus Birth Cohort (2008) Perinatal Epidemiology Research Unit. Aarhus University Hospital, Skejby.

Walsh, D. (2007) *Evidence-based care for normal labour and birth: a guide for midwives*, pp. 108–9. London, Routledge.

Webb, S., Parsons, M., Toozs-Hobson, P. (2007) The role of specialised birth plans for women with previous third or fourth degree obstetric anal sphincter injuries (OASIS). *MIDIRS* 17(3), 353–4.

Yiannouzis, K. (2002) Describing perineal trauma: the development of an assessment tool. Are you sitting comfortably? Issues around perineal trauma. *RCM Midwives Journal* 5(9), 300–1.

5 Examination of the newborn baby at birth

Caroline Rutter

Introduction

The journey of the newborn baby from the dark, warm security of the mother's uterus to the stark reality of extra-uterine life has been described as the most dramatic physiological event that can occur in a human's life (Mercer and Erikson-Owens, 2010). While the midwife's role in overseeing this physiological adaptation is paramount, of equal importance is ensuring respect for the 'state of sanctity' of the mother–baby relationship (Davies and Richards, 2008). The benefits of delayed cord clamping and skin-to-skin contact are discussed in Chapter 1. Observations should be as non-invasive as possible to support this mutually beneficial mother–baby contact throughout the early hours of newborn life.

The initial neonatal examination is performed soon after the birth, and should not take long. A more detailed newborn examination will also be offered later, within 72 hours of birth, by a qualified healthcare professional: midwife, paediatrician or neonatal practitioner (NIPE, 2012). RCM (2008) guidelines stress that 'routine delivery ward practice' should not interfere with mother–baby interaction and emphasise kindness, respect, gentle handling and lack of excessive noise. Much of the examination can be performed while the mother is holding or feeding her baby. General

The Midwife's Labour and Birth Handbook, Third Edition. Edited by Vicky Chapman and Cathy Charles.
© 2013 John Wiley & Sons, Ltd. Published 2013 by John Wiley & Sons, Ltd.

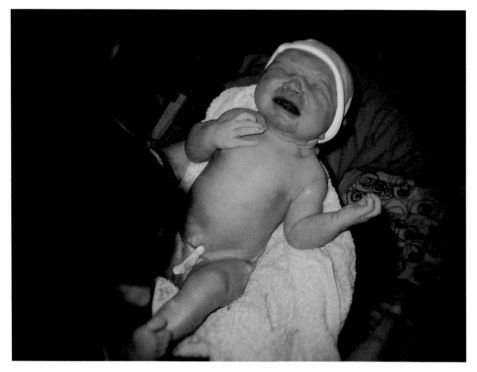

Fig. 5.1   Baby Amber being examined on a midwife's lap after home birth.

observation of the baby's condition and behaviour is as important as formal systematic assessment.

Involve the parents; explain the process and let them ask questions and explore their new baby. Any neonatal assessment is an opportunity for parent education and health promotion (Demott *et al.*, 2006; NHS QIS, 2004). If you suspect an abnormality explain simply and clearly and contact a senior paediatrician: this may require transfer from home or midwifery-led birthing centre. How this situation is handled and how information is provided to parents regarding congenital abnormality can have a lasting effect (Kerr and McIntoch, 1998; Williamson, 2004).

The midwife's assessment of the baby at birth

Most babies are born responding well. These should be received immediately by their mother for uninterrupted skin-to-skin contact (see page 25). Occasionally, a baby may have an obvious problem requiring a prompt response. The Apgar score is one method of assessing the baby's condition following birth (Table 5.1). It is well established but not uncritically accepted; some suggest abandoning it, or replacing it with a more objective precise measure (Patel and Beeby, 2004; O'Donnell *et al.*, 2007). It may be helpful for deciding if resuscitation is required, but cannot determine the cause or prognosis of any hypoxic episode. If a baby's condition causes concern then analyse cord bloods for a clearer picture of the degree/duration of any labour hypoxia.

Table 5.1   Apgar score.

Score	0	1	2
Colour	Blue or pale	Body pink, limbs blue	Pink
Respiratory effort	Absent	Irregular gasps	Strong cry
Heart rate	Absent	<100 bpm	>100 bpm
Muscle tone	Limp	Some limb flexion	Strong active movements
Reflex irritability	None	Grimace or sneeze	Cry

Apgar score is normally assessed at 1 and 5 min. Some like to record a 10 min score.
The 1 min score is often low: babies often recover quickly and have a good 5 min score.
A poor 5 min score is more indicative of a baby with real problems requiring active resuscitation.
Score at 5 min: 8–10, normal; 5–7, mild asphyxia; ≤4, severe asphyxia.

Colour

Caucasian babies should appear pink at birth, often with bluish extremities (peripheral cyanosis) for several hours following delivery. Babies with darker skins tend to have a much paler version of their parents' skin tone with lighter extremities.

Possible problems

- **Blueness around the mouth and trunk (central cyanosis)** may indicate a respiratory/cardiac problem. Darker skin babies can look greyish white when cyanosed. For cyanosis: give oxygen, assess respiratory effort and heart rate, consider pulse oximetry, summon paediatrician, initiate resuscitation if required (see Chapter 18).
- **Very pale baby.** Consider infection (Kenner and Wright-Lott, 2007), cardiac anomalies, anaemia, hypoxia or shock; initiate resuscitation if necessary.
- **Facial congestion.** Petechiae (tiny broken capillary blood vessels) appear as a blue/mauve rash or discoloured skin of the face and head; caused by increased pressure on the head and chest during birth, possibly after precipitous labour, tight nuchal cord or shoulder dystocia. Lips and mucous membranes are pink. Facial congestion is usually unproblematic and should not be confused with a more generalised rash resulting from serious clotting disorders or congenital infections e.g. toxoplasmosis, meningitis, herpes (Henley, 2010).
- **Plethoric baby.** Red skin colouration may indicate excessive red blood cells (polycythaemia), possibly following a large transfusion of placental blood, e.g. twin-to-twin transfusion.
- **Jaundice** at birth, or within the first 24 hours, is abnormal and serious. Causes include haemolytic disease/rhesus incompatibility or congenital infection.

Respirations and cry

Not all newborns breathe immediately at birth nor do all cry, particularly if the birthing environment is calm, quiet and relaxed. Anecdotal reports suggest that water birth babies may be slow to breathe, but if the cord is unclamped and still pulsating at >100 bpm, the baby is probably receiving a good oxygen supply. However, some babies appear inconsolable at birth. Once settled skin-to-skin with its mother the baby will usually relax and stop crying, often opening its eyes and with patience will eventually root towards the breast.

Possible problems

- Persistent tachypnoea (respirations >60/min at term), grunting, nasal flaring or sternal recession are signs of respiratory distress. Causes include infection, prematurity, meconium aspiration and cardiac problems. Refer to a paediatrician.
- A baby who does not breathe following attempted inflation breaths may require gentle suction of mucus or meconium. Excessive secretions may indicate oesophageal atresia.
- A distinctly high-pitched or 'irritable' cry may indicate pain, cerebral irritation, metabolic abnormalities or drug withdrawal (Lumsden, 2011).

Heart rate

Use a stethoscope or palpate a baby's heartbeat by placing two fingers on the chest directly over the heart, or hold the base of the umbilical stump. Normal neonatal heart rate (HR) is 110–160 bpm.

Possible problems

- *Bradycardia* (HR < 100 bpm) may result from hypoxia. With adequate respiration the HR can recover quickly. If <60 bpm cardiac massage will be necessary (see Chapter 18).
- *Tachycardia* (HR > 160 bpm) may indicate a healthy response to a hypoxic episode. Again with adequate respiration it can recover quickly. It can however indicate infection or a respiratory/cardiac problem. Refer to paediatrician if it persists.

Muscle tone

The newborn should have good muscle tone and normal reflexes and responses, e.g. opening eyes and responding to external stimuli and touch. A floppy baby with poor muscle tone or reflex response may have experienced significant hypoxia, or have a congenital abnormality, e.g. Down's syndrome.

Measurements of the newborn

Weight

Following skin-to-skin contact and feeding the baby should be weighed. The parents may wish to observe and take photographs. Ideally use electronic scales for greatest accuracy, zeroed after positioning a warm towel (Figure 5.2).

A baby weighing <2.5 kg is considered low birth weight; and <1.5 kg is very low birth weight. Ethnic-origin-specific weight charts avoid inappropriately labelling a baby small for dates (Chung *et al.*, 2003). A macrosomic (large) baby is 4–4.5 kg or >90th centile for gestational age.

Both small babies, due to prematurity or intrauterine growth restriction (IUGR) and macrosomic babies are at risk of hypoglycaemia, so blood glucose testing should be considered (Newel *et al.*, 1997; Holmes, 2010).

A baby born at <37 weeks is classified as preterm. Some babies may be both preterm and small for dates: these are at higher risk of problems, as IUGR may indicate placental insufficiency.

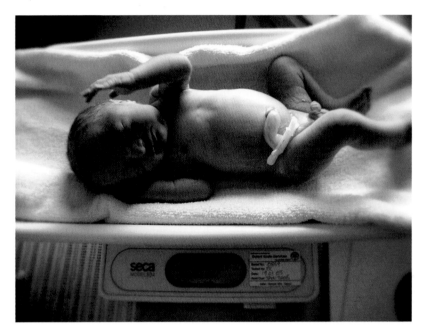

Fig. 5.2   Place something soft on the scales.

Length

Measuring length at birth is not always recommended. Whilst growth is an important indicator of a child's health and well-being (DoH, 2009; CGF, 2009) the latest World Health Organization (2009) growth charts are for use from two weeks of age.

If length *is* measured, Jokinen (2002) recommends waiting at least one hour after birth: the baby may remain in a fetal position for some hours (NICE, 2007). Tape measures are somewhat unreliable (Wilshin *et al.*, 1999); a roll-up mat may be better (Jokinen, 2002). A term baby's length is typically 48–55 cm (Seidel *et al.*, 2006).

Head circumference

Measure the occipitofrontal circumference of the head (page 45): normally 32–37 cm at term (McDonald, 2008). Some advise waiting until the head has regained its shape following birth, and advise a specifically designed metric insertion tape (Fry, 2002; McDonald, 2008).

Vitamin K prophylaxis

Vitamin K is essential for the formation of prothrombin, which enables blood to clot. Haemorrhagic disease of the newborn (HDN) or vitamin K deficiency bleeding (VKDB) is a rare, potentially fatal, disorder associated with low vitamin K levels. HDN/VKDB usually occurs in the first week of life: common bleeding sites are gastrointestinal, cutaneous, nasal and circumcision (Puckett and Offringa, 2000). Late-onset bleeding (1 week to 8 months) may indicate liver disease or malabsorption and is potentially more dangerous (Hey, 2003b).

Vitamin K administration at birth significantly reduces the incidence of haemorrhagic disease (Puckett and Offringa, 2000).

Incidence and facts

- HDN/VKDB affects:
  - 1 in 17 000 babies without vitamin K prophylaxis.
  - 1 in 25 000 to 1 in 70 000 in babies after a single oral 1–2 mg dose at birth.
  - 1 in 400 000 after a single intramuscular (IM) injection at birth (Puckett and Offringa, 2000).
- Babies most at risk are premature, unwell or have had traumatic deliveries.
- The Department of Health recommends vitamin K for all newborn babies: more than 97% of UK babies receive it.

Vitamin K controversy

Doubt exists as to the optimal level of newborn vitamin K. Wickham (2000) suggests that a 'low' level is physiologically normal and desirable. Cranford (2011) suggests that physiological, as opposed to medicalised, birth, supports the newborn's innate clotting system. In the early days and weeks following birth, babies build up a vitamin K supply from feeding. Totally breastfed babies are slightly more prone to late-onset haemorrhagic disease. Vitamin K is added to artificial milk. Wickham (2000) proposes that the research suggesting that breast milk is low in vitamin K was conducted when feeds were restricted in length and frequency, resulting in reduced intake of fat-rich colostrum and hindmilk (where fat-soluble vitamin K is mostly found). Term breastfed babies may be at risk mainly if early intake is limited or poor (Palmer, 1993; Hey, 2003b). Over 50% of babies developing late-onset HDN have an underlying cause, e.g. malabsorption or liver disease (Puckett and Offringa, 2000).

There is debate over IM versus oral administration (Hey, 2003a). IM administration, although more effective, is invasive, so parents may refuse it. Also some time ago Golding *et al.* (1992) suggested a tentative link between IM vitamin K and childhood leukaemia. Whilst further studies showed no association (Fear *et al.*, 2003) parents still express concerns. Some clinicians argue that vitamin K is more important for babies who have experienced difficult births (e.g. forceps) and recommend selective administration (McNinch, 2010).

Oral preparations are more expensive, more poorly absorbed, rely on parent compliance and may affect babies with undiagnosed cholestasis (Sutor *et al.*, 1999).

In conclusion, NICE (2006) recommends vitamin K for newborns, preferably IM or, if not, orally. Give parents clear evidence-based information so they can make an informed choice (Demott *et al.*, 2006; MIDIRS, 2005).

Top-to-toe check

Each midwife will have a system for checking the newborn baby (e.g. 'top to toe and front to back'). Minimise naked exposure so the baby stays warm. Most of the check can be done with the baby in the mother's arms or in a cot or on the bed near her.

Table 5.2   Types of neonatal infection.

Neonatal infection	Neonatal signs and symptoms at birth	Neonatal diagnosis and treatment
Cytomegalovirus (CMV) a herpes virus: commonest congenital infection in the developed world	Often initially asymptomatic 10–15% petechiae/jaundice 40–58% adverse outcomes, e.g. neurodevelopmental, hearing loss (CMV infection in utero is the leading cause of congenital deafness)	Urine, saliva or blood cultures Few treatments, occasionally antivirals
Group B streptococcus (GBS) bacterium: commonest UK cause of severe early newborn infection	RDS, septicaemia Prompt referral essential as baby can deteriorate rapidly	If known: intrapartum antibiotic prophylaxis significantly reduces risk, or antibiotics to baby at birth Diagnosis via blood cultures, possible lumbar puncture (for meningitis) Prophylactic antibiotics whilst awaiting results Babies may require ventilatory support
Rubella: congenital rubella syndrome (CRS) virus rare in developed countries due to vaccination programmes	Transient congenital problems: lymphadenopathy, low birth weight, hepatosplenomegaly, hepatitis, jaundice, thrombocytopenic purpura, petechiae and 'blueberry muffin' lesions Permanent 'problems': deafness, cataracts, learning difficulties, diabetes	Cultures: stools or cerebrospinal fluid Isolation is required Treatment depends on symptoms
Chicken pox Varicella zoster virus – many women immune through childhood infection	If **early pregnancy** fetal infection often transient/ asymptomatic, but 2–3% develop varicella syndrome: skin lesions, skeletal abnormalities, cataracts, encephalitis and/or neurological damage	If late pregnancy, i.e. maternal infection 5 days prebirth to 2 days postbirth there is a 30% neonatal mortality rate: these babies should receive varicella-zoster immune globulin (VZIG)
Toxoplasmosis parasite acquired through contaminated food or handling animal faeces, especially cats	Often initially asymptomatic; sometimes rash, jaundice, thrombocytopenia, enlarged liver, pneumonia, hydrocephalus, microcephaly, microphthalmia	Blood test Antibiotics (possibly up to one year) with eye examination & scan for brain damage
Syphilis bacterial infection rare in developed countries	Often initially asymptomatic; occasional palm/sole skin lesions, fever, eye infection, jaundice, rhinitis, osteitis, anaemia, thrombocytopenia	Blood test, placental histopathology, lumbar puncture Antenatal blood screening and treatment reduces transplacental transmission
Gonorrhoea bacterial infection: 50% infected women will be asymptomatic	(Usually asymptomatic in pregnancy but risk of premature labour) Congenital/early onset ophthalmia neonatorum: purulent discharge and lid swelling, leading to corneal hazing & blindness	Eye swab culture Antibiotics
Herpes simplex virus (HSV) 85% neonatal HSV occurs during labour, so CS recommended if active maternal lesions (Davies & Anderson, 2008)	Often vague: prematurity, low birth weight, fever, encephalitis, eye infection, skin blisters/lesions, although often asymptomatic until aged 5–21 days	Lumbar puncture (often initially negative) Acyclovir (antiviral) treatment
Listeria bacterial infection carried by 5% population	Granulomatous rash on baby/ placenta, RDS and pneumonia	Blood and CSF culture, placental examination. Antibiotics
Chlamydia trachomatis bacterial infection, usually asymptomatic in pregnancy	Up to 50% exposed babies become infected, usually conjunctivitis: untreated can cause blindness Occasional pneumonia	Blood tests, eye/nose swab culture Antibiotics

Head

Newborn babies can have misshapen heads. Reassure parents that moulding (overriding skull bones) and caput succedaneum (scalp oedema) are common and the shape quickly returns to normal. Cephalhaematoma (bleeding beneath the cranial periosteum causing unilateral swelling) is not usually present at birth but develops hours/days later. Inform the parents it may take several weeks to resolve and may contribute to jaundice but is not usually serious.

Face

Abnormal facial appearance, e.g. a prominent narrow/flat forehead or asymmetry may indicate various conditions including palsy, Edward's, Down's or Turner's syndromes. Baston and Durward (2010) recommend seeing both parents before commenting on any unusual appearance as the baby may simply have inherited familial traits.

Eyes

Note position, shape and symmetry. Discharge or inflammation <24 hours after birth could indicate chlamydia or gonococcal infection (Table 5.2). Other infections, e.g. staphylococcal usually occur several days after birth. Check for cataracts (cloudy cornea). Translucent irises may indicate albinism. Subconjunctival haemorrhages (red areas on the sclera/conjunctiva) are common, due to birth pressure, and usually resolve in days.

Ears

Tags or dimpling while usually of no significance and sometimes familial, occasionally indicate renal problems, so always refer. Low-set ears may indicate disorders, e.g. Patau's/Down's syndrome.

Mouth

Check the mouth for problems, e.g. congenital teeth, which may need removing. A short, square or heart-shaped tongue may indicate a tight frenulum, i.e. tongue tie (ankyloglossia). Some babies may need a simple procedure to cut the frenulum (frenectomy), especially if interfering with breastfeeding.

To check for a cleft palate, insert a clean finger and move the pad across the roof of the mouth (Figure 5.3), and/or inspect with a light which may reveal a sub-mucous cleft, not easily felt. Undetected clefts can cause feeding, and later speech, difficulties. Suspect cleft palate if milk comes from the nose while feeding (if not vomiting) (Martin and Bannister, 2003).

A cleft lip may be unilateral or bilateral, almost unnoticeable or extensive. Surgery is normally required. Cleft lip or palate may be associated with other congenital abnormalities including Pierre Robin's syndrome.

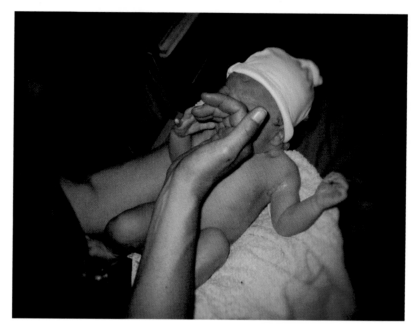

Fig. 5.3   Finger inspection for cleft palate.

Neck

Shortness, webbing or folds of skin on the back of the neck may indicate chromosomal abnormalities, e.g. Turner's syndrome.

Chest and abdomen

There should be two nipples. Breast enlargement is common in both boys and girls; the breasts may even secrete a little milk. Sternal recession, particularly with other respiratory distress signs e.g. nasal flaring, grunting or tachypnoea, should be reported to a paediatrician. Check for fractures: move the fingers along the clavicles feeling for irregularities.

The abdomen should feel soft. Report hernias. Protrusions at the base of the umbilicus may indicate exomphalos (herniating bowel). Check that the umbilical clamp is secure. The cord should have one vein and two arteries; a single artery occurs in 1% of singletons and 5% of twins: 20% of these babies have abnormalities, e.g. cardiovascular, gastrointestinal, renal or multiple anomaly syndromes (Beall and Ross, 2012).

Genitalia

Note size, position and any skin pigmentation. Darker-skinned parents may have babies with a darker scrotum or labia. In cases of ambiguous gender avoid guessing the baby's sex, as an incorrect guess can cause great distress. Indeterminate gender is a complex area and very stressful for the parents. Sometimes a paediatrician can clearly determine the gender by palpating penile tissue and gonads. More complex cases require genetic and endocrine blood tests, possibly scanning for ovaries, usually including specialist referral. This can take weeks. Blood is often taken for congenital adrenal hyperplasia (CAH) screening, another cause of ambiguous genitalia, possibly repeated several weeks later as initial results are not always conclusive. CAH is a serious condition which can be life-threatening; treatment is lifelong.

Baby boys

The size of the penis varies. Locating the urethral orifice may reveal hypospadias (1:300 male babies), where the urethral meatus opens on the undersurface of the penis (Hypospadias UK, 2011) Babies with hypospadias should not be circumcised, as skin may be needed for surgical repair later. Note any passage of urine, as dribbling could indicate urethral blockage: surgery may be indicated to prevent renal damage.

Gently examine the scrotal sack for the presence/absence of testes; if absent they usually descend by six weeks. Document their presence: they may move out of the scrotal sac later and be incorrectly diagnosed as undescended.

A large, swollen scrotum (hydrocele) is fairly common, not serious in the newborn, and resolves spontaneously over following months.

Baby girls

The labia/clitoris can look large in preterm and small-for-dates newborns but excessive size could suggest indeterminate sex; testes can sometimes even be felt beneath the 'labia'.

A mucus vaginal discharge, possibly blood-tinged, may persist for several days. Reassure parents this is due to maternal hormone withdrawal and is normal.

Anus

Check the presence and location of the anus. If positioned anteriorly it may be associated with malformation of the rectum (Baston and Durward, 2010). Document passage of meconium.

Back and spine

Run a finger down the spine to feel for hidden swellings or indentations. Spina bifida can be found anywhere from the neck to the coccyx. Any neurological damage occurs below the level of the lesion:

- Spina bifida occulta: often visible as a dimple. Often asymptomatic/insignificant.
- Meningocele: a sac covers the spinal cord. Some degree of disability often results.
- Myelomeningocele: spinal nerves are exposed. This is the most serious form.

Limbs

Limbs should look symmetrical. Check fingers and toes for webbing or overlapping, deformed, fused, missing or extra digits. These can be hereditary or indicate various syndromes. In-utero amniotic bands may cause fused, malformed or missing digits and are associated with club foot, cleft problems and haemangioma. A single palmar crease may indicate Down's syndrome.

Talipes presents as the foot appearing internally rotated at the ankle. If the foot can be palpated back into position, this is talipes equinovarus ('positional talipes') which resolves spontaneously. If not this 'structural talipes' requires physiotherapy, splinting and occasionally surgery. Most babies do well after treatment and grow up able to walk and run normally (STEPS, 2006).

Skin

Birthmarks may be found; some are more obvious than others: see Box 5.1. Parents can be naturally distressed at large or visible birthmarks, e.g. facial, and want information on permanence and/or treatment. Document and discuss other features, e.g. hyperpigmented macule (formerly 'Mongolian blue spot'), rashes, bruising and birth trauma.

Box 5.1   Birthmarks and skin discolouration.

Hyperpigmented macule (formerly known as Mongolian blue spot)
- Bluish pigmentation over the sacrum/back, occasionally shoulders and limbs.
- Completely benign; tends to fade within a year.
- More common in babies with dark skin; occasionally in pale skin.
- Documentation is important, as parents may be accused later of bruising their baby.

Stork marks (naevus simplex)
- Pink/purple pressure marks, usually on face and nape of neck.
- A third of babies have these; they are benign and fade within a year.

Port wine stain/capillary haemangioma
- Deep dense bluish-purple permanent mark present at birth; tends to grow with the baby.
- Cosmetic coverage may be sufficient but laser therapy is available.

Pigmented naevus
- Permanent birthmark often extensive; may have hair growing through it.
- Excision and skin grafting possible if area is not too large.

Strawberry naevus
- Pink/purple raised areas of blood-filled capillaries. Not obvious at birth; develop in the early days of life.
- Most resolve by 8 years; normally left alone but laser treatment or surgery possible.

Neonatal infection

The fetus and newborn baby have several factors which protect against infection:

- The placenta and membranes protect against most bacteria, although not viruses.
- Passive immunity via vaccination or exposure; as immunoglobulin G (IgG) passes through the placenta.
- Vernix caseosa acts as a protective 'surface microbicidal shield' (Levy, 2007).
- Breastfeeding provides antibodies for passive immunity.

Despite these factors, neonates are considered born immunocompromised due to their immature immune systems, and at greater risk of infection than at any other time (Stables and Rankin, 2011).

Paradoxically, the main routes of infection are aligned to the protective factors mentioned above:

- Transplacental route: viruses (rubella, cytomegalovirus, varicella, HIV), parasites (toxoplasmosis), bacteria (listeria: one of very few transplacental bacteria) and malaria.
- Ascending and intrapartum route: especially after prolonged rupture of membranes, e.g. group B streptococcus (GBS), E. coli, pseudomonas, listeria, gonococcus, hepatitis B, candida albicans, chlamydia trachomatis.
- Postpartum route, i.e. breastfeeding, environmental (including hospital-acquired infection: midwives have a key role in prevention), e.g. staphylococcus aureus. Prime areas are eyes, fingernails, umbilicus, mucous membranes and skin, which is fragile at birth and susceptible to damage by instrumental delivery or fetal scalp electrode (Levy, 2007; Paterson, 2010).

Antenatal/intrapartum risk factors for infection

- Low birth weight: the most important risk factor for sepsis (Isaacs and Moxon, 1999)
- Preterm birth (often caused by maternal infection) – another very vulnerable group
- Prolonged and/or premature rupture of membranes
- Known maternal infection, e.g. GBS
- Maternal pyrexia/tachycardia in labour +/− fetal tachycardia/pathological CTG
- Offensive liquor and/or 'smelly' baby
- Thick/fresh meconium-stained liquor
- Maternal substance abuse

General signs and symptoms

See Table 5.2 for types of infection.

Infections vary from superficial to life-threatening: many present with similar symptoms which may be subtle. Be vigilant and refer promptly if suspicious.

- Respiratory/circulatory: tachypnoea/apnoea, sternal recession, grunting, tachycardia, pallor, pyrexia/hypothermia
- Behaviour/tone: irritability, high-pitched cry, jitteriness (low blood sugar), poor/excessive tone, lethargy, unresponsiveness
- Other: rashes, jaundice, swollen abdomen, purulent eyes, bulging fontanelle.

Neonatal observations will vary according to type and level of infection and local policy, but should include temperature, apex beat, respiratory rate, and observation of colour, sternal recession, nasal flaring and possibly blood sugar estimation. Oxygen saturation monitoring may be helpful – see algorithm page 295 for normal saturation for a newborn baby.

Breastfeeding (and/or expressed breastmilk) should be encouraged throughout any treatment for maximum health benefits (NICE, 2012).

Giving upsetting news to parents

In resource-rich countries where women are offered antenatal screening and scans to detect problems, the birth of a baby with an anomaly can come as a profound shock to the parents. Feelings are often contradictory: love and protectiveness mixed with revulsion and guilt. Many people ask 'why us?'; unable to understand why their baby is physically imperfect when the rest of the world seems full of perfect, healthy children. Their reactions may be akin to grieving, as they mourn the loss of an anticipated perfect baby before acceptance and attachment to the 'imperfect' one is possible.

For the midwife, the birth of a baby with a problem can also be an unexpected shock. The midwife may feel useless and lost for words or ways to make things better. Parents will take their cue from the midwife; if he/she can sound positive without being unrealistic, then they will be more likely to accept their baby. The midwife may need to tell the parents immediately of a visible/obvious problem at birth, or refer to a paediatrician for an opinion, who may then break the news to the parents.

There is a wealth of seminal work about loss and grief over a baby with a congenital abnormality, whether identified antenatally or when a 'perfect' addition to the family had been expected (Solnit and Stark, 1961; Khubler-Ross, 1973; Drotar *et al.*, 1975; Johnston, 2003). However, Davies and Anderson (2008) state that despite an abundance of literature identifying good practice, discussion of abnormality/disability is often poorly handled by professionals.

Robb (1999) suggests that there is no perfect way of giving upsetting news. However, a few simple guidelines, sensitively followed, can mitigate some of the distress. Williamson (2004) discusses the disempowerment felt at the birth of a child with problems. Some of the most important factors from the parents' perspective when upsetting news is being given include:

- Provide privacy.
- Keep it simple: be honest. Avoid jargons or euphemisms. Be prepared to repeat.
- Show empathy but do not lose control.
- Talk to parents together whilst holding their baby; do not try to cover up a visible abnormality.
- Avoid blaming the parents.
- Don't be afraid of silence: it allows parents to consider information and form questions.
- Do not take away all hope: say something positive.
- Personalise the information: use the baby's name if he/she has one.
- If you don't know the answer to a question, do not guess: get a senior paediatrician.
- Recognise and acknowledge feelings the parents may have, e.g. anger.
- Make appropriate referrals and ensure early follow-up.
- Written information, support groups and contact numbers are important, but they are no substitute for giving time and explanations.

(Robb, 1999; Williamson, 2004; Webb and Lomax, 2011)

All health professionals should have training in breaking bad news (Farrell *et al.*, 2001). Robb (1999) suggests midwives should practise role play with colleagues. Midwives often are not involved regularly enough to feel proficient at it. Parents are usually shocked and only remember pieces of what they are told. However, they do remember who told them and if it was handled positively or not (Robb, 1999).

It is important to recognise the power of language used in emotive situations and that an individual's perception of what is normal or abnormal, or what is 'bad news', depends on personal, philosophical, societal and cultural beliefs and experiences (Davies and Anderson, 2008). Bainbridge (2009) suggests the use of terms like 'negative' and 'normal' when reporting screening results reinforces parental perceptions of the perfect child, and should be reviewed. Providing sensitive therapeutic care for families where anomalies present at birth can be demanding and challenging, as well as rewarding. Peer and supervisory support should be encouraged for midwives involved in such difficult and emotional aspects of their work.

Useful contacts

Contact a Family. UK charity providing information and support to parents of disabled children. www.cafamily.org.uk

Department of Health (2010) *The Pregnancy Book*. www.dh.gov.uk
This has a useful contacts section for many support groups.

Newlife Foundation for Disabled Children. www.newlifecharity.co.uk

References

Bainbridge, L. (2009) Not quite perfect! Diagnosis of a minor congenital abnormality during examination of the newborn. *Infant* 5(1), 28–31.

Baston, H., Durward, H. (2010) *Examination of the Newborn: A Practical Guide*, 2nd edn. London, Routledge.

Beall, M. H., Ross, M. G. (2012) Single umbilical artery. *Umbilical cord complications*. http://emedicine.medscape.com/article/262470-overview.

CGF (Child Growth Foundation) (2009) Growth Assessment Recommendations. http://www.childgrowthfoundation.org/.

Chung, J. H., Boscardin, W. J., Garite, T. J. (2003) Ethnic differences in birth weight by gestational age: a partial explanation for the Hispanic epidemiologic paradox? *American Journal of Obstetrics and Gynecology* 189(4), 1058–62.

Cranford, M. (2011) Vitamin K: Did nature get it right? *Midwifery Today* (98), 28, 66.

Davies, L., Anderson, J. (2008) Congenital abnormality: screening, diagnosis and communication. In Davies, L., McDonald, S. (eds) *Examination of the Newborn and Neonatal Health: a Multidimensional Approach*, pp. 197–220. London, Elsevier.

Davies, L., Richards, R. (2008) Maternal and newborn transition: adjustment to extrauterine life. In Davies, L., McDonald, S. (eds) *Examination of the Newborn and Neonatal Health: a Multidimensional Approach*, 107–26. London, Elsevier.

Demott, K., Bick, D., Norman, R. *et al.* (2006) *Clinical Guidance and Evidence Review for Postnatal Care: Routine postnatal care of recently delivered women and their babies*. London, National Collaborating Centre for Primary Care and RCOG.

DoH (Department of Health) (2009) *Healthy Child Programme: pregnancy and the first five years of life*. London, DoH.

Drotar, D., Baskiewiez, A., Irvin, N. (1975) The adaptation of parents to the birth of an infant with a congenital malformation: a hypothetical model. *Paediatrics* 56, 710.

Farrell, M., Ryan, S., Langrick, B. (2001) 'Breaking bad news' within a paediatric setting: an evaluation report of a collaborative education workshop to support health professionals. *Journal of Advanced Nursing*, 36(6) 765–75.

Fear, N., Roman, E., Ansell, P., Simpson, J., Day, N., Eden, O. (2003) Vitamin K and childhood cancer: a report from the UK Childhood Cancer Study. *British Journal of Cancer* 8(7), 1228–31.

Fry, T. (2002) Measuring newborns: yes, size does really matter. *Midwives Journal* 5(7), 220–1.

Golding, J., Greenwood, R., Birmingham, K., Mott, M. (1992) Childhood cancer, intramuscular vitamin K and pethidine given in labour. *British Medical Journal* 305, 341–6.

Henley, J. (2010) Birth Injury. In Lumsden, H., Holmes, D. (eds.) *Care of the Newborn by Ten Teachers*, pp.146–58. London, Hodder Arnold.

Hey, E. (2003a) Vitamin K – can we improve on nature? *MIDIRS* 13(1), 7–12.

Hey, E. (2003b) Vitamin K – what, why and when. *Archives of Disease in Childhood Fetal and Neonatal Edition* 88(2), 80–3.

Holmes, D. (2010) Transition to extrauterine life. In Lumsden, H., Holmes, D. (eds) *Care of the Newborn by Ten Teachers*, pp.11–22. London: Hodder Arnold.

Hypospadias UK. (2011) www.hypospadiasuk.co.uk/

Isaacs, D., Moxon, E. (1999) *Handbook of Neonatal Infections: a practical guide*. London, WB Saunders.

Johnston, P. (2003) *The Newborn Child*, 9th edn. Edinburgh: Churchill Livingstone.

Jokinen, M. (2002) Measuring newborns: does size really matter? *Midwives Journal* 5(5), 186–7.

Kenner, C., Wright-Lott, J. (2007) *Comprehensive Neonatal Care: An Interdisciplinary Approach*, 4th edn. London, Saunders.

Kerr, S., McIntoch, J. (1998) Disclosure of disability: exploring the perspectives of parents. *Midwifery* 14, 225–32.

Khubler-Ross, E. (1973) *On Death and Dying. Social Science*. New York, Tavistock.

Levy, O. (2007) Innate immunity of the newborn: basic mechanisms and clinical correlates. *Nature Reviews. Immunology*. [online] 7, 379–390 http://www.nature.com/nri/index.html

Lumsden, H. (2011) Examination of the newborn. In Lumsden, H., Holmes, D. (eds) *Care of the Newborn by Ten Teachers*, pp. 34–50. London, Hodder Arnold.

Martin, V., Bannister, P. (eds) (2003) *Cleft Care – A Practical Guide for Health Professionals on Cleft Lip and/or Palate*. Salisbury, Academic Publishing Services.

McDonald, S. (2008) The practical examination of the newborn. In Davies, L., McDonald, S., (eds) *Examination of the Newborn and Neonatal Health: a Multidimensional Approach*, pp. 7–38. London, Elsevier.

McNinch, A. (2010) Vitamin K deficiency bleeding: Early history and recent trends in the United Kingdom. *Early Human Development* 86 (1), 63–65.

Mercer, J., Erickson-Owens, D. (2010) Evidence for neonatal transition and the first hour of life. In Walsh, D., Downe, S. (eds) *Essential Midwifery Practice: Intrapartum Care*. Chichester: Wiley-Blackwell.

MIDIRS (2005) *Informed choice for professionals: Vitamin K: the debate and the evidence, No. 18*. Bristol: MIDIRS.

Newel, S. J., Miller, P., Morgan, I., Salariya, E. (1997) Management of the newborn baby: midwifery and paediatric perspectives. In Henderson, C., Jones, K. (eds) *Essential Midwifery*, 229–64. London, Mosby.

NHS QIS (NHS Quality Improvement Scotland) (2004) *Best Practice Statement for Routine Examination of the Newborn*. Edinburgh: NHS QIS.

NICE (National Institute for Health and Clinical Excellence) (2006) *Routine Postnatal Care of Women and Their Babies.* www.nice.org.uk

NICE (2007) *Clinical Guideline 55: Intrapartum Care.* www.nice.org.uk

NICE (2012) *Antibiotics for Early-onset Neonatal Infection: antibiotics for the prevention and treatment of early-onset neonatal infection.* www.nice.org.uk

NIPE (NHS Newborn and Infant Physical Examination Programme) (2012) http://newborn physical.screening.nhs.uk/

O'Donnell, C. P., Kamlin, C. O., Davis, P. G. (2007) Interobserver variability of the 5-minute Apgar score. *Journal of Pediatrics* 149(4), 486–89.

Palmer, G. (1993) *The Politics of Breastfeeding.* London, Pandora.

Patel, H., Beeby, P. J. (2004) Resuscitation beyond 10 minutes of term babies born without signs of life. *MIDIRS* 14(3), 391–3.

Paterson, L. (2010) Infection in the newborn period. In Lumsden, H., Holmes, D. (eds) *Care of the Newborn by Ten Teachers*, 115–16. London, Hodder Arnold.

Puckett, R. M., Offringa, M. (2000) Vitamin K for preventing haemorrhagic disease. *Cochrane Library*, Issue 4. Oxford, Update Software.

Robb, F. (1999) Congenital malformations: breaking bad news. *British Journal of Midwifery* 7(1), 26–31.

RCM (Royal College of Midwives) (2008) Practice Guidelines. *Immediate Care of the Newborn. Evidence-based guidelines for midwifery-led care in labour.* London, RCM.

Seidel, H. M., Rosenstein, B. J., Pathak, A., McKay, W. H. (eds) (2006) *Primary Care of the Newborn*, 4th edn. Philadelphia: Saunders Elsevier.

Solnit, A., Stark, M. (1961) Mourning and the birth of a defective child. *Psychoanalytic Study of the Child.* 16, 523–37.

Stables, D., Rankin, J. (2011) (eds) *Physiology in Childbearing with Anatomy and Related Biosciences*, 3rd edn. Edinburgh, Balliere Tindall.

STEPS (2006) *National Association for Families of Children with Congenital Abnormalities of the Lower Limbs.* www.steps-charity.org.uk

Sutor, A. H., von Kries, R., Cornelissen, E. A. M., McNinch, A. W., Andrew, M. (1999) Vitamin K deficiency bleeding in infancy. *Thrombosis and Haemoststasis* 81, 456–61.

Webb, D., Lomax, A. (2011) Chromosomal and genetic problems: giving feedback to parents. In Lomax, A. (2011) *Examination of the Newborn. An evidence-based guide*, pp. 179–200. Chichester: Wiley-Blackwell.

Wickham, S. (2000) Vitamin K: a flaw in the blueprint. *Midwifery Today* 56, 39–41.

Williamson, A. (2004) Breaking bad news: a parent's perspective. *Midwives* (4)170–1.

Wilshin, J., Geary, M., Persaud, M., Hindmarsh, P. (1999) The reliability of newborn length measurement. *British Journal of Midwifery* 7(4), 236–9.

World Health Organization, United Nations Children's Fund (2009) *WHO Child Growth Standards and the Identification of Severe Acute Malnutrition In Infants and Children. A Joint Statement by the WHO and the United Nations Children's Fund.* Geneva, WHO.

6 Home birth

Janet Gwillim and Cathy Charles

Introduction

There is no place like home.

A home birth can be a deeply personal fulfilling experience for the woman, her partner and family.

Until recent years home birth was the natural place of delivery. From the 1940s onwards there has been a trend towards hospital birth without any evidence of its superiority, culminating in the Peel report (DoH, 1970) which stated that the safest place for all women to give birth was in hospital. This biased approach has been vigorously challenged by many, and in the light of positive evidence the Department of Health and NICE now recommend that all women are advised that they can choose from an obstetric unit (OU), midwife-led unit or home birth (DoH, 1993, 2004, 2007; NICE, 2007; BECG, 2011). The *Birthplace* Study (BECG, 2011) showed overall risks for low-risk women planning home birth in England were low, although there was a very slightly increased neonatal risk for first time births.

The subject of home birth still elicits strong feelings in many mothers, midwives and obstetricians; Walsh (2010) reports a resignation from one of the NICE team over the subject of place of birth. It is the midwife's duty of care to provide support and care for the woman who chooses a home birth, even if the woman's pregnancy is considered to be outside normal parameters (NMC, 2004).

In an ideal world the midwifery service would be flexible enough to provide home assessment for most low-risk women, whether planning a home birth or not. Then the

The Midwife's Labour and Birth Handbook, Third Edition. Edited by Vicky Chapman and Cathy Charles.
© 2013 John Wiley & Sons, Ltd. Published 2013 by John Wiley & Sons, Ltd.

woman could decide whether to stay at home or go to a birthing centre/hospital at that point. This flexibility has been achieved by many independent midwives and in some NHS trusts, e.g. Northampton (O'Connell *et al.*, 2001) where home birth rates have risen accordingly. Sadly, at present this ideal situation remains something of a dream for most trusts.

Incidence and facts

- Planned home birth for low-risk women results in a higher likelihood of a normal birth, with fewer interventions (NICE, 2007; BECG, 2011).
- Neonatal/maternal outcomes worldwide for planned home births appear favourable compared to hospital births (Fullerton and Young, 2007) although they are difficult to measure due to the self-selected population choosing home birth.
- In the UK adverse neonatal/maternal outcomes at home appear similar to hospital birth for multiparous women (BECG, 2011).
- In the UK nulliparous women planning home birth have very slightly worse neonatal mortality/morbidity outcomes than in obstetric units (OU), although the risks still remain extremely low: 1:110 (home) versus 1:190 (hospital): an increased risk of 1.75 (BECG, 2011).
- Up to two thirds of women are suitable for home birth (DoH, 2007); however, the UK home birth rate is 2–3% with wide geographical variation (BirthChoiceUK).
- Up to 74% of pregnant women in England say home birth was mentioned by staff as an option (CQC, 2010).
- All women should be given full information on booking on the options of hospital, birthing centre or home birth (DoH, 1993, 2007; NICE, 2007), and be aware that they do not have to decide until later in pregnancy and can change their mind if they wish.
- Women with significant health risks are usually advised to deliver in an obstetric unit (NICE, 2007) but it remains their choice.
- Some health trusts have financial/staffing restraints which create difficulties providing home birth cover (RCOG and RCM, 2007) but home birth is actually a cheaper option than hospital birth (Schroeder *et al.*, 2012).

Benefits of home birth

Sense of security. A woman is likely to be more relaxed in her familiar surroundings at home with her partner, and perhaps children, around her. She is more likely to feel experience greater privacy and feel more in control of events.

Fewer interventions. Birth is more likely to be active and unassisted, as women planning home birth are less likely to be induced, and receive fewer other interventions, i.e. augmentation of labour, epidural, episiotomy and instrumental/caesarean section (CS) delivery (NICE, 2007). Waterbirth is more likely (BECG, 2011).

Reduced infection risk. The woman and baby avoid proximity to other mothers/babies so have a lower risk of hospital-acquired infection.

Continuity of care. There is more chance of having a known midwife (Allen *et al.*, 1997), although this depends very much on the way maternity services are organised in a particular area. Continuity cannot always be guaranteed.

Breastfeeding. The woman is more likely to breastfeed (NBTF, 1997) although the reason for the correlation is unclear; possibly those who choose to breastfeed also choose home birth.

Feeling of well-being. Women are less likely to suffer from postnatal depression (Mind, 1995) and are more likely to report a postitive birth experience.

Home birth is cheaper! Midwifery time/mileage involved in a home birth may seem that one group of women are getting special care at the expense of others. This accusation is often made when the maternity service is under financial restraint. *Birthplace* study evidence shows otherwise:

Average cost of birth

£1,066   births planned at home
£1,435   births in freestanding midwifery units
£1,461   births in midwifery units alongside hospitals
£1,631   births in hospital obstetric units

> 'The potential for cost savings could make offering women more choice an attractive option for the NHS' (Schroeder *et al.*, 2012).

Home birth on-call/staffing/mileage costs are outweighed by the higher cost of increased interventions in hospital, such as epidurals, caesareans and hospital postnatal care, not to mention less quantifiable costs resulting from breastfeeding failure, such as readmission, treatment for jaundice, depression and increased infection risk.

Issues to consider before choosing home birth

Home birth is not for everyone. Some women/partners might worry about children or neighbours overhearing the birth, making a mess on beds and carpets and fear of something going wrong. Those people will be more relaxed in hospital and that is the right decision for them.

Possible delay. In the event of a sudden emergency it will take longer to access specialist care than in an acute unit, and the outcome may consequently be worse. In England 46% of primigravidae and 12% of multigravidae transfer from home to hospital (BECG, 2011). While most transfer for slow progress, not usually an emergency, some degree of delay is inevitable and this should not be glossed over, especially if the nearest acute unit is some distance away.

'Unsuitable client'. Some women with a higher risk pregnancy may choose home birth, sometimes because of a previous traumatic experience in hospital. Many benefit from the relaxed environment, but sometimes all the relaxation in the world will not change a high-risk pregnancy into a low-risk one. Even the most enthusiastic home birth midwife will occasionally have a woman on the caseload who is not ideally suited for home birth. See Box 6.1.

Attending home births

Home births should be provided by midwives who are confident and competent, and who believe that home is an appropriate place for birth. Midwives who do not truly

Box 6.1 Action if you are worried about a woman's suitability for home birth.

'If you judge that the type of care a woman is requesting could cause significant risk to her or her baby, then you should discuss the woman's wishes with her; providing detailed information relating to her requests, options for care, and outlining any potential risks, so that the woman may make a fully informed decision about her care. If a woman rejects your advice, you should seek further guidance from your supervisor of midwives to ensure that all possibilities have been explored and that the outcome is appropriately documented. The woman should be offered the opportunity to read what has been documented about the advice she has been given. She may sign this if she wishes. You must continue to give the best care you possibly can, seeking support from other members of the health care team as necessary.'

Midwives Rules and Standards (NMC, 2004).

have a home birth philosophy risk providing a 'hospital birth at home' (Edwards, 2000). Inexperienced midwives may require support from more experienced colleagues until they have built up their confidence and understanding. Home birth study days and workshops are usually inspiring, offering the opportunity to sharing knowledge and experience.

A good philosophy is not enough. All midwives, especially those who practise in the community, need to keep their skills and emergency drills up to date: as a minimum **breech birth** and **shoulder dystocia** manoeuvres, **cannulation**, **PPH management** and **basic resuscitation** of adults and babies.

Personal safety checklist

- Know your destination and how to access the house/flat. Communicate this information to colleagues.
- Obtain adequate information *before* you set off, e.g. directions and landmarks, full address and postcode – and client landline/mobile numbers, in case you get lost! Technology is great; e.g. satellite navigation for a car/mobile, online maps and trip planners like Googlemaps. But don't rely solely on technology; mobile signals and batteries can fail. Carry an Ordnance Survey and A–Z map.
- Suggest the woman displays something eye-catching, e.g. Christmas lights in the garden to catch the attention at night.
- Have a system in place for informing your colleagues of your whereabouts both day and night. Many midwife teams keep central records of staff car details, e.g. make/colour of car, registration, etc.
- Inform other relevant people, e.g. labour suite coordinator, supervisor of midwives, GP, should they need/wish to be involved.
- If you feel threatened going somewhere, take a colleague.
- Ensure mobile battery is charged, torch charged and car fuelled.

Supervision issues

A supervisor of midwives (SOM) can be a helpful resource for a home birth, and can help the midwife identify personal and professional development needs (NMC, 2011). A SOM can be an advocate for the mother too: providing help for a woman who has had a home birth 'refused'. Build up a good rapport with your SOM; keep them informed of impending births and discuss cases, especially if you have concerns about a high-risk mother requesting home birth. If necessary a SOM may attend the birth as well, to support the midwife.

Midwives working outside the NHS also need supervision and support. They may be independent, working as a midwife teacher or employed by a GP practice. These midwives may or may not have links with an NHS trust and may practise to different protocols.

Preparing for a home birth

Home visit

It is helpful to visit the house by 36 weeks, so the midwife and mother can discuss birth plans and clarify any uncertainty. Some equipment may be left at the house at this stage. This is usually a pleasant occasion; the mother is likely to be excited and hopeful. She needs to know who and when to call, and to plan for several possible scenarios. Be positive but realistic: consider practical points; who would look after your children if you had to transfer? Will you need to switch on the immersion heater early to ensure you have enough hot water for your birthing pool?

Environmental planning/risk assessement

Increasingly midwives may complete a form, sometimes a so-called 'risk assessment'; identifying key issues, e.g. distance from hospital, mobile coverage, electrical/trip hazards, number of steps, dangerous dog, etc. If a water birth is planned, access to water and drainage may need to be considered. Planning and risk assesssment can be a helpful exercise, allowing midwives and prospective parents to identify and minimise problems, but the language used may make the mother feel midwives are regarding her home birth as a hazardous exercise. A good midwife will use this document appropriately as a simple tool, not something to dominate the preparations, and will remain positive and encouraging about the forthcoming birth.

Equipment preparation

For equipment list see Boxes 6.2 and 6.3. The list appears endless, but if equipment is always separated into the appropriate bags/boxes then colleagues become familiar with it. It is then much easier to find something quickly. Keep equipment stocked, in working order and in date.

Preparation by the mother

It is helpful if the woman can make these preparations.

- **Protective coverings.** Carpets can be protected if desired by a large sheet of thick polythene (easily available from builders' merchants) with a layer of padding on top, e.g old sheets or blankets. Soft furnishings, e.g. bed/settee, may be protected by a shower curtain as this is softer and less noisy than polythene. Everything can be burnt or taken to the hospital incinerator afterwards. A home-made birthing pad can be made with plastic, newspaper and towels if wished, although plenty of inco sheets should be available in the birthing kit.

Box 6.2   Midwifery equipment.

Labour and birth bag	**Antenatal/postnatal bag**	**Emergency bag**
Delivery pack (small community pack) – some units combine delivery/suture packs	Thermometer	IV giving set × 3 (clear fluids and blood)
Suture pack (small suture pack) and suture material	Sphygmomanometer	Grey/large bore cannulae × 4
Tampon	Pinards	Selection of small cannulae
Urethral catheter & bag	Doppler device	Three-way tap
Amnihook	Urine testing strips	Plaster & IV fixing dressing
Sterile gloves	Tape measure	Sterile gloves
Unsterile gloves	Baby scales	Unsterile gloves
Inco pads/sanitary towels	Label for drug additives	Razor
Water based vaginal lubricating jelly	Stitch cutters	Pinards
Baby labels (some parents wish to have these) Syringes and needles	Scissors	Plastic apron
Blood bottles *full blood count, group and save, & Kleihauer/Coombs for rhesus-negative women*	Plastic apron	Inco pads/sanitary towels
Drugs/IV fluids (see Box 6.4)	Sterile gloves	Blood bottles for haemoglobin, cross-matching and forms
Plastic aprons	Unsterile gloves	IV fluids
Rubbish bag	Glycerine suppositories	Normal saline
	Speculum	Hartmann's solution
	Water-based vaginal lubricating jelly	Gelofusine/haemaccel
	Swabs for culture	Essential resuscitation equipment (see Box 18.2 on page 294)
	Torch	
	Neonatal screening test kits	
	Paperwork for pathology laboratory and notes	
	Blood bottles	
	Sharps container	

Box 6.3   Drugs and gases carried by the midwife.

Syntometrine®
Syntocinon® 10 IU (also 40 IU for PPH)
  Ergometrine
  Oxytocics can be kept for about 1 year in high temperatures. Advisable to discard every 6 months (Chua et al., 1993)
  Lidocaine/lignocaine 1% 20 ml
  Antacid, e.g. ranitidine in case of hospital transfer
  Neonatal IM/oral vitamin K
  Naloxone hydrochloride for baby if using pethidine
  Diclofenac suppositories (after suturing)
Gases
  Entonox
  Oxygen

- **Refreshments and home comforts.** Plenty of drinks and snacks. Pillows, duvet, flannels, bowls, towels for hot/cold compresses, TENS machine, music, massage oils, beanbag, birth ball and candles.
- **Birthing pool** if desired. See Chapter 7 for more details on home waterbirth.
- **Warm birthing environment.** Ensure house heated in winter. Baby blankets, clothes and nappies. Hot water bottle to warm whatever the woman has chosen to wrap her baby in at birth.

- **Pethidine:** rarely used at a home birth, but if the woman wishes she should get it prescribed by her GP and dispensed ready for use. It is her property so the midwife cannot remove it from the house afterwards, but suggest it is destroyed with the woman as your witness prior to your departure.
- **Childcare backup.** Some women want their other children in the house for the birth; others prefer not, as children may become bored, demanding or distressed. Also contingency plans should be made in case of long labour/transfer.

Care in labour

The woman and family are at the centre of care, which should be given *sensitively*. The midwife should support the woman's decision, and continue to support her if she changes her mind or needs hospital admission. It is an honour to be asked to attend a home birth and the midwife should respond accordingly.

Early labour

- **First call.** When the woman contacts you to say she thinks she may be in labour, listen and decide whether to visit. For independent midwives distance may play its part, as she may not live nearby, and it may be appropriate to stay once the decision is made to visit. Once you arrive, perform a full check (see Chapter 1). Watch for a while to see how the contractions are progressing before offering a vaginal examination. Think to yourself: 'Is a vaginal examination necessary?' Discuss the woman's plans with her again now that she has started labouring.
- **Advice.** Encourage her to call if her waters break or (if already ruptured) the colour changes, there is heavy bleeding, stronger contractions or any concerns. Document your findings and actions.
- **Communicate.** Arrange a time to phone/return unless she calls you back earlier.
  If you have agreed a return time, and are running late, keep her informed. You may need to return several times before she needs you to stay. Staying when you are not required does not help a labouring woman and family.

Labour

- **Blend into the background.** Most women labour well when they remain in their own environment, in a position they have chosen, with their family/friends. Stand back and enable the woman to labour. Do not dominate the situation. It is her day and *she* is going to birth *her* baby, not the midwife.
- **Equipment.** Try not to have all the equipment in the birthing space; keep it handy perhaps just outside the room. The woman may feel threatened seeing all the 'emergency' equipment ready, as if problems are expected. A discreet newborn resuscitation area in a corner is sensible. If the baby requires ventilation the mother could be asked to move towards the area or the ambubag brought to the mother, so the baby can remain attached to its umbilical cord.

- **Care in labour:** see Chapter 1. Discuss any deviation from normal with the woman and her partner, and record in the notes. Encourage her to drink and empty her bladder frequently. Avoid artificial rupture of the membranes due to the potential complications associated with this intervention, although it can be justifiable as a last resort for a slow labour before planning to transfer a woman to a consultant unit (see also Chapter 9 Slow progress).

The birth

- **Second midwife/designated second professional.** Call your back-up colleague before they are needed urgently. This is an area of slight controversy; some NHS Trusts require two midwives to attend a home birth. Others allow a maternity care assistant/support worker to be the second person (Feedback, 2011). Independent midwives have challenged the routine of having a second professional at all home births, suggesting that a second person can affect the dynamics of the relationship with the woman, and only call for back-up if they have a specific concern. If a second colleague attends, leaving the door on the latch is sensible so the woman is not disturbed. The second colleague could perhaps remain just outside the room, so as not to intrude.
- **The birth.** Providing the woman feels in control and well supported, a home birth can be a deeply personal experience for her and her partner. Enable the woman to birth her own baby, to make as much noise as she wishes and to lift her baby to her breast and to discover the sex. Give her time to do this; do not overcrowd her but just quietly observe until she is ready to speak.
- **The third stage.** See Chapter 1 for physiological/active management. It is probably true to say that more women who choose home birth choose to deliver their placenta physiologically. The placenta is the woman's property and she may want to keep it. If not a placenta bin/bag will be required for transporting it to the hospital incinerator.
- **After the third stage.** The woman may want to celebrate in a variety of ways. She may want to remain very quiet and together with her partner, or she may want to enjoy champagne with her family and friends or share the moment with her other children. She may also be very hungry and want lots of tea and toast. Whatever she chooses, respect her wishes.
- **Prior to leaving the house.** Midwives normally remain in the house after the third stage until the woman and the midwife feel happy that the time has come for the midwife to leave. During this time weighing, measuring and examining the baby can be performed, offering vitamin K, completing the notes and having a cup of tea.
- **On leaving.** Make sure that the woman's uterus is well contracted and her lochia is not excessive. Ensure she has passed urine, or arrange to call her back later to check. Give the woman/family a contact number for any problems/questions and arrange the next midwife visit. NHS midwives will need to complete hospital paperwork/computer details. Replenish equipment. Inform relevant colleagues that the woman and baby are safely delivered.

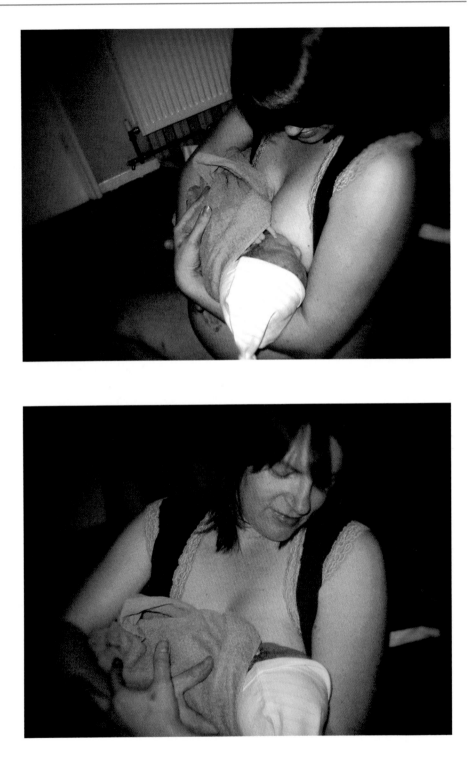

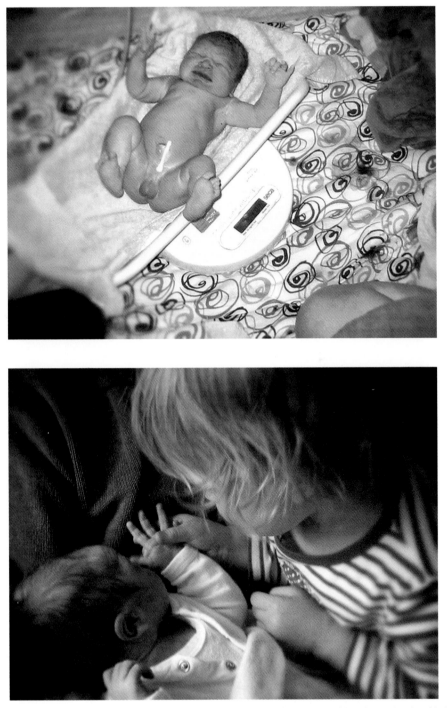

Many thanks to Sue for allowing us to use the beautiful photos of her home birth of baby Amber.

Possible transfer to hospital

When things do not go according to plan during labour or after the birth, transfer may be indicated (see Box 6.4). Around 46% of UK primigravidae and 12% of muligravidae transfer from planned home birth to hospital in labour/postnatally (BECG, 2011).

Box 6.4   Possible problems requiring transfer to hospital.

Vaginal loss
- Heavily bloodstained liquor or frank bleeding
- Offensive smelling liquor
- Significant meconium, e.g. thick/tenacious dark green or black staining, or lumps

Fetal heart rate (FHR)
- FHR less than 110 or greater than 160 bpm
- Deceleration after a contraction
- Persistent bradycardia/tachycardia

Position/presentation of baby
- Posterior and/or asynclitic position with no progress
- Malpresentation: e.g. breech, face, brow

Maternal observations
- Pyrexia
- Persistent tachycardia
- Raised blood pressure

Pain
- Request for further analgesia
- Unusual pain in labour

Choice
- Woman changed her mind

Dilatation
- No progress for a length of time
- Swollen anterior lip of cervix for a long time

Postpartum
- Third/fourth-degree tear
- Retained placenta
- Postpartum haemorrhage
- Maternal collapse

Baby
- Difficult resuscitation
- Respiratory distress, e.g. grunting, sternal recession, nasal flaring
- Abnormal movements, e.g. poor tone, jitteriness, fitting
- Any condition causing concern

Remember that the woman does not *have* to transfer. If you have a good relationship with her and her partner and they know you would suggest the transfer to them unless you were worried, they are unlikely to refuse. Ensure they understand the situation, and document your explanation.

Use your judgement. If the woman is very near, or in, the second stage, especially is if she is multigravid, it may not be possible or safe to move to hospital before the birth.

Non-emergency transfer to hospital

The usual non-urgent reasons for transfer are slow labour progress and/or epidural request. The mother may be calm but fed up with waiting, or conversely very distressed. Think: 'Can she travel by car or is an ambulance needed?' If you need to summon an ambulance non-urgently, in some trusts you may be asked to call a different number and grade the urgency level, e.g. within the hour/two hours. With increasing service pressure a non-emergency ambulance may take a long time to arrive, so it may be preferable to travel by car (not the midwife's) in a a calm non-emergency situation: consider following the car/ambulance to the hospital in your own car, depending on the needs of the woman.

Emergency transfer to hospital

- **Dial 999 (Europe 112).** Ask the partner to do this if you are busy; request a paramedic ambulance. It should be dispatched immediately but the control operator will ask other questions.
- **Directions.** If complex perhaps hand the phone to the partner, who will probably explain better. Finding a house, especially at night, can be tricky. Consider sending someone outside to flag down the ambulance.
- **Consider calling a second midwife/designated professional** – especially if potential ambulance delay. It may be difficult if you are busy controlling bleeding or resuscitating the baby. The partner could make the call, or dial and hold a mobile for you to speak into.
- **Inform delivery suite coordinator.** The co-ordinator will assess the situation, get a room prepared and inform the relevant people, e.g. senior obstetrician, paediatrician, theatre, neonatal intensive care unit (NICU). Working as a team inside and outside the hospital counts. Remember to keep communicating.
- **Record keeping.** Write everything down as contemporaneously as possible – and remember to take the notes with you!
- **Equipment.** Take any relevant equipment e.g. emergency bag, resuscitation equipment. Leave anything non-essential to be collected later.
- **Consider antacids.** Some transfer protocols include a dose of antacid, e.g. ranitidine in preparation for possible surgery.
- **Consider IV access/fluids and take bloods (crossmatch, group and save).** IV fluids may be advisable, e.g. for fetal distress to increase maternal circulation and save time at the hospital, or essential, e.g. for PPH. Paramedics are usually wonderful at cannulation if time is tight.
- **Escort the woman.** Go with her in the ambulance, if the situation is an emergency or birth is imminent, leave the car and get a lift/taxi back to the house later. The hospital will pay the fare.

The woman and her partner may be extremely upset with the decision to transfer to hospital, even if it is entirely their decision. Explain that neither of them have failed; language like 'failure to progress' and 'maternal distress' does not help parents.

It may be helpful to debrief carefully afterwards, preferably by the attending midwife, using the notes. Women/partners may feel traumatised, or conversely look back on the experience positively. Some mothers report that the part of the labour which took place at home was a happy memory in an otherwise complicated labour/birth: 'At least we had a chance ... we lost nothing by trying: we ended up in hospital, which is where we would have been had we opted for that in the first place.' (Karen, quoted by Hill, 2011).

Home birth problems

Born before arrival (BBA) at home. A term BBA is usually just a precipitate straightforward birth, although occasionally a baby delivers quickly because there is a problem, e.g. placental abruption. When reviewing the statistics for home births, make sure that unplanned BBAs are not included, as these can affect outcomes.

The main risks of unattended births are PPH, retained placenta and neonatal heat loss.

Often the parents were not planning home birth, and may be shocked, frightened and unsure what to do. Usually just congratulations and soothing are required. Make sure the baby is not cold: skin-to-skin contact, a hat and a warm blanket over the outside are usually sufficient. The midwife may need to deliver the placenta. An ambulance crew may have arrived first; they are usually well trained, but sometimes the cord has been unnecessarily clamped and cut (see Chapter 1 for optimal third stage management). Ambulances occasionally carry syntometrine, but not always. It would be very helpful if ambulance staff were trained **not** to clamp and cut the cord when an oxytocic has not been given (Loughney *et al.*, 2006). The midwife should decide what to do about this unsatisfactory mix of physiological and active management! Either go ahead and give syntometrine, and continue with active management, or remove the maternal clamp and await physiological delivery.

Decide whether hospital admission is advisable, e.g. a history of fresh thick meconium-stained liquor. The mother may not agree to transfer; if so ensure she understands the implications and knows how to recognise adverse signs, e.g. respiratory difficulty, and document all discussions. Preterm babies are often well at birth, but can deteriorate rapidly (see Chapter 13). Skin-to-skin contact/kangaroo care is ideal for transfer and physiologically preferable to an incubator (Christensson *et al.*, 1998), but it may be tricky: some ambulance trusts discourage transferring 'unsecured' babies. Safety laws state that the driver takes responsibility for transferring a baby to hospital (DoT, 2006).

Unplanned/undiagnosed home breech. It can be something of a surprise for a midwife to arrive to find the breech presenting and descending. A breech baby can deliver rapidly, particularly in a multigravida, and quick descent is often uncomplicated. If it is too late for transfer, all the midwife can do is summon help and get on with the birth. Consider an upright postion (see Chapter 14). Breech babies are more likely to be temporarily shocked at birth and may need some basic resuscitation (see Chapter 18).

Summary

- Know your destination and keep colleagues informed of your whereabouts.
- Keep equipment stocked, in date and in working order.
- Care as per normal labour (Chapter 1).
- Minimise interventions with potential complications, e.g. ARM.
- Stand back; do not dominate the couple's space. Let the woman labour.
- Consider calling a second colleague for the birth.
- Discuss and document any need for hospital transfer fully with woman and partner.
- In an emergency call an ambulance, and, if transferring, inform labour ward coordinator.

Useful contacts

Association for Improvements in Maternity Services (AIMS). www.aims.org.uk
Finding a doula. www.doula.org.uk
Home birth. www.homebirth.org.uk and www.birthchoice.com
Independent Midwives Association (IMA). www.independentmidwives.org.uk
National Childbirth Trust (NCT). www.nct.org.uk
Royal College of Midwives (RCM). www.rcm.org.uk

References

Allen, I., Bourke, Dowling, S., Williams, S. (1997) *A Leading Role for Midwives?* London, Policy Studies Institute.

BECG (Birthplace in England Collaborative Group) (2011) Perinatal and maternal outcomes by planned place of birth for healthy women with low risk pregnancies: the Birthplace in England national prospective cohort study. *British Medical Journal* 343:d7400 www.npeu.ox.ac.uk/birthplace

BirthChoice UK www.birthchoiceuk.com

Care Quality Commission (CQC) (2010) *Maternity Services 2010.* www.cqc.org.uk

Christensson, K., Bhat, G. J., Amadi, B.C., Eriksson, B., Hojer, B. (1998) A randomized study of skin-to-skin versus incubator care for rewarming low risk hypothermic neonates. *The Lancet* 352, 1115.

Chua, S., Arulkumaran, S., Adaikan, G., Ratnam, S. (1993) The effect of oxytocics stored at high temperatures on postpartum uterine activity. *British Journal of Obstetrics and Gynaecology* 100, 874–5.

DoH (Department of Health) (1970) *Peel Report.* London, HMSO.

DoH (Department of Health) (1993) *Changing Childbirth. Report of the Expert Maternity Group.* London, HMSO.

DoH (2004) *National Service Framework for Children, Young People and Maternity Services*, 27–9. London, DoH.

DoH (2007) *Maternity Matters.* London. DoH.

DoT (2006) *Think Road Safety Leaflet.* www.thinkroadsafety.gov.uk

Edwards, N. (2000) Women planning homebirths: their own views on their relationships with midwives. In Kirkham, M. (ed.) *The Midwife-Woman Relationship*, pp. 55–91. London: Macmillan.

Enkin, M., Keirse, J. N. C., Renfrew, M. J., Neilson, J. P. (1995) *A Guide to Effective Care in Pregnancy and Childbirth*, 2nd edn. Oxford, Oxford University Press.

Feedback (2011) Your published views – Homebirth. *Midwives* 5, 6.

Fullerton J., Young, S. (2007) Outcomes of planned home birth: an integrative review. *Journal of Midwifery and Women's Health* 52, 323–33.

Hill, A. (2011) Home Birth: 'What the hell was I thinking?' *The Guardian* 16 April (34).

Loughney, A., Collis, R., Dastgir, S. (2006) Birth before arrival at delivery suite: associations and consequences. *British Journal of Midwifery* 14(4), 204–8.

Mercer, J., Erikson-Owens, D. (2010) Evidence for neonatal transition and the first hour of life. In Walsh, D., Downe, S. (eds) *Intrapartum Care*. Oxford, Wiley-Blackwell.

NBTF (National Birthday Trust Fund) (1997) *Home Births – The Report of the 1994 Confidential Enquiry* (Chamberlain, G., Wraight, A. and Crowley, P., eds). Lancaster, NBTF Parthenon Publishing.

NICE (2007) *Clinical Guideline 55: Intrapartum Care*. London, NICE. www.nice.org.uk

Nicolson, P. (1995) *Postnatal Depression – Psychology Science and the Transition to Motherhood*. London, MIND.

NMC (Nursing and Midwifery Council) (2004) *Midwives Rules and Standards* London, NMC. www.nmc-uk.org

NMC (Nursing and Midwifery Council) (2011) *Standards for the Preparation and Practice of Supervisor of Midwives*. London, NMC. www.nmc-org.uk

O'Connell, S., Williams, B., Richley, A. (2001) Feeling right at home *Midwives* 2, 28–9.

RCOG and Royal College of Midwives (RCM) (2007) *Joint Statement No. 2*, April. www.rcog.co.uk

Schroeder, E., Petrou, S., Patel, N., Hollowell, J., Puddicombe, D., Redshaw, M., Brocklehurst, P. on behalf of the Birthplace in England Collaborative Group (2012) *Cost effectiveness of alternative planned places of birth in woman at low risk of complications: evidence from the Birthplace in England national prospective cohort study. BMJ* 344 doi: 10.1136/bmj.e2292.

Walsh, D. (2010) Birth Environment. In Walsh, D., Downe, S. (eds) *Intrapartum Care*. Chichester: Wiley-Blackwell.

7 Water for labour and birth

Cathy Charles

Introduction

Labour and/or birth in water can be a wonderfully relaxing experience for a mother and baby. Deep-water immersion in labour became popular in the 1970s, when women relaxing in water unexpectedly gave birth and it was realised that fears about drowning were unfounded (Odent, 1983). In this respect research has followed, rather than preceded, practice. Water immersion and water birth appear to be safe, and women repeatedly express high levels of satisfaction when surveyed (Cluett and Burns, 2009).

NICE (2007), the Royal College of Midwives and the Royal College of Obstetricians and Gynaecologists (RCM/RCOG, 2007) all recommend that the opportunity to labour in water should be available to all healthy women with uncomplicated pregnancies. The National Service Framework (DoH, 2004) requires that 'all staff have up to date skills and knowledge to support women who choose to labour without pharmacological intervention, including the use of birthing pools' and 'wherever possible, allow access to a birthing pool with staff competent in facilitating water births'. It should be a service requirement to provide continuing professional development for midwives on water births (RCM, 2000). Assisting birth in water should be regarded as a core midwifery competence not an arcane alternative therapy.

The Midwife's Labour and Birth Handbook, Third Edition. Edited by Vicky Chapman and Cathy Charles.
© 2013 John Wiley & Sons, Ltd. Published 2013 by John Wiley & Sons, Ltd.

Sadly some midwives seem to dislike water births, sometimes inventing rather lame excuses, and some hospitals have pools sitting virtually unused. Some suggest that only midwives who enjoy water birth should be involved, because they are likely to be positive and more supportive. However, potentially a woman may arrive on a delivery suite to be told: 'Sorry, there's no one on tonight who can do water births'. Also, midwives ignorant of water births may be placed in a dangerous position if called upon to assist at a pool birth in the home, birthing centre or acute unit, especially in an emergency. *All* midwives should be able to assist at a water birth.

Facts

- 95% of UK Trusts claim to offer water for labour, but only around 11% of women appear to labour in a pool (this may be an underestimate as recording of intermittent pool use is erratic); only 3% deliver in water (Healthcare Commission, 2008). Some birth centres have water birth rates of up to 80% (NICE, 2007).
- In the Republic of Ireland only three centres offer labour in water and no maternity unit offers water birth (Murphy-Lawless, 2011).
- There is still a shortage of appropriately experienced midwives in the UK (Garland, 2010).
- NICE (2007) recommend that warm water immersion should be offered to all straightforward labouring women: having the birth itself in water is optional.

Benefits of warm water immersion

Research into water immersion/birth is not easy. Researchers may not clearly distinguish between shallow- or deep-water immersion, and/or confuse *labour* in water with *birth* in water. The much-revered randomised controlled trial is not well suited to this subject (Jowitt, 2001), as women prefer to choose options in labour if and when they are ready for them. Being pressured into or denied water immersion/birth following the opening of a brown envelope (even though a woman may have consented to this in principle) may raise anxiety levels and affect labour progress. Practice also varies between professionals: some believe in a 'hands-off' water birth while others do not. Research should, therefore, be interpreted with caution. NICE (2007), for example, feels that the evidence supports water immersion in labour, but does not prove or disprove the benefits of actual birth in water.

Benefits include:

- **Relaxation.** Water offers a peaceful, secure environment, which helps the woman to relax, leading to;
- **Beneficial labour hormone levels** including endorphins and oxytocin, with reduced catecholamine secretion so reducing pain perception (Odent, 1983; Ockenden, 2001), leading to;
- **Less analgesia** needed (Burns, 2001; Cluett and Burns, 2009; da Silva *et al.*, 2009). This also saves money: water is cheap.
- **Buoyancy effects:** the woman can move freely to try positions like squatting, which also can be sustained for longer than on dry land.
- **Backache** appears to be eased (Nightingale, 1996).

- **Reduced perineal trauma.** Women incur similar/less overall perineal trauma including fewer episiotomies. There is no difference in third/fourth degree tears (Bodner *et al.*, 2002; Otigbah *et al.*, 2000; Cluett and Burns, 2009).
- **Postpartum haemorrhage (PPH)** rates appear similar or lower in women having water births, although again further research is needed (Garland, 2006). This is interesting because many water birth third stages are physiological. Other authors have suggested that PPH risk may be increased since warm water may reduce the contractility of uterine muscle (Richmond, 2003), but since the uterus is at body temperature anyway, it is hard to follow the logic of this.
- **Slow progress** may be improved (yes, really!) by water immersion (Cluett *et al.*, 2004).
- **Shorter first stage of labour and similar 5 min Apgar scores** following use of a water birth pool (Cluett and Burns, 2009).
- **No increased neonatal infection or NICU admission** according to Cochrane review (Cluett and Burns, 2009). In 1993 one baby born in a home spa bath died from *Legionella* pneumonia which was later isolated from the bath (Nagai *et al.*, 1993). Unlike most birthing pools, spa baths have inaccessible recesses, making them unsuitable for water births.
- **Gentle birth for the baby.** The sight of a baby calmly opening its eyes for the first time with its body still in water, before it has even breathed, is magical to behold. This smooth transition from uterine to extrauterine life is likely to be more gentle for a baby than the sudden cold shock of dry land birth.

Possible risks of warm water immersion

- **Premature gasping.** There are anecdotal accounts of babies developing post-birth respiratory distress secondary to water inhalation (Nugyen *et al.*, 2002), but these are not backed up by larger studies. Babies do not appear to gasp or inhale water unless severely hypoxic. Due to fears of premature gasping in cold water, researchers originally suggested the water should be around body temperature (Johnson, 1996). Harper (2002) challenges this, describing healthy babies born in cold sea as low as 24°C.
- **Hyperthermia (overheating).** Fetal temperature is 0.5°C higher than normal (37°C) maternal temperature. If the mother becomes pyrexial, however, there will be a greater relative difference in the mother's and baby's temperatures, i.e. the baby will get considerably hotter and will take longer to cool down (Charles, 1998). If the mother becomes significantly overheated in the pool, the baby can become excessively hot and become severely asphyxiated (Rosevear *et al.*, 1993), so maternal temperature must be monitored.
- **Maternal infection.** CEMACH (2004) suggested water birth risks faecal contamination of the perineum and genital tract, but evidence is weak.
- **Snapped cord.** As in any birth this occasionally happens (Crow and Preston, 2002) but is easily dealt with (see later in chapter).
- **Slow progress.** Some women find that if they enter the pool very early in labour and/or stay in for a long time then labour can slow down. This is probably due to the reduced gravity effect, which is known to aid labour progress. The risk may have been overstated since it is easily reversible: i.e. get out of the pool and mobilise.

A woman who is very distressed and feeling out of control in early labour may find a period of water immersion an ideal way of relaxing and regaining some control. She also may not want a vaginal examination (VE) prior to entering the pool. Prescriptive restrictions on when a woman should enter the water and how long she should stay in are therefore unhelpful (Garland, 2006). It is just a question of being vigilant to the frequency and strength of contractions, and responding appropriately.

Interestingly, water immersion may actually help some women with slow progress, possibly due to its relaxing effect, reversing the stress response which inhibits contractions (Cluett *et al.*, 2004).

- **Midwifery back pain.** This is sometimes an excuse cited by midwives who do not feel comfortable with water birth. In fact, there is rarely any need to lean over the side of the pool, except perhaps briefly to perform a VE. Think about a low stool for sitting alongside the pool: FH auscultation can be performed without performing gymnastics. One of the joys of water is that it stops clinicians interfering with the birth process. Like so many labour situations, try to sit on your hands and avoid continually leaning over to peer at the perineum. As discussed later, the birth itself should be 'hands off'.

Criteria for labouring in water

Each unit/trust will have its own criteria for labouring in water but care should be individualised to meet women's requests. Ultimately, the woman makes the decision when she has been presented with all the information.

Criteria may include the following:

- Maternal request.
- Normal, term pregnancy from 37 weeks (RCM, 2000).
- Singleton, cephalic presentation (RCM, 2000).
- Any opioid (e.g. pethidine) given >2 hours ago and the woman is not drowsy (NICE, 2007).
- Arguably, most situations where intermittent monitoring is being performed. If the woman is not having electronic fetal monitoring (EFM), even if clinicians do not agree with her decision, there are few arguments against water immersion in labour.

Relative contraindications

- **Infection.** This is a contentious area, since many trusts are unhappy to 'permit' water birth for women with infections, e.g. HIV, hepatitis B, MRSA and group B strep. There is no definitive answer to this. Remember that many women have infections we know nothing about, so practise universal precautions. Whilst body fluids obviously cannot be so well contained when birth occurs in water, one might speculate that concentrated blood splash injuries might be fewer, since (a) blood is diluted in large volumes of water; (b) the birth is usually 'hands off': a sudden gush of fluid will be dispersed in the water, rather than splashing the midwife's face; and (c) the baby may be partially cleansed of maternal body fluids as it delivers through the water.
- **Pyrexia.** Any pyrexial woman should be advised to leave the pool due to risk of infection and fetal hyperthermia (Charles, 1998). She will probably feel hot and uncomfortable anyway.

- **Prolonged rupture of membranes.** There is supposedly an ascending infection risk, but since NICE (2007) do not exclude a bath with prolonged rupture of membranes one might question the logic.
- **High body mass index.** Larger women may benefit from the buoyancy effects, allowing them to take up otherwise awkward positions, e.g. kneeling, but there is a fear that very large women may be difficult to 'extract' from the pool in an emergency. This is probably an overstated risk, since the requirement to lift a woman from the pool is rare. Think about a back up plan, however, if possible. If a hoist is available make sure you are familiar with its use.
- **Need for electronic fetal monitoring.** It is technically possible to monitor continuously during water immersion as waterproof cardiotocography (CTG) leads are available (Zanetti-Dallenbach *et al.*, 2007) and EFM by telemetry is increasingly used in some hospitals. Some midwives may be horrified at the idea of a water pool being invaded in this way and worry that this may lead to far more unnecessary CTG monitoring. It is however an option which may enable some 'high risk' women to access a pool. Alternatively ask if she would consider as a compromise getting out for an occasional CTG trace. She has every right to refuse.
- **Heavy bleeding/thick meconium liquor.** Both may cause/indicate fetal distress which could cause a baby to gasp prematurely, so water is not advisable. CTG/closer monitoring is recommended. Thin/old meconium is less concerning and may not need continuous CTG (NICE, 2007), so logically there is no reason to exclude water immersion.
- **Oxytocin augmentation.** Despite reports of women with an oxytocin infusion labouring successfully in pools (H. Ponette, website; Zanetti-Dallenbach *et al.*, 2007), this is unusual UK practice at present.
- **Previous caesarean section.** If a woman has chosen to have intermittent auscultation for her vaginal birth after caesarean (VBAC) labour, there is no reason to exclude her from water immersion. A number of enlightened units now provide water immersion/birth for VBAC women (Garland, 2006). Since women do not use epidural anaesthesia in water, they may possibly be more aware of the pain of uterine dehiscence/rupture.
- **Multiple birth/breech.** There are anecdotal accounts of breech and water births, e.g. German midwife Cornelia Enning and Belgian obstetrician Herman Ponette (see Useful contacts); however, such accounts must be read critically. Ponette also protects the perineum, controls the head and even occasionally clamps and cuts the cord underwater: highly questionable practices.

Preparation

Pools are available in many shapes and sizes, fixed or portable. Fill deeply so the woman's abdomen is covered and she is comfortably buoyant. Garland (2010) wonders why midwives who complain their trusts do not provide adequate facilities cannot instead use portable pools. Imagination and flexibility overcome most barriers.

Water temperature

There is no clear evidence on optimal pool temperature and local guidelines vary. Burns and Kitzinger (2001) suggest 35–37°C for first stage and 37°C for second stage and birth. NICE (2007) recommends ≤37.5°C. Anderson (2004), however, suggests the mammalian capacity for thermostasis ensures that women will be uncomfortable if they are too hot or cold and agrees with Harper (2002) who says: 'There is no reason for midwives ... to worry over keeping the water at a set temperature other than the mother's physical comfort', but ensure the mother does not become pyrexial (Charles, 1998). The RCOG and RCM support this approach (RCOG/RCM, 2007). Surface temperature is cooler than deeper down, so stir the water well to mix it before measuring the temperature. Hot water may need to be added periodically.

Cleansing

Local infection control policies should cover water birth (RCM, 2000). Following use, the pool should be rinsed of debris and cleaned with a chlorine-releasing agent effective against HIV and hepatitis B and C (Burns and Kitzinger, 2001). Running hospital pool taps for 5 minutes every day may minimise infection risk (Woodward and Kelly, 2004). Consider running the taps for a while prior to filling the pool, particularly if the pool is not frequently used. Mobile pools normally have a single-use disposable liner.

Equipment

- Thermometer for water temperature.
- Waterproof fetal heart doppler device.
- Lift/aid to get the woman out of the pool in an emergency (if available).
- Gauntlet gloves and eye protectors (not all midwives use these).
- Small mirror for visualising progress when pushing, e.g. the Howes mirror (see useful contacts).
- Low stool/steps for pool access. The midwife may sit on this too.
- Plenty of towels, preferably warmed.
- Portable Entonox or extended tubing to reach the pool.
- Sieve and bowl for collecting faeces.

Water birth at home

Some NHS trusts rent out pools, and many companies offer pool hire (see end of chapter). Alternatively a home-made tub can be constructed, including:

- Pool liner (available from water birth companies).
- Submersible pond pump for emptying the pool (available from garden centres). Alternatively jugs or bowls can be used, but these are extremely time-consuming: both staff and birth partners will have better things to do after the birth than spending an hour emptying the tub.
- Plastic sheeting matting (available from garden centres/builders merchants) to cover carpets.

A trial run is advisable. Filling a large pool takes time and can quickly drain a domestic hot water tank. Plan how to maintain a good supply, e.g. when labour starts set the thermostat to continuous heating, and/or consider switching on the immersion heater to the hot water cylinder. Used water should preferably drain down a toilet.

Beware of the danger of water and electricity. Trailing leads and lamps are dangerous. Always have a charged torch to hand.

A structural survey of the floor is rarely indicated, but think about where the pool is to be placed. When filled it can weigh up to 850 kg so may be best on the ground floor. Birth pool companies are usually very helpful and have a wealth of experience and literature about home water birth.

Labour care

(See also Chapter 1)

First stage of labour

- **Check the woman's temperature** hourly.
- **Allow her to drink freely** to avoid dehydration as water immersion may have a diuretic effect (Ockenden, 2001) and exposed areas of the body will sweat. Encourage birth partners to drink and do the same yourself: humid pool rooms can be enervating for everyone.
- **Measure and record the water temperature**. Frequency may vary with local guidelines; typically every 30–60 minutes. As discussed earlier, there is no reason for rigid guidelines as long as the pool is <37.5°C: adjust to the woman's comfort.
- **VEs** are usually performed with relative ease in the pool.

Second stage of labour

- **Keep lights as low as possible** (within the bounds of safety) and voices quiet.
- **Monitor maternal and fetal well-being** as per normal labour.
- Consider a **second midwife** present for the birth (this is policy in some areas). However, as with all births, try to ensure they do not 'break the spell' and interrupt the birth process. A quiet presence in the background is usually enough.
- **Check water temperature again:** do not exceed 37.5°C.
- **Viewing the perineum.** If it is really necessary and the woman does not mind, or wants to see for herself, submerge a mirror (e.g. the Howes mirror) to visualise progress. It should be easily cleanable or disposable. Do not constantly peer at the perineum. Think: 'what does this achieve?'
- **Have a 'hands off' approach to delivery.** It is thought that touching the fetal head underwater may stimulate the baby to try to breathe, although there is no evidence for this. Usually, there is no need for 'hands on'.
- **Let the head deliver.** The woman will usually tell you (not necessarily in coherent words!) or she may instinctively put her hands down to touch. Sometimes there is a small cloud of blood/liquor as the head pops out. You may be able to see the dark head underwater.
- **Do not check for cord.**
- **Don't expose the baby's head to air.** Once the head is visible, if the woman raises herself out of the water exposing it, suggest she remains out of the water to avoid the risk of premature underwater gasping (RCM/RCOG, 2007). Just standing should suffice: she does not necessarily need to climb out of the pool.
- **Await the next contraction.** The woman will usually then birth the baby. Occasionally a little help may be needed to release the shoulder, but assist only if really necessary. If she wishes, encourage the woman to bring her baby to the surface herself.
- If the woman is on all fours, pass the baby underwater through (not around) her legs and bring it gently up to the surface in front of her.

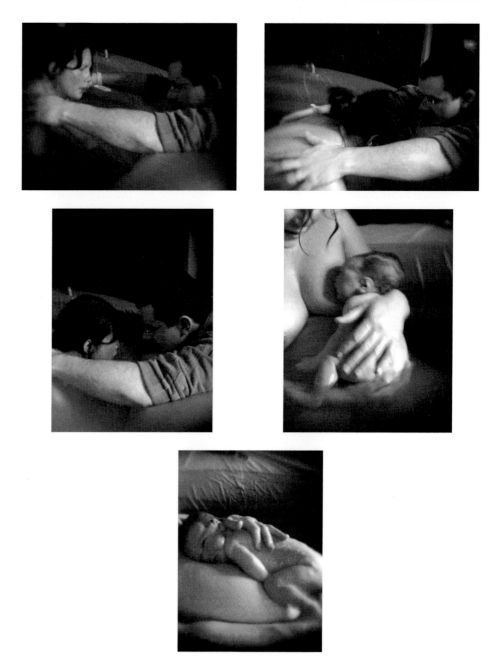

Photos by kind permission of Tor and Steve who had a wonderful VBAC home water birth of their baby daughter Daisy.

- **Water babies do not always cry** or breathe instantly (Wickham, 2005). Be calm, and check the baby's colour; if unsure place your fingers on its chest to feel the heart rate. The baby may open its eyes, look around and move calmly even though it is not breathing. This can be disconcerting, but is rarely a problem: remember if the cord is pulsating, the baby is getting oxygen. If you are concerned, lift the baby's body briefly into the cool air; this will usually stimulate baby to breathe.
- **Ensure the cord is left attached and pulsating.** This may continue for some time. It is sensible to check that the cord is intact, as a snapped cord can be a life-threatening emergency for the baby if unnoticed (Crow and Preston, 2002). (See below under the heading 'Possible problems'.)

Third stage of labour

It is not usually necessary to leave the pool to deliver the placenta unless the woman wishes. If she chooses to remain in the water, keep the baby warm by submerging its body in the water: only its face needs to emerge.

Some women within a few minutes of birth are ready to climb out of the water, which can be by this point a little murky and uninviting. Often the water is just cloudy until the placenta has delivered, but: 'birth pools can sometimes look like a shark attack in a toilet' (http://www.homebirth.org.uk/water.htm).

- **Physiological third stage.** Watch, wait and do nothing (see Chapter 1). Austin *et al.* (1997) cite one isolated case where a water birth baby developed polycythaemia, presumably through a large placental transfusion. Odent (1998) suggests that cold air would stop the umbilical cord pulsating sooner on dry land (as cold encourages vasoconstriction) and that warm water may delay this. This is a good point, but the above case is only one case in thousands of uneventful water births. It can also be argued that placental blood at birth has benefits (see delayed cord clamping/milking the cord, page 28). Midwives should be guided by the woman's preference.
- **Active management.** Opinion is divided whether the woman should stay in the pool for an actively managed third stage. Some would argue that physiological third stage in the pool is more appropriate than active management which is an unnecessary intervention (Garland, 2010). If she does want this, however, ask her to lift her leg out of the water and cleanse with an alcohol swab prior to giving the oxytocic, or give in the arm. *Do not give the injection underwater* as this risks infection. Consider delayed cord clamping (see page 28). Controlled cord traction with fundal guarding is quite possible in pools, but ensure that you are happy to do this, and watch your back. If in doubt, suggest the woman leaves the pool.
- **Estimated blood loss.** This is not always easy, although many midwives are adept at assessing the colour of the water: there is usually a moderate visible bleeding as the placenta separates, which tends to sink to the bottom of the tub around the woman. If in doubt, ask her to leave the pool.

Possible problems

In any emergency, home or hospital, call for assistance immediately.

Most common reasons to leave the pool

In a large study by Burns (2001), 47% of primigravidae left the pool while 53% remained for the birth. Water was consistently rated positively irrespective of whether the woman stayed in the pool for birth or not. As discussed earlier, some midwives readily find spurious reasons to suggest the woman leaves the pool, while others are much more positive and flexible. Reasons might be:

- **Slow progress in the first stage** (see Chapter 9 for suggestions to resolve this). Getting out may help the 'gravity effect' to kick in, but once contractions are stronger always consider re-entering the pool.
- **Slow progress during the second stage of labour.** This may often be rectified by the woman leaving the pool or standing up in it, perhaps with one foot up on a stool to widen the outlet. As the baby starts to descend she can get back in the pool for the birth. It may take some time to increase contraction strength. Make sure she does not get cold.
- **Personal choice.** A few women do not enjoy being in the water so do not stay. Others decide to get out just before giving birth.
- **Additional analgesia.** While women using the pool are less likely to need additional analgesia (Garland and Jones, 2000; Burns, 2001; Cluett and Burns, 2009), some women do request additional pain relief, e.g. pethidine/epidural so need to leave the pool.
- **Change in the baby's condition.** Evidence of fetal compromise, e.g. fresh meconium or abnormal fetal heart changes.
- **Change in the mother's condition**, e.g. bleeding, pyrexia or hypertension.

Cord entanglement

Most babies will easily deliver with the cord around the neck/body without the need for any intervention (ARM, 2000). You cannot tell if the cord is holding the baby back until the baby fails to deliver. If this happens, confirm the presence of a cord by gentle touch. In the rare eventuality that the cord will not slip over the head, *do not clamp and cut it underwater* but proceed as follows:

- Get the woman out of the water quickly. Standing up may be sufficient, but be ready to catch the baby if necessary.
- Once out of the water, if the baby really will not deliver due to cord entanglement apply two clamps to the cord and cut between them; this can be very awkward if the cord is very tight. Remember you have now cut off the baby's oxygen supply, so birth should be imminent or the baby may be compromised.
- Deliver the baby outside the water.
- Never submerge a baby's face once it has come out of the water.

Snapped cord

This rare event is usually uneventful if recognised quickly. However, it is sometimes difficult to visualise a snapped cord due to cloudy water or the position of the baby. Several cases where the problem has gone unnoticed have had serious neonatal consequences (Crow and Preston, 2002).

Always lift the baby carefully into the mother's arms avoiding pulling on a short cord (Garland, 2010).

If the cord snaps, grasp the baby's end of the cord quickly to prevent blood leakage. Apply a clamp securely. Assess the baby and if necessary inform a paediatrician. Post-birth neonatal haemoglobin may be advised.

Shoulder dystocia

If the shoulder fails to deliver ask the woman to stand up, perhaps with one foot on the pool side/step to widen the pelvic outlet. If this does not help, then the woman must get out of the tub immediately. This in itself often rotates the baby in the pelvis and spontaneous birth may occur. See Chapter 17 for management of shoulder dystocia.

Postpartum haemorrhage

A little bleeding occurs as the placenta separates. Be concerned however if you see a large fresh bleed spreading through the water, quickly turning it maroon. Ask the woman to leave the pool or quickly drain it. See page 262 for PPH management.

Loss of consciousness

Very unusually a woman may collapse: usually just a simple faint. It is surprisingly easy to hold a woman who has fainted in the pool, as the water supports her weight and you can hold her head and shoulders comfortably above water. Women tend to recover without ill effects. For a more serious collapse you will require help, preferably several people, to lift her out. Use a lifting aid or hoist, if available and you have time. At home, enlist the birth partner's help. Practise hypothetical emergency situations with colleagues. See Chapter 17 for more information.

The unresponsive baby

The procedure to follow for an unresponsive baby is to:

- Clamp and cut the cord.
- Transfer the baby in a warm towel to the resuscitaire (or prepared area at a home birth).
- Dry the baby vigorously.
- See Chapter 18 for neonatal resuscitation.

Summary

- Maintain a quiet, relaxed atmosphere.
- Encourage plenty of fluids.
- Keep water temperature comfortable; <37.5°C for second stage.
- Monitor maternal temperature hourly and water temperature every 30–60 min.
- Suggest leaving the pool for a while if slow progress.
- *Hands off* at birth if possible.
- Water babies are often slow to breathe, especially if cord still pulsating.
- Physiological or active management can be conducted in the pool.

Useful contacts

Active Birth Centre www.activebirthcentre.com

Association for Improvements in the Maternity Services (AIMS) www.aims.org.uk

Cornelia Enning (German midwife who champions water birth) www.hebinfo.de/(website in German but possible to use online translation; good pictures)

Dr Herman Ponette (Belgian obstetrician with a medicalised approach to water birth, but still very interesting) www.helsinki.fi/~lauhakan/whale/waterbaby/p0.html

Howes birth mirror www.kentmidwiferypractice.co.uk/howes-birth-mirror/
Shaped, narrowish birth mirror made from high polished metal. Easily cleanable and useful to see around corners!

Recommended reading

Garland, D. (2010) *Waterbirth: An Attitude to Care*, 2nd edn. London, Palgrave Macmillan.

References

Anderson, T. (2004) Time to throw the waterbirth thermometer away? *MIDIRS Midwifery Digest* 14(3), 370–74.

ARM (Association of Radical Midwives) (2000) ARM Netalk: Checking for cord. *Midwifery Matters*, 87, 28–30.

Austin, T., Bridges, N., Markiewicz, M., Abrahamson, E. (1997) Severe polycythaemia after third stage of labour underwater. *The Lancet* 350, 1445–7.

Bodner, K., Bodner-Adler, B., Wierrani, F., Mayerhofer, K., Fousek, C., Niedermayr, A., *et al.* (2002) Effects of water birth on maternal and neonatal outcomes. *Wiener Klinische Wochenschrift* 114(10–11), 391–5.

Burns, E. (2001) Waterbirth. *MIDIRS Midwifery Digest* 11 (3, Suppl. 2), 10–13.

Burns, E. and Kitzinger, S. (2001) *Midwifery Guidelines for Use of Water in Labour*. Oxford Centre for Health Care Research and Development, Oxford Brookes University.

CEMACH (Confidential Enquiry into Maternal and Child Health) (2004) *Why Mothers Die 2000–2002. The sixth report of confidential enquiries into maternal deaths in the United Kingdom*. CEMACH, London.

Charles, C. (1998) Fetal hyperthermia risk from warm water immersion. *British Journal of Midwifery* 6(3), 152–6.

Cluett, E., Burns, E. (2009) Immersion in water in labour and birth. *Cochrane Database of Systematic Reviews*, Issue 2.

Cluett, E., Pickering, R., Getliffe, K., St George Saunders, N. J. (2004) Randomised controlled trial of labouring in water compared with standard augmentation for management of dystocia in the first stage of labour. *British Medical Journal* 328(7), 314–8.

Crow, S., Preston, J. (2002) Cord snapping at a waterbirth delivery. *British Journal of Midwifery* 10(8), 494–7.

da Silva, F. M., de Oliveira, S. M., Nobre, M. R. (2009) A randomised controlled trial evaluating the effect of immersion bath on labour pain. *Midwifery* 25(3), 286–94.

DoH (Department of Health) (2004) *National Service Framework for Children, Young People and Maternity Services*, pp. 27–9. London, DoH.

Garland, D. (2006) 'On the crest of a wave' completion of a collaborative audit. *MIDIRS* 16(1), 81–5.

Garland, D. (2010) *Waterbirth: An Attitude to Care*. Basingstoke, Palgrave Macmillan.

Garland, D., Jones, K. (2000) Waterbirth: supporting practice through clinical audit. *MIDIRS* 10(3), 333–6.

Harper, B. (2002) Taking the plunge: re-evaluating water temperature guidelines. *MIDIRS* 12(4), 506–8.

Healthcare Commission (2008) *Towards Better Births: a review of maternity services in England*. London: Commission for Healthcare Audit and Inspection. www.healthcarecommission .org.uk/_db/_documents/Towards_better_births.pdf

Johnson, P. (1996) Birth under water – to breathe or not to breathe. In Lawrence Beech, B. (ed.) *Waterbirth Unplugged. Proceedings of the First International Water Brith Conference*, pp. 31–3. London, Books for Midwives Press.

Jowitt, M. (2001) Problems with RCTs and midwifery. *Midwifery Matters* 91, 9–10.

Murphy-Lawless, J. (2011) 'Ceiling caves in': the current state of maternity services in Ireland *MIDIRS* 21(4), 446–51.

Nagai, T., Sobajima, H., Iwasa, M., Tsuzuki, T., Kura, F., Amemura, J., Watanabe, H. (1993) Neonatal sudden death due to *Legionella* pneumonia associate with water birth in a domestic spa bath. *Journal of Clinical Microbiology* 41(5), 2227–9.

Otigbah, C. M., Dhanjal, M. K., Harmsworth, G., Chard, T. (2000) A retrospective comparison of water births and conventional vaginal deliveries. *European Journal of Obstetrics and Gynecology and Reproductive Biology* 91(1) 15–20.

NICE (National Institute for Health and Clinical Excellence) (2007) *Clinical Guideline 55: Intrapartum Care*. London, NICE.

Nightingale, C. (1996) Water and pain relief – observations of over 570 waterbirths at Hillingdon. In Lawrence Beech, B. (ed.) *Waterbirth Unplugged. Proceedings of the First International Water Birth Conference*, pp. 63–9. London, Books for Midwives Press.

Nugyen, S., Kuschel, C., Teele, R., Spooner, C. (2002) Water birth – a near drowning experience. *Pediatrics* 110, 411–3.

Ockenden, J. (2001) Waterbirth. *The Practising Midwife* 4(9), 30–2.

Odent, M. (1983) Birth under water. *The Lancet* 2, 1476–7.

Odent, M. (1998) Use of water during labour – updated recommendations. *MIDIRS* 8(1), 68–9.

Rosevear, S., Fox, R., Marlow, N., Stirrat, G. (1993) Birthing pools and the fetus. *Lancet* 342, 1048–9.

RCM (2000) The use of water in labour and birth. *RCM Midwives Journal* 3(12), 374–5.

RCM (2005) *Evidence Based Guidelines for Midwifery Led Care in Labour: Midwifery Practice Guideline No 1*. www.rcm.org.uk

RCOG (Royal College of Obstetricians)/RCM (2007) *Immersion in Water During Labour and Birth*. Joint statement 1. London, RCOG.

Richmond, A. (2003) Theories surrounding waterbirth *The Practising Midwife* 6(2), 10–13.

Wickham, S. (2005) Is the Apgar a flexible friend? *Practising Midwife* 8(7), 35.

Woodward, J., Kelly, S. (2004) A pilot study for a randomised controlled trial of waterbirth versus land birth. *BJOG: An International Journal of Obstetrics and Gynaecology* 111(6), 537–45.

Zanetti-Dallenbach, R., Lapaire, O., Maertens, A., Holzgreve, W., Hosli, I. (2007) Water birth: more than a trendy alternative. *Obstetrical and Gynaecological Survey* 62(4), 222–3.

8 Malpositions and malpresentations in labour

Vicky Chapman

Introduction

The most common presentation for a baby to be born is vertex, with the occiput positioned anteriorly. Sometimes, however, the vertex is awkwardly positioned or does not present first. Malpositions and malpresentations commonly cause slow labour progess, sometimes ending in obstructed labour, and preventing normal birth. Complications include deep transverse arrest, cord prolapse, fetal heart concerns, operative delivery and increased maternal and neonatal morbidity (Chadwick, 2002; Coates, 2002; Gardberg *et al.*, 2011). Good midwifery care can help women get through these complicated labours, and/or identify when things really are not going to progress. This chapter explores the different malpositions and malpresentations, associated midwifery care and possible outcomes.

Definitions

Malposition

Normally the fetal head (vertex) is well flexed, so the smallest head diameter, the suboccipitobregmatic (see Figure 2.2, page 45) passes down the birth canal. A *malposition*

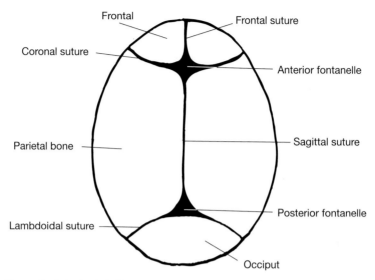

Fig. 8.1　The vault of the fetal skull.

is the vertex in an abnormal position, so the skull diameter presenting to the pelvic opening is greater than normal. The head is either

- Asynclitic, where the fetal head is tilted laterally so that the parietal bone presents first (Figure 8.1), or
- Deflexed, often resulting from the occipitoposterior (OP) position (Figure 8.2).

Malpresentation

If the leading part (denominator) of the fetus is anything other than vertex, a *malpresentation* exists, i.e. breech (see Chapter 14), face, brow, or shoulder presentation (Figures 8.3, 8.4, 8.5, 8.6).

Incidence

- Persistent malpositions/malpresentations (Gardberg *et al.*, 2011)
  - occipito posterior 5.2%
  - breech 3.1%
  - face 0.1%, brow 0.14%; shoulder/transverse lie 0.12%.

Facts

- Fetal head position changes are common during labour, with the final fetal position established close to delivery (Lieberman *et al.*, 2005).
- Ultrasound scanning is more accurate at diagnosing OP and other malpositions than digital vaginal examination alone (Souka *et al.*, 2003; Chou *et al.*, 2004; Kawabata *et al.*, 2010).

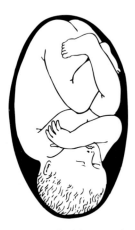

Fig. 8.2   Occipitoposterior position.

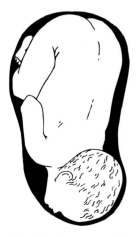

Fig. 8.3   Face presentation.

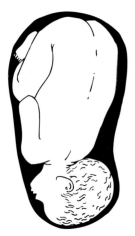

Fig. 8.4   Brow presentation.

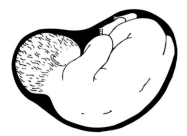

Fig. 8.5   Transverse lie/shoulder presentation.

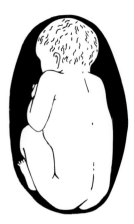

Fig. 8.6   Breech presentation (see Chapter 14 for more information).

- Labour with a malposition/malpresentation is likely to be slower and more painful, so women will need a great deal of support and positive encouragement.
- Epidurals may encourage rotation to OP position at delivery, reducing the spontaneous birth rate (Lieberman *et al.*, 2005).
- Shoulder presentation is the most serious malpresentation in labour and constitutes an obstetric emergency.
- Midwives at home/birthing centres need to be vigilant for presentations, positions or complications which may necessitate obstetric unit transfer. Advanced second stage occurrence/diagnosis may make transfer less feasible or safe.

Occipitoposterior position

This is the most common malposition. The fetus lies with its back against the mother's, the occiput in the posterior part of the pelvis with the head deflexed. Maternal and newborn outcomes are often worse and psychological trauma is more common (Simpkin, 2010).

Two thirds of persistent OP positions develop as a malrotation from occiptoanterior (OA) to OP during labour (Gardberg *et al.*, 1998; Gardberg *et al.*, 2004). This has been confirmed in several studies using serial USS in labour. Coates (2002) suggests that midwifery thinking does not reflect this, as many midwives commonly believe OP positions establish during pregnancy. Mobilisation and upright postures may hold the key to avoiding this complication in labour (Figures 8.7, 8.8, 8.9, 8.10, 8.11).

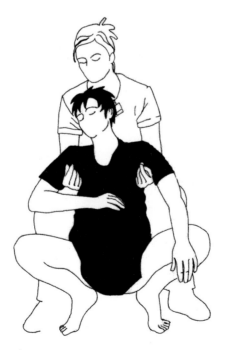

Fig. 8.7 Supported squat.

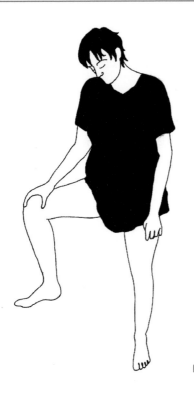

Fig. 8.8   Asymmetrical posture.

Fig. 8.9   Pelvic press. Simkin and Archeta (2005) describe this in the following way: the woman squats with her birth partner kneeling behind her. The partner places the flats of the hands over the woman's iliac crests and presses them very firmly towards each other during a contraction. Within three to four contractions there should be some evidence of rotation or descent. Do not try this if the woman has an epidural or if this causes any joint pain. Many women with backache find the pelvic press eases their back pain.

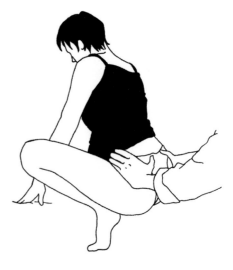

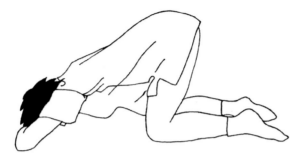

Fig. 8.10   Knee-chest position.

Fig. 8.11   Asymmetrical posture. Postures like this can be useful for poorly positioned babies, e.g. OP or asynclitism. Give the woman plenty of reassurance and encourage her to try different positions to see which she finds most effective.

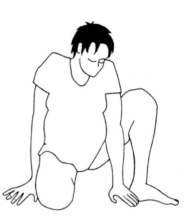

Incidence and facts

- OP has a 15% prevalence in labour but most rotate: only 5% persist at birth (Gardberg and Tuppurainen, 1994).
- OP is more common in primigravidae but also more likely to recur in women who've had a previous OP delivery, suggesting pelvic shape has an influence (Gardberg *et al.*, 2004).
- Persistent OP has a greater impact on labour in primigravid women (Gardberg *et al.*, 2004):
  - Slower painful 'dystocic' labour
  - Increased instrumental and caesarean section (CS) delivery
  - More perineal and anal sphincter trauma.
- OP is more likely to have adverse fetal effects (Cheng *et al.*, 2006):
  - Abnormal fetal heart rate (FHR) and meconium stained liquor in labour
  - Increased birth trauma
  - 5-minute Apgar <7, acidotic blood gases, admission to neonatal intensive care and longer hospital stay
- Fraser *et al.* (2002) found increased risk of difficult delivery in women with epidurals who started second stage with a high head/OP.

Diagnosis

Abdominal palpation. The fetal back is against the maternal spine, creating a dip around the woman's umbilicus which marks the space between the baby's arms and legs. The FHR is clearest far over to the side of the uterus (Sutton, 2000). The woman may find abdominal palpation deeply uncomfortable as she has to lie back, causing intense back pain/discomfort.

Vaginal examination (VE) may confirm the anterior fontanelle in the anterior of the vagina if the head is deflexed (which it often is) but can also detect the posterior fontanelle posteriorly if there is reasonable flexion. Caput and moulding may also be present and make the diagnosis of landmarks on the fetal skull difficult.

Ultrasound scan (USS) is more accurate than digital VE in determining cervical dilatation, station and fetal position (Chou *et al.*, 2004; Souka *et al.*, 2003; Kabawata *et al.*, 2010). VE for position may be incorrect in one third of cases in the first stage of labour (particularly <7 cm) and incorrect in two thirds of second stage cases (Souka *et al.*, 2004; Kabawata *et al.*, 2010). Non-OA positions are even less accurately diagnosed (Souka *et al.*, 2004, Chou *et al.*, 2004; Kabawata *et al.*, 2010). USS is not always routinely available in hospitals, only rarely in birth centres and never at home.

Manual rotation from OP to OA

Evidence suggests manual rotation (MR) of the fetal head to OA improves spontaneous delivery rate. Manual rotation has become a neglected skill which requires no technology or instrumentation (AAFP, 2012).

Successful manual rotation appears to reduce the risk of instrumental/CS delivery, severe perineal laceration, postpartum hemorrhage and chorioamnionitis (Simkin, 2010). The number of rotations attempted to avert one CS was four (Shaffer *et al.*, 2011). The latter study found an increased cervical laceration risk, but Le Ray *et al.* (2007) study found greater success if rotation was undertaken at full dilatation; theoretically this could reduce the risk of cervical trauma.

Le Ray *et al.*, 2007, found that rotation for failure to progress quadrupled the trauma risk in comparison with prophylactic rotation.

Failed manual rotation was associated with a higher CS rate than was success (58.8% of failed rotation, compared with 3.8% successful). Out of all vaginal deliveries following attempted rotation, all failed rotation babies remained OP while all those successfully rotated remained OA (Le Ray *et al.*, 2007).

Midwives performing MR is something of a grey area: it is hard to know how often it is performed. Some midwives do it covertly, whilst performing a VE, through fear of criticism from colleagues, as there seems to be a pervasive belief that only obstetricians can perform it. The AAFP (2012) suggest a midwife should discuss with her supervisor of midwives prior to starting to practice MR. Others may feel this is disempowering and an unnecessary formalising the procedure.

Technique

Ensure the woman understands what you are about to do, and has consented. As the procedure can be extremely uncomfortable, consider extra analgesia, e.g. Entonox.

Think: wedge, flex, rotate

- Reconfirm the position. *Do not attempt if you are uncertain*: you may do more harm than good.
- Gently insert fingers to the posterior area of the pelvis, behind the occiput. Use left hand for ROP and right for LOP (AAFP, 2012).
- The fingers replicate and enhance the levator sling, acting like a wedge to flex the head. Exert steady pressure on the occiput to flex the fetal head: DO NOT apply pressure to the fontanelle.
- Try to rotate the head, using for purchase any palpable fontanelle/suture, avoiding direct fontanelle pressure. Some clinicians grasp the head with the thumb as well and pronate the hand (like closing a book).
- Rotate ROP clockwise and LOP anticlockwise. Encourage rotation during a contraction with the mother pushing, as this will enhance natural flexion and rotation mechanisms (AAFP, 2012).

Characteristics of OP labour and birth

- **Deep back pain** during labour, more intense during contractions (Sutton, 2000; RCM, 2008).
- **Contractions can be irregular**, often coupling, with a lengthy gap before the next; labour is often long and protracted (Sutton, 2000; Simkin and Ancheta, 2005).
- **Involuntary pushing is more common** before full dilatation and can be very distressing. Walmsley (2000), however, suggests that a premature urge to push, common in OP position, may be physiologically desirable because it forces the presenting part to flex, then rotate, optimising its position prior to full dilatation. Opinions vary between midwives as to whether early pushing should be discouraged in OP position due to fear of causing an odematous cervix (RCM, 2008); there is no evidence to support or refute either option.
- **Second stage labour progress can be slow** due to the wide diameter of the presenting part, which also causes gaping of the vagina before the vertex is visible.

Midwifery care

Some authors stress that there is not always a 'quick fix' solution for the OP baby. Walmsley (2000) suggests that the most effective midwifery intervention may be preparing the woman for a labour of indeterminate length and providing good midwifery support.

While manual rotation has, as discussed, shown positive results, 87% of OPs rotate naturally to OA for birth (Gardberg and Tuppurainen, 1994). It takes time for a baby to rotate naturally from OP to OA; labour is usually longer and progress can be slow. The woman's general condition, ability to cope and wishes are all important factors. Huge support, praise and encouragement are necessary to help her cope and keep a positive frame of mind.

- **Eat and drink** as desired to avoid dehydration and ketoacidosis.
- **Empty the bladder regularly**.

- **Avoid ARM.** Some authors suggest that, if labour is slow, rupturing the membranes can be detrimental as it encourages sudden descent, which may possibly preclude the baby from rotating into a more favorable position and predispose the baby to a deep transverse arrest (Chadwick, 2002, citing El Hata, 1996).
- **Syntocinon infusion** may be beneficial especially for the second stage. OP positions usually have poor head to cervix application, resulting in less effective contractions, poor progress and reduced opportunity for rotation to OA. While augmentation may be beneficial it should not be automatic and should be discussed with the woman.

What may help?

- **Heat** can be applied locally to the woman's lower back by the use of a hot water bottle or a microwavable heat pack (Simkin and Ancheta, 2005).
- **Warm water submersion** is comforting and assists postural changes through buoyancy. Cluett and Burns (2009, Cochrane review) found water reduced labour duration and the need for pharmacological pain relief and epidural – all of which may benefit a women facing an OP labour.
- **Firm, lower back massage** or direct pressure centrally over the sacrum as directed by the woman can help ease discomfort.
- **Pelvic press** can bring relief as it alters the shape of the pelvis and may help the baby to shift its head and descend (Figure 8.9) (Simkin and Ancheta, 2005).
- **Abdominal lifting** may improve fetal alignment and relieve backache. The woman places her hands under her abdomen and lifts it up during a contraction while keeping her knees slightly bent and her pelvis tilted forward (Simkin and Ancheta, 2005).
- **An epidural** may bring welcome relief and help the woman continue with a difficult labour. It may, however, complicate and prolong an OP labour and increase the risk of a difficult instrumental delivery (Fraser *et al.*, 2002).

Mobilisation and upright postures

Historically midwives have advocated all fours and non-supine postures for OP labour. Sutton (2000) suggests 'as a rule of thumb; when a woman's knees are lower than her hips she allows ample room in her pelvis for the baby to enter'. Women should benefit from adopting positions of comfort, being assisted to following their own instincts, inclinations and personal comfort.

- **Mobilising** encourages greater contractions, prevents dystocia and increases spontaneous births (Lawrence *et al.*, 2009).
- **Swaying the hips** from side to side, stepping on and off a small stool or marching on the spot are advocated by some.
- **All fours/kneeling/forward leaning postures** (Figures 8.10, 8.11, 8.12, 8.13) usually bring the greatest relief from back pain and are commonly promoted by midwives (RCM, 2008). All fours reduces pain, improves women's feelings of control and comfort, and if tried specifically in OP labour improves rotation to OA and reduces instrumental delivery rate (Stremler *et al.*, 2005).

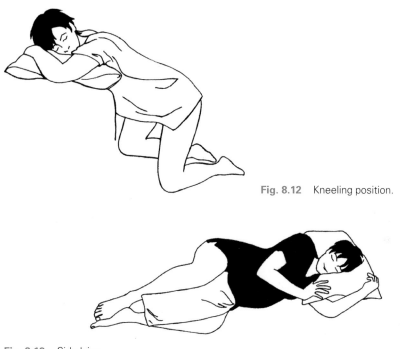

Fig. 8.12   Kneeling position.

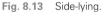

Fig. 8.13   Side-lying.

- **Lying on alternate sides** is useful for tired women or those with an epidural. Sutton (2000) recommends that if the baby is left occipitoposterior (LOP), the woman lies on her left side, and if the baby is right occipitoposterior, she lies on her right side. This, she suggests, facilitates rotation of the fetal trunk and occiput with the aid of gravity to pull into the correct position (see also Figure 8.13). One study confirmed Sutton's side lying approach converted more OP to OA, with improved birth outcomes (Wu *et al.*, 2001).
- **Avoid semi-recumbent or sitting back postures.** Conversely, some women adopt for pushing a 'flat on the back' legs abducted position (Figures 8.14 and 8.15). Providing the fetal heart is satisfactory, and this is what the woman wants to do, then this may well flatten the spine and be the ideal position for the woman.

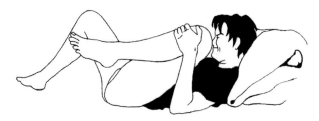

Fig. 8.14   On back with one leg raised.

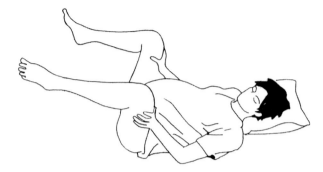

Fig. 8.15 Lithotomy style, or lying back, with legs supported, possibly on lithotomy poles, can be useful to move a stuck baby. This position can be uncomfortable for some women and disempowering if not used sensitively and appropriately. Prolonged lying in this position also risks aortocaval occlusion.

Face presentation

See Figures 8.3 and 8.16.

When the face presents the head is hyperflexed so the occiput is in contact with the fetal back and the mentum (chin) is the denominator. A face presentation can develop from an OP position during the second stage of labour (Chadwick, 2002). Most face presentations are mentoanterior and are usually unproblematic. Mentoposterior is uncommon and is rarely deliverable vaginally (Gaskin, 2002; AAFP, 2012) because the fetal neck is shorter than the maternal sacrum, and therefore cannot stretch to the hollow of the sacrum (Chadwick, 2002). 30% of mentoposterior presentations rotate to mentoanterior. Most authors report increased adverse morbidity from face and brow presentations e.g. FHR abnormalities, meconium-stained liquor and lower Apgar scores (Bhal *et al.*, 1998; Bashiri *et al.*, 2008).

Incidence and facts

- 0.1–0.2% of vaginal births (AAFP, 2012).
- Over 50% are diagnosed during the second stage of labour (Bhal *et al.*, 1998).
- Shaffer *et al.* (2006) found that face presentation was more prevalent in prematurity and in women of black ethnicity, possibly due to pelvic shape.
- Associated factors include prematurity, polyhydramnios, fetal malformations (e.g. anencephaly) and previous CS.
- Gaskin (2002) identifies a short cord as a contributory factor.

Characteristics of a face presentation

- Usually high presenting part (Gaskin, 2002).
- Facial features can be felt. The mouth and two molar prominences can be felt as a triangle. Confirm the chin and mouth carefully to exclude a brow presentation. Take care not to damage the baby's eyes on VE (Chadwick, 2002).
- First-stage cervical dilatation may be slower in a face presentation but second-stage mentoanterior progress is usually good (Gaskin, 2002).

Midwifery care

Spontaneous mentoanterior vaginal delivery usually occurs with relative ease (AAFP, 2012). See Figure 8.16. Such births are uncommon and may attract an audience; it is the midwife's duty of care to protect the woman's privacy and stop uninvited people from coming into the room. Prepare and reassure the parents that their baby may have a bruised and swollen face at birth but it will improve significantly in the hours and days following birth.

- Manipulation to convert the presentation to OA or the use of a fetal scalp electrode or ventouse is contraindicated in face presentation (AAFP, 2012).
- Oxytocin augmentation is usually avoided (AAFP, 2012).
- At birth be prepared: there could be a tight, entangled or short umbilical cord and, although unlikely, anencephaly is a possibility.

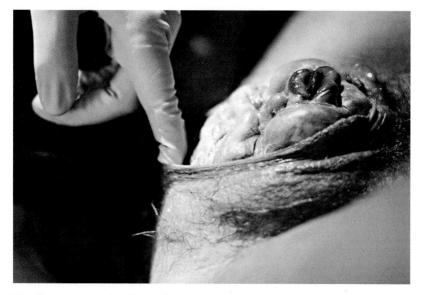

Fig. 8.16 Face presentation birth. *Photo by doula and birth photographer Kali Shanti Park (www.mamamatters.com).*

Brow presentation

A brow presentation is an *unstable presentation* and will usually convert to a face or vertex presentation prior to birth (AAFP, 2012). The baby's head is partially extended, with the widest diameter (mentovertical) presenting (see Figure 2.2, page 45): consequently a persistent brow can prove very difficult to birth but vaginal delivery is possible (Gaskin, 2002). AAFP (2012) suggests more guardedly that a brow is undeliverable under 'normal conditions' and requires a small baby or a roomy pelvis.

The cord may be wrapped around the baby's neck several times in brow presentations (Gaskin, 2002). FHR abnormalities, meconium-stained liquor and lower Apgar scores are more likely (Bhal *et al.*, 1998; Bashin *et al.*, 2008).

Incidence and facts

- 0.2% of vaginal births (AAFP, 2012).
- Over 50% diagnosed/occur during second stage (Bhal *et al.*, 1998).
- More common in primigravidae.

Characteristics of a brow presentation

- Labour may be slower, more difficult and felt by the woman as a 'back pain' labour (Gaskin, 2002).
- VEs can be difficult to interpret due to oedema and the unfamiliarity of the presenting features (AAFP, 2012):
  - Anterior fontanelle and frontal sutures can be felt on one side of the pelvis, orbital ridges on another; the eyes and root of the nose may also be felt (Chadwick, 2002).
  - The presenting part is usually very high and the presenting diameter feels unusually large (Gaskin, 2002).

Midwifery care

Gaskin (2002) suggests that the pelvic press (see Figure 8.9) during the second stage of labour, as well as adopting an upright or squatting posture, will improve the chances of a spontaneous birth. If the head does not convert to a vertex presentation and becomes obstructed, a CS is required (AAFP, 2012).

Transverse lie (shoulder presentation)

Shoulder presentation is undeliverable vaginally and occurs when the baby lies transverse with the shoulder as the denominator (acromion process/dorsum). See Figure 8.5.

External cephalic version (ECV) may be successful. Some doctors then attempt a controlled ARM. However, this is risky; cord prolapse or rupture of the cord with the amnihook can occur with an unengaged presenting part. Once in labour internal poladic version can be difficult as the uterus shapes around the baby (AAFP, 2012).

Incidence and facts

- 1.7% babies are transverse 36–40 weeks (Nassar *et al.*, 2006) while 0.3% remain transverse at delivery (AAFP, 2012).
- Most shoulder presentations occur in multigravid women.
- Predisposing factors include multiple pregnancy, polyhydramnios, placenta praevia, macerated fetus, prematurity, weak abdominal muscles and uterine abnormality (Coates, 1999).

Characteristics of a transverse lie/shoulder presentation

- The uterine shape appears wide, fundal height is lower than expected and the head is palpable on one side, buttocks on the other, and usually nothing in the pelvis

(AAFP, 2012). The lie is occasionally oblique but it usually becomes transverse during labour (Coates, 1999).

- VE (contraindicated in placenta praevia) will detect a high presenting part and sometimes the distinctive pattern of the ribs may be felt or the shoulder, arm or hand.

Midwifery care

The midwife who detects a shoulder presentation *during labour* should summon help. If at home, or birthing centre, immediate transfer to hospital is indicated. In an emergency it may be necessary for the midwife to attempt external and, if necessary, internal cephalic version (AAFP, 2012). Only perform a VE if placenta praevia has been excluded.

External cephalic version. Attempted ECV, even if labour has started, can often be successful. AAFP (2012) notes that a second twin presenting transverse at full dilatation can be turned easily, as the uterus is initially relaxed and accommodating following first twin delivery.

Internal cephalic version is often considered hazardous for the baby, and CS is often the preferred option. However, internal version may be undertaken, this requires the clinician to perform a VE, grasp the baby's feet and pull the baby into a breech position.

Indications for immediate CS

- Cord prolapse
- Rupture of membranes
- Unsuccessful ECV
- Long labour (uterine rupture is a serious complication)

Breech presentation

See Figure 8.6.
This is covered in depth in Chapter 14.

Summary

- Malpositions
  - Tend to result in longer labours, backache, increased intervention and maternal/ neonatal morbidity.
  - Try upright postures, positive reassurance and give huge support.
  - **Internal manual rotation** from OP to OA in second stage, has potential as a useful intervention.
- Malpresentations (non-vertex presentations)
  - Sometimes associated with prematurity, short/entangled cord, fetal malformations.
  - Often slow labour, back pain, higher risk of fetal distress.
  - **Mentoanterior** is usually an uneventful but unusual delivery.

- ○ **Brow** or **mentoposterior** *may* rotate during second stage; if not unlikely to be deliverable vaginally.
- ○ A labour shoulder presentation constitutes an emergency and cannot deliver vaginally.

References

AAFP (American Academy of Family Physicians) (2012) *Advanced Life Support in Obstetrics.* Course Syllabus Manual. AAFP, Leawood, Kansas.

Bashiri, A., Burstein, E., Bar-David, J., Levy, A., Mazor, M. (2008) Face and brow presentation: independent risk factors. *Journal of Maternal and Fetal Neonatal Medicine* 21(6), 357–60.

Bhal, P. S., Davies, N. J., Chung, T. (1998) A population study of face and brow presentation. *Journal of Obstetrics and Gynaecology* 18(3), 231–5.

Chadwick, J. (2002) Malpositions and presentations. In Boyle, M. (ed.) *Emergencies Around Childbirth*, pp. 76–9. Abingdon, Radcliffe Medical Press.

Cheng, Y. W., Shaffer, B. L., Caughey, A. B. (2006) The association between persistent occiput posterior position and neonatal outcomes. *Obstetrics and Gynecology* 107(4), 837–44.

Chou, M. R., Kresier, D., Taslimi, M., Druzin, M. L., El-Sayed, Y. Y. (2004) Vaginal versus ultrasound examination of the fetal head position during the second stage of labor. *American Journal of Obstetrics and Gynecology* 191, 521–4.

Cluett, E. R., Burns, E. (2009) Immersion in water in labour and birth. *Cochrane Database of Systematic Reviews*, Issue 2.

Cluett, E. R., Pickering, R. M., Getliffe, K. (2004) Randomised controlled trial of labouring in water compared with standard of augmentation for management of dystocia in first stage of labour. *BMJ* 328(7435), 314. www.bmj.com

Coates, T. (1999) Malpositions of the occiput and malpresentations. In Bennett, R., Brown, L. K. (eds) *Myles Textbook for Midwives*, 13th edn, pp. 507–37. Edinburgh, Churchill Livingstone.

Coates, T. (2002) Malpositions and malpresentations of the occiput: current research and practice tips. *MIDIRS Midwifery Digest* 12(2),152–4.

Fraser, W. D., Cayer, M., Soeder, B. M., Turcot, L., Marcoux, S. (2002) Risk factors for difficult delivery in nulliparas with epidural analgesia in second stage of labor. *American Journal of Obstetrics and Gynecology* 99(3), 409–18.

Gardberg, M., Tuppurainen, M. (1994) Persistent occiput posterior presentation – a clinical problem. *Acta Obstetrica et Gynaecologica Scandinavica* 73, 45–7.

Gardberg, M., Laakkonen, E., Salevaara, M. (1998) Intrapartum sonography and persistent occiput posterior presentation: a study of 408 deliveries. *Obstetrics and Gynecology* 91, 746–9.

Gardberg, M., Stenwall, O., Laakkonen, E. (2004) Recurrent persistent occipito-posterior position in subsequent deliveries. *BJOG: An International Journal of Obstetrics and Gynaecology* 111(2), 170–1.

Gardberg, M., Leonova, Y., Laakkonen, E. (2011) Malpresentations – impact on delivery. *Acta Obstet Gynecol Scand.* 90(5), 540–2.

Gaskin, I. M. (2002) Unusual presentations and positions. *Spiritual Midwifery*, 4th edn. Summertown, Tennessee, The Book Publishing Co.

Kawabata, I., Nagase, A., Oya, A., Hayashi, M., Miyake, H., Nakai, A. Takeshita, T. (2010) Factors influencing the accuracy of digital examination for determining fetal head position during the first stage of labour. *Journal of Nippon Medical School* 77(6), 290–5.

Lawrence, A., Lewis, L., Hofmeyr, G. J., Dowswell, T., Styles, C. (2009) Maternal positions and mobility during first stage labour. *Cochrane Database of Systematic Reviews*, Issue 2.

Lieberman, E., Davidson, K., Lee-Parritz, A., Shearer, E. (2005) Changes in fetal position during labor and their association with epidural analgesia. *Obstetrics and Gynecology* 105(5), 974–98.

Le Ray, C., Serres, P., Schmitz, T., Cabrol, D., Goffinet, F. (2007) Manual rotation in occiput posterior or transverse positions: risk factors and consequences on the cesarean delivery rate. *Obstetrics and Gynecology* 110(4), 873–9.

Nassar, N., Roberts, C. L., Cameron, C. A., Olive, E. C. (2006) Diagnostic accuracy of clinical examination for detection of non-cephalic presentation in late pregnancy. *BMJ* 333, 578.

RCM (Royal College of Midwives) (2008) *Persistent Lateral and Posterior Fetal Position at the Onset of Labour. Midwifery Practice Guideline*, 4TH edn. London, RCM.

Shaffer, B. L., Cheng, Y. W., Vargas, J. E., Laros, R. K., Caughey, A. B. (2006) Face presentation: predictors and delivery route. *American Journal of Obstetrics and Gynecology* 194(5), 10–12.

Shaffer, B. L., Cheng, Y. W., Vargas, J. E., Caughey, A. B. (2011) Manual rotation to reduce caesarean delivery in persistent occiput posterior or transverse position. *Journal of Maternal-Fetal and Neonatal Medicine* 24(9), 65–72. http://informahealthcare.com/doi/abs/10.3109/14767051003710276

Simkin, P., Ancheta, R. (2005) *The Labour Progress Handbook*, 91. Oxford, Blackwell Publishing.

Simkin, P, (2010) The fetal occiput posterior position: state of the science and a new perspective. *Birth* 37(1), 61–71.

Smyth, R. M. D., Allderd, S. K., Markham, C. (2007) Amniotomy for shortening spontaneous labour. *Cochrane Database of Systematic Reviews*, Issue 4.

Souka, A. P., Haritos, T., Basayiannis, K., Noikokyri, N., Antsaklis, A. (2003) Intrapartum ultrasound for the examination of the fetal head position in normal and obstructed labor. *Journal of Maternal and Fetal Neonatal Medicine* 13, 59–63.

Stremler, R., Hodnett, E., Petryshen, P., Stevens, B., Weston, J., Willan, A. (2005) Randomised controlled trial of hands knees positioning for occipitoposterior position in labour. *Birth* 32(4), 243–51.

Sutton, J. (2000) Occipito posterior positioning and some ideas about how to change it. *The Practising Midwife* 3(6), 20–2.

Walmsley, K. (2000) Managing the OP labour. *MIDIRS Midwifery Digest* 10(1), 61–2.

Wu, X., Fan, L., Wang, Q. (2001) Correction of occipito-posterior by maternal postures during the process of labor. *Zhonghua Fu Chan Ke Za Zhi* 36(8), 468–9. In Chinese, available in English.

9 Slow progress in labour

Vicky Chapman

Introduction

> *'Labours wax and wane in intensity and progress: there is no 'right length' for a labour. One should be on the lookout for any clinical indications that might suggest fetal distress or other concerns but a longer labour need not, of itself, be seen as a problem'* (RCM Campaign for normal birth, 2005).

Labour is a complex process in which psychological and physiological events are intertwined and inseparable. Some women by nature have longer labours than others. Sometimes slow progress is more serious and indicates a significant problem. The midwife must recognise and refer those labours running into trouble, and avoid unnecessary intervention in labours which are simply progressing slowly but surely.

Current parameters for 'normal' labour duration have been defined and imposed on labouring women by obstetricians from a time where practice 'served organisational and management priorities' rather than evidence, and when the views of women were not considered important (RCM, 2005). Diagnosis of slow progress often marks the transfer from 'normality' and 'midwifery care' to one of 'obstetric management' (Cluett *et al.*, 2004). This may cause cultural friction between two different philosophies of care and may result in a sense of powerlessness in midwives and childbearing women to challenge obstetric control in 'normal' birth. This chapter is dedicated to critiquing and offering solutions to assist a labour that doesn't follow a medically defined time frame.

The Midwife's Labour and Birth Handbook, Third Edition. Edited by Vicky Chapman and Cathy Charles.
© 2013 John Wiley & Sons, Ltd. Published 2013 by John Wiley & Sons, Ltd.

Incidence and facts

- The diagnosis of slow progress (dystocia) is subjective; it affects mainly primigravidae (Cluett *et al.*, 2004) and statistics vary between practitioners and units (Crowther *et al.*, 2000; Walsh, 2010). In some UK hospitals up to 57% of nulliparous women receive syntocinon augmentation (Mead, 2007).
- Approximately 50% of women judged to have slow labour will progress equally well with or without oxytocin (Keirse *et al.*, 2000).
- Oxytocin augmentation for slow progress (compared with no/delayed treatment) shortens labour by approximately 2 hours but does not affect caesarean section (CS) rates (Bugg *et al.*, 2011) or instrumental delivery rates (Frölich, 2011).
- Encouraging women to mobilise and remain upright during labour enhances contractions and shortens labour duration by an average of one hour (Lawrence *et al.*, 2009).
- Continuous one-to-one midwifery or female companion support shortens labour, increases spontaneous birth rate, reduces intervention and improves neonatal outcomes and maternal satisfaction (Hodnett *et al.*, 2011).
- Routine ARM in labour is unhelpful; for nulliparae with slow progress it may shorten labour, although it does not reduce the need for oxytocin augmentation (Smyth *et al.*, 2007).
- Some care adversely affects labour duration: restricted mobility, non-private environment, sedative analgesia or epidural, poor labour support (all discussed later).
- Warm water submersion is effective at reducing labour duration as well as having other clinical benefits (Cluett and Burns, 2009).

Prolonged labour

'A defining feature of the last fifty years of labour care has been the preoccupation with the pathology of labour length, so much so that it has become an orthodoxy in intrapartum approaches across the world' (Walsh, 2007).

How slow is too slow?

Ermerging evidence suggests that normal labour progress does not always follow a linear model, formerly suggested by Friedman, and reflected in the standard labour progress curve (Zhang *et al.*, 2002). Walsh (2010) cites Winter and Duff (2010) who refer to labour as 'orderly chaos', reflecting the variability of labour rhythms. New voices, evidence and ways of thinking are emerging about what is normal for any particular labour (Walsh, 2010):

- Midwives practising automomously have observed that some labours slow then resume without complications (Walsh, 2010).
- Cervical dilation is often slower than 0.5 cm/hour in earlier active labour (nulliparas) and faster in more advanced active labour for all parities (Zhang *et al.*, 2010; Neal *et al.*, 2010).
- Slow progress from 7 cm should be observed carefully (Zhang *et al.*, 2002).

Assessing progress in labour and the partogram

Midwives use a variety of methods to assess progress: see Chapter 1, pages 11–12. VEs are the most commonly accepted method, but they can be subjective, inaccurate and remain unevaluated by research (see Chapter 2).

The cervicogram/partogram evolved from Friedman's work on mean time limits for cervical dilatation (Walsh, 2000a) and offers an immediate visual impression of the woman's overall physical condition with alert/action lines based on mean dilatation. Partograms may be beneficial where midwives are caring for several women and shifts change regularly. NICE (2007) recommends its use, with a 4-hour action line (which, as discussed later, may be inappropriate for many labours).

A Cochrane review could not recommend routine cervicogram/partogram in standard labour care but suggested its removal would be 'difficult' and meet resistence (Lavender *et al.*, 2008).

Obstructed labour

Obstruction is rare in the developed world. Failure of the presenting part to descend in spite of uterine contractions manifests itself ultimately not as *slow progress* but *no progress*. Obstruction may be caused by cephalopelvic disproportion (CPD) and/or abnormal lie, position or presentation.

What really distinguishes *delay* from *obstruction* are the following; unfortunately seen too often in developing countries:

- No further descent of the presenting part
- Fetal rate rate (FHR) abnormalities
- Formation of a rigid retraction band: 'Bandl's ring'
- Maternal pyrexia and tachycardia.

Complications include bladder damage (often indicated by bloodstained urine), fistulae (usually nulliparous women), ruptured uterus (usually multigravid women), fetal death, maternal shock and sepsis, leading to maternal death.

Causes of a prolonged labour

Slow progress can be normal for an individual or have one/several causes.

Physical causes

- **Fetal malposition or malpresentation:** see Chapter 8.
- **Cephalopelvic disproportion.** Previous uncomplicated delivery of a baby of similar weight is the most reliable predictor of pelvic adequacy. CPD is not easily predictable but is usually determined during labour if there is lack of descent of the presenting part (Crowther *et al.*, 2000) with increased caput and moulding. Predisposing factors include maternal diabetes, a macrosomic baby and malpresentation/malposition.

Less common physical causes

Usually these problems will have been identified and discussed prior to labour:

- **Pelvic anomalies:** fractured pelvis, significant weight-bearing problems, e.g. from lower limb amputation, spina bifida and spinal injury.
- **Cervical problems** may arise following cervical surgery, e.g. previous cone biopsy. The internal os can feel rough to the touch and the cervix tight and unyielding for a prolonged period, commonly during the latent phase. Simkin and Ancheta (2005) anecdotally suggest contractions of great intensity may be required to overcome the initial resistance, following which dilatation usually occurs.

Analgesia choice

- **Epidural anaesthesia** offers total pain block but also increases the risk of malrotation delay in the first and second stage with associated increased interventions (Lieberrman *et al.*, 2005). Epidural rates vary dramatically between units, suggesting that it is not women who always choose this form of analgesia but those who 'care' for them. If dystocia is to be prevented, alternative methods of pain relief should be explored first and epidural reserved for those women who genuinely request it.

Stress response and emotional dystocia

'In a typical hospital environment, women are disturbed at every turn – with machines, intrusions, strangers, and a pervasive lack of privacy ... Together these fears contribute in powerful ways to the release of stress hormones, moving women into an attitude of physiologic fight or flight. On an intellectual level, a woman may believe that the hospital is a safe, protected environment, but her body reacts quite differently' (Lothian, 2004).

- **Stress hormones** interact with beta-receptors in the uterine muscle to inhibit contractions, slowing labour down (Cluett, 2000). This is most evident in primigravidae arriving for the first time on labour ward, where their anxiety response causes their labour to temporarily stop.
- **Environmental stressors:** for more information on preparing a good birth environment see Chapter 1.
- **Psychological stress and anxiety** can be stimulated by many factors. Some women may have a phobia or fear of pain or childbirth; others may have previously endured a traumatic delivery or be victims of childhood sexual abuse (Simkin and Ancheta, 2005).

Prolonged latent phase

The latent phase of labour can last several days (Burvill, 2002). In the absence of problems, it requires no medical intervention other than effective explanations, reassurance and support (see Chapter 1).

Women admitted earlier in labour have higher CS rates (Rahnama *et al.*, 2006). Use of triage facilities, early labour assessment centres and home assessment have all been shown to reduce interventions including time spent on labour ward, augmentation, analgesia use and epidurals, with a modest increase in spontaneous vaginal birth; women are more likely to report an improved birth experience (Lauzon and Hodnett, 2001; Spiby *et al.*, 2008; Hodnett *et al.*, 2008).

Midwifery care

A prolonged latent phase can leave the woman exhausted and demoralised, doubting her body's ability to continue to labour without problems. Midwives often consider 'nigglers' to not be in real labour rather than women in need of midwifery reassurance and kind support. Midwives have a vital role in helping women cope by validating their experienced pain and confirming the normality of the slow process, as well as offering information and support. In one study, women reported the time they spent at home in early labour difficult to manage; reporting a state of continual agitation and constant worry about the journey to hospital (Nolan, 2011).

Spiby *et al.* (2008) explored how best to provide advice to women in early labour about when to come to hospital. Women wanted *prolonged contact with midwives* in early labour and were dissatisfied when their anxieties were not resolved during telephone conversations. This study also found that midwives encountered tensions in trying to encourage women to stay at home in early labour without appearing to deny them hospital admission.

- Women benefit from their midwife giving them *time*; perhaps sitting quietly with them through several contractions, chatting, *offering empathic acknowledgement of the pain*, giving reassurance.
- Women in the latent stage who eat and drink and get good rest and sleep in the preceding 24 hours are more likely to have a shorter labour, independent of other factors e.g. malposition, birthweight and maternal age (Dencker *et al.*, 2010).
- Offer practical ideas for coping with contractions:
  - Simple analgesia.
  - Soaking in a warm bath, massage, hot water bottle.
  - Distractions and keeping busy, e.g. going for a walk, cooking, watching a film.

For a minority of women this phase is abnormally prolonged and too painful to bear, sometimes due to a malposition, e.g. occipitoposterior (OP). They can become exhausted, nauseated, dehydrated and desperate. Stronger analgesia may be necessary. Pethidine may offer some respite, allowing the woman to relax and doze. Epidural analgesia in the latent phase (cervix 1–4 cm), does not prolong labour nor increase the CS rate in nulliparous women compared with epidural at >4 cm (Wang *et al.*, 2009). Never forget the benefits of deep water immersion at any, even the latent, phase of labour: it may give 'time out' for the woman to get herself together.

Prolonged active first stage

The active phase should see contractions increasing in frequency, strength and pain. It can be useful to ask 'Do the woman's contractions seem the same or more frequent, and more painful, than an hour ago?' While some women with slow progress may feel exhausted and demoralised, and welcome assistance, others will be coping well, 'gone into themselves', oblivious to the passing of time. A 'wait and see' course of action may be all that is required.

A prospective study of 26 838 labours found that the active labour phase did not start until 5 cm of cervical dilation in multigravidae and even later in nulliparous women (Zhang *et al.*, 2010). Time progressing from one centimetre to the next decreased as labour advanced (from 1.2 hours at 3–4 cm to 0.4 hours at 7–8 cm in nulliparas). Nulliparous women had the longest and slowest labour curve; multigravid women of varying parities had very similar curves. Zhang *et al.* suggest a 2–hour threshold for diagnosing labour arrest may be too short before 6 cm dilation, whereas a 4-hour limit may be too long after 6 cm.

Midwifery care

Good one-to-one midwifery support, encouraging comfortable positions, soaking in warm water, breathing and relaxation, massage and touch, will both encourage pain-relieving endorphin release and improve labour progress. Directly ask the woman if anything is worrying her. Sharing information, explanations and offering possible solutions for specific anxieties can help. Avoid offering 'empty' reassurances: 'Don't worry about that, you'll be fine' will do little to address her anxieties and even unintentionally suggest that the matter has been discussed and is somehow resolved.

Midwives control the environment: ensure lights are dim, doors and curtains drawn. Maintain privacy, keep interruptions to a minimum and encourage the woman's partner to offer massage and support. It can be useful to also address simple physical issues: is she hungry or thirsty, when did she last pass urine, has she tried mobilising/upright postures?

In some cases, e.g. malposition, simple mobilisation and accepting that progress will be slower will help (see Chapter 8).

(1) If appropriate try the interventions in Box 9.1 to increase contractions.
(2) If natural interventions do not help, then further intervention is necessary:
  • Consider ARM (see Chapter 2)
  • VE 2 hours after ARM to check progress (NICE, 2007)
(3) If this does not increase labour NICE (2007) advises:

> When delay in the established first stage of labour is confirmed in nulliparous women, advice should be sought from an obstetrician and the use of oxytocin should be considered. The woman should be informed that the use of oxytocin following spontaneous or artificial rupture of the membranes will bring forward her time of birth but will not influence mode of birth or other outcomes.' They should be also aware that oxytocin increases pain and the risk of hyperstimulation and continuous monitoring of the fetal heart is recommended.

Following assessment the obstetrician may decide to:

• Wait and see
• Recommend oxytocin infusion (with further VE after 4 hours), possibly with further analgesia (NICE, 2007): see Box 9.2
• Offer continuous electronic fetal monitoring (EFM) (NICE, 2007)
• Proceed to CS if:
  ○ Oxytocin is contraindicated
  ○ No further labour progress
  ○ FHR concerns.

Box 9.1   Interventions to improve labour progress.

Support	• Continuous female labour support reduces labour duration, improves maternal/neonatal outcomes and increases maternal satisfaction (Hodnett *et al.*, 2011).
	• Lay attendants like doulas, or family/friends can also provide warmth, comfort and care (Simkin & Ancheta, 2005).
Mobilisation & position changes	• Mobilising & upright positions during labour enhance contractions and reduce labour duration, epidural use, episiotomy and instrumental delivery (Gupta *et al.*, 2012; Lawrence *et al.*, 2009; RCM, 2010).
	• Upright positions help align pelvic bones and pelvic shape/capacity, optimising a 'good fit' between baby and pelvis (Simkin & Ancheta, 2005).
	• Squatting and kneeling significantly widen the pelvic outlet (Borrell and Fenstrom, 1957; Russell, 1982).
	• Even if the woman is tired, supported upright positions are possible and more comfortable than semi-recumbent.
Comforting touch	• Massage, stroking, hand holding, and close contact increase endogenous oxytocin production, thereby stimulating contractions (Simkin and Ancheta, 2005).
	• Give partners 'permission' to get in close and hold the woman; encourage attendants to offer comfort and massage and provide privacy for this.
	• Touch is very personal; some women do not like it. Use this simple intervention with care.
Acupressure	• Acupressure remains unevaluated, but it is simple, harm free and may do good.
	• Press firmly for 10–60 seconds over the tibia (4 fingers width up from inner ankle bone) or to the Hoku point on the back of the hand (where the metacarpal bones of thumb and index finger meet). It may feel tender but worth repeating several times if necessary (Simkin and Ancheta, 2005).
Nipple stimulation	• Releases natural oxytocin which enhances contractions (Kavanagh *et al.*, 2005).
	• Give privacy if required.
	• Some may decline due to embarrassment or discomfort.
Water/ hydrotherapy	• Stimulates oxytocin and endorphin release (Ockenden, 2001).
	• Prolonged immersion may slow labour (Odent, 1998) but easily reversed by leaving the pool.
	• Water is as effective as pharmacological augmentation in nulliparas with dystocia and reduces epidural use (Cluett *et al.*, 2009). See Chapter 7.

Box 9.2   Use of oxytocin.

• Oxytocin is firmly established in labour ward culture as routine practice for managing 'longer than average' labours.
• It shortens labour by approximately 2 hours but does not affect CS/instrumental rate (Bugg *et al.*, 2011; Frölich, 2011).
• It may achieve cervical dilatation without improving the outcome (NICE, 2007).
• Women should be closely observed for hyperstimulation.
• Continuous EFM is recommended (NICE, 2007).
• Women describe oxytocin as unpleasant and more painful and would prefer to try without it when next giving birth (Keirse *et al.*, 2000).
• Regime for oxytocin administration: see page 315.

Prolonged second stage

Upright maternal birthing position, non-active pushing and avoiding arbitrary second stage time limits improve the spontaneous vaginal birth rate (Walsh, 2000b; Gupta *et al.*, 2012). There is some evidence that second stage >3 hours increases maternal risk of morbidity (Cheung *et al.*, 2004), and >4 hours increases the risk of more severe perineal trauma, PPH and infection (Myles and Santolaya, 2003). A longer second stage increases the vaginal delivery rate, reduces CS rate and has no adverse effect on neonatal morbidity (Myles and Santolaya, 2003).

Terminating a straightforward but slow second stage with an instrumental delivery (a painful and traumatic experience for a women) contributes to maternal morbidity and does not benefit infant outcomes (Sleep *et al.*, 2000; Walsh, 2000b).

Reassess

- NICE (2007) recommend offering a VE after an hour of active second stage, to assess rotation and descent:
  - Refer multigravidae for obstetric opinion if birth not imminent.
  - Offer primigravidae support and encouragement, amniotomy (if membranes intact) and consider further analgesia/anaesthesia. If not delivered after another hour (i.e. 2 hours of active second stage) refer to an obstetrician.

Assessing progress

- Increased moulding and caput may appear misleadingly like descent, so always check descent by abdominal palpation (WHO, 2003).
- A total lack of progress in the presence of good contractions indicates possible obstruction. Refer to an obstetrician.
- Consider fetal position and station at the onset of the second stage. These factors will help decide the timing of further VE and any obstetric review (NICE, 2007).

Referral

An obstetrician will assess by VE and palpation and may recommend the following:

- 'Wait and see' if birth is approaching
- Consider oxytocin (with EFM)
- Instrumental delivery in the labour room (see Chapter 10) or trial of forceps/ventouse in theatre
- CS if no descent at all with pushing.

NICE (2007) diagnoses second stage delay as:

- 2 hours of active second stage for a nulliparous woman: instrumental delivery recommended after 3 hours.
- 1 hour of active second stage for a parous woman: instrumental delivery recommended after 2 hours.

- Women with epidurals are recommended to delay pushing for an hour unless urge present or vertex visible: if so, instrumental delivery recommended after 4 hours.

Checklist for slow progress

- Is the cervix fully dilated?
- Is the woman's bladder full?
- Does she have a genuine urge to push? Is she experiencing a latent second phase of labour? If so, pause and await events.
- Is she pushing effectively (see Chapture 1)? For ideas when pushing with an epidural see page 155.
- Is she lying down? If so, help her to change position and get upright.
- Are contractions adequate? Contractions with a long gap between them mean the second stage will be longer: take this into account if augmentation is not being used. For inadequate or incoordinate contractions see Box 9.1.

Problem solving

For malpositon/malpresentation see Chapter 8.

Anxiety. The imminent arrival of the baby may trigger anxieties in the woman ranging from worries about the baby to a fear of pain and tearing (Simkin and Ancheta, 2005). You may not be able to alleviate her fears, but acknowledge them and offer plenty of praise and reassurance, particularly when she is pushing.

Holding back. A woman who is tense, frightened or inhibited needs quiet, privacy and a relaxed focus away from her perineum and towards her well-being.

Keep the atmosphere calm, mellow and relaxed. Avoid stimulating the autonomic nervous system with unnecessary noise, lights, distractions, 'white coats' and interruptions. Refrain from shining a spotlight on, or staring at, the woman's perineum with every contraction. If appropriate suggest she goes and sits privately on the toilet to push for a while; give her the call bell and be ready close by.

Maternal exhaustion. Unlike a woman who is inhibited and holding back, a tired, demoralised woman may benefit from stimulation: refreshments, a cool flannel, some music, a position change, a breeze via an open window, and for sleepy, tired supporters to rally round, brighten up, wake up and give support.

Abdominal lifting. The woman herself lifts her bump upwards during a contraction, which may shift an impacted head (Simkin and Ancheta, 2005). Lemay (2000) and Parry (2003) similarly describe this: the mother adopts the knee-chest (Figure 8.10, page 135) or side-lying (Figure 8.13, page 139) position and tries to literally pull/draw her baby up to her neck for a few pushes. It may be worth a go!

Midwife exhaustion. We have all been there after a long night with a primip: exhausted and desperate for our warm bed. A slow second stage can leave tired midwives tempted to call the obstetrician in order to get the baby delivered. Such exhaustion does not always have an easy answer, but asking an energetic trusted colleague to assist you or relieve you to get something to eat and sit down for ten minutes will help refresh your batteries.

Survivors of childhood sexual abuse. It may help to focus the women in the present, offering gentle reassurance that what they feel is their baby soon to be born. Chapter 2 provides information on counteracting, and not re-enacting, abuse.

Effective positions for a slow second stage

General mobilisation or upright and frequent position changes should help poor contractions and aid fetal descent.

- **Frequent change of position** is a simple intervention and yet can be the solution to delay in the second stage.
- **A supported squat, kneeling or asymmetrical postures** can prove beneficial in malpositions/asynclitism (see pages 133–140). Radiological evidence illustrates that the pelvis moves and widens during birth and outlet diameters can increase by nearly a third in squatting/ kneeling positions (Borrell and Fenstrom, 1957; Russell, 1982).
- **Encouraging the woman to 'climb'** on, over and off the bed a couple of times, or step on and off a low stool (try stairs at home – an old midwifery trick). This may cause a stuck baby to move its position and free the lumbar spine.
- **Lithotomy position.** It is not uncommon for women prepared for an instrumental delivery to spontaneously deliver when their legs are abducted and placed in lithotomy: see page 140. This position should be used sensitively and with caution as it has potential risks to the mother (including risk of DVT, aortocaval occlusion and perineal trauma). It is bad for midwives' backs to support women's legs on their hips and it can put stress on the woman's pelvis.

Epidural anaesthesia is associated with an increase in instrumental deliveries; however, spontaneous vaginal births with epidurals have been attributed to:

- **Delayed pushing** for around 1 (NICE, 2007) or 2 hours, or until the head is visible at the introitus (Fraser *et al.*, 2000; Roberts *et al.*, 2004).
- **Maternal position.** Second-stage duration is shorter, and instrumental delivery is less likely if the woman in the second stage adopts an upright, all fours or side lying position compared to a semi-recumbent position (Downe *et al.*, 2004; Roberts *et al.*, 2005).
- **Urinary retention** can result from an epidural, and a full bladder can impede progress; consider a catheter.
- **Direction.** Women who have a dense block may need direction and encouragement as to when and how to push. Let the contraction build so they don't push too early, then encourage their pushing effort. Offer positive feedback when they push effectively.
- **Do not let the epidural wear off** as it does not improve the rate of spontaneous birth and is distressing for the woman (NICE, 2007).
- **Reassess.** If there is slow progress after an hour or two of pushing:
  - Consider a VE and abdominal palpation for reassessment of descent/progress.
  - Refer to an obstetrician for review if necessary.

Summary

Slow progress in labour

- Mostly affects primigravidae – evidence suggests current parameters for 'normal' progress may be incorrect.

- Preoccupation with strict time definitions in labour are not evidence based.
- There is no clinical evidence to support any general benefits from a shorter labour.
- Prevention of dystocia is better than cure.

Factors that slow labour

- Hospital practices:
  - immobility and semi-recumbent postures
  - stressful birth environment ('fight or flight'): noise, bright lights, lack of privacy
  - lack of continuity of carer, staff changes
- Epidural anaesthesia
- Malposition/malpresentation (see Chapter 8)
- Large baby, CPD, pelvic injury, previous cervical surgery.

Interventions that help progress

- Continuous presence and support from the midwife or other female support
- Mobilisation, upright postures, position changes
- Comforting touch
- Nipple stimulation
- Hydrotherapy/warm bath/water tub
- Oxytocin.

Recommended reading

Simkin, P., Ancheta, R. (2005) *The Labor Progress Handbook.* Oxford, Blackwell Publishing.

Walsh, D. (2007) Rhythms in the frst stage of labour. *Evidence Based Care for Normal Labour: a guide for midwives*, pp. 29–43. London, Routledge.

Zhang, J., Troendle, J., Mikolajczyk, R. (2010) The natural history of the first stage of labour. *Obstetrics and Gynaecology* 115(4), 705–10.

References

Borrell, U., Fenstrom, I. (1957) The movements of the sacroiliac joints and their importance to changes in the pelvic dimensions during parturition. *Acta Obstetrica et Gynaecologica Scandinavica* 36, 42–57.

Bugg, G. J., Siddiqui, F., Thornton, J. G. (2011) Oxytocin versus no treatment or delayed treatment for slow progress in the first stage of spontaneous labour. *Cochrane Database of Systematic Reviews.* 6;(7):CD007123.

Burvill, S. (2002) Midwifery diagnosis of labour onset. *British Journal of Midwifery* 10(10), 600–5.

Cheung, Y., Hopkins, I., Caughey, A. (2004) How long is too long: does a prolonged second stage of labour in nulliparous women affect maternal and neonatal morbidity? *American Journal of Obstetrics and Gynaecology* 191:933–8.

Cluett, E. (2000) The onset of labour. 2: implications for practice. *The Practising Midwife* 3(7), 16–19.

Cluett, E. R., Burns, E. (2009) Immersion in water in labour and birth. *Cochrane Database of Systematic Reviews*, Issue 2.

Cluett, E. R., Pickering, R. M., Getliffe, K. (2004) Randomised controlled trial of labouring in water compared with standard of augmentation for management of dystocia in first stage of labour. *BMJ* 328(7435), 314. www.bmj.com

Crowther, C., Enkin, M., Keirse, M. J. N. C., Brown, I. (2000) Monitoring progress in labor. In Enkin, M., Keirse, M. J. N. C., Neilson, J., *et al.* (eds) *A Guide to Effective Care in Pregnancy and Childbirth*, 3rd edn, pp. 281–8. Oxford, Oxford University Press.

Dencker, A., Berg, M., Bergqvist. L., Lilja, H. (2010) Identification of latent phase factors associated with active labor duration in low-risk nulliparous women with spontaneous contractions. *Acta Obstet Gynecol Scand.* 89(8), 1034–9.

Downe, S., Gerrett, D., Renfrew, M. J. (2004) A prospective randomised trial on the effect of position in the passive second stage of labour on birth outcome in nulliparous women using epidural analgesia. *Midwifery* 20(2), 157–68.

Fraser, W. D., Marcoux, S., Klauss, I., Douglas, J., Goulet, C., Boulvain, M. (2000) Multicenter, randomized, controlled trial of delayed pushing for nulliparous women in the second stage of labor with continuous epidural analgesia. The PEOPLE (Pushing Early or Pushing Late with Epidural) Study Group. *American Journal of Obstetrics and Gynecology* 182(5), 1165–72.

Frölich, M. (2011) Oxytocin for slow progress in the first stage of spontaneous labour is not associated with different rates of caesarean or assisted delivery compared with no treatment or delayed use in second stage. Systematic review. *Evidence Based Medicine* doi:10.1136/ebm.2011.100183 ebm.bmj.com

Gupta, J. K., Hofmeyr, G. J., Shehmar, M. (2012) Position in the second stage of labour for women without epidural anaesthesia. *Cochrane Database of Systematic Reviews*, Issue 5.

Hodnett, E. D., Stremler, R., Willan, A. R., Weson, J. A., Lowe, N. K., Simpson, K. R., Fraser, D., Gafni, A. (2008) Effect on birth outcomes of a formalised approach to care in hospital labour assessment units: international, randomised controlled trial. *BMJ.* 28;337:a1021. doi: 10.1136/bmj.a1021.

Hodnett, E. D., Gates, S., Hofmeyr, G. J., Sakala, C., Weston, J. (2011) Continuous support for women during childbirth. *Cochrane Database of Systematic Reviews*. Issue 2.

Kavanagh, J., Kelly, A., Thomas, J. (2005) Breast stimulation for cervical ripening and in-duction of labour. *Cochrane Database of Systematic Reviews*, Issue 3.

Keirse, M. J. N. C., Enkin, M. W., Lumley, J. (2000) Social and professional support in childbirth. In Enkin, M., Keirse, M. J. N. C., Neilson, J., Crowther, C., Duley L., Hodnett, E., Hofmeyr, J. (eds) *A Guide to Effective Care in Pregnancy and Childbirth*, 3rd edn, pp. 247–54. Oxford, Oxford University Press.

King, M., Bewes, P. C., Carns, J., Thornton, J. (1999) Online edition. *Primary Surgery: Non-Trauma*, Vol. 1. Oxford Medical Publications. www.meb.uni-bonn.de/dtc/primsurg

Lauzon, L., Hodnett, E. D. (2001) Labour assessment programs to delay admission to labour wards. *Cochrane Database of Systematic Reviews*. Issue 3.

Lawrence, A., Lewis, L., Hofmeyr, G. J., Dowswell, T., Styles, C. (2009) Maternal positions and mobility during first stage labour. *Cochrane Database of Systematic Reviews*. Issue 2.

Lemay, G. (2000) Pushing for first time Moms. *Midwifery Today*. http://www.midwifery today.com/articles/pushing.asp.

Lieberman, E., Davidson, K., Lee-Parritz, A., Shearer, E. (2005) Changes in fetal position during labour and their association with epidural analgesia. *Obstet Gynecol* May;105 (5 Pt 1):974–82.

Lothian, J. (2004) Do Not Disturb: the importance of privacy in labor. *Journal of Perinatal Education. Lamaze publication.* 13(3), 4–6.

Mead, M. (2007) Midwives perspectives in 11 UK maternity units. In Downe, S. (ed.) *Normal Childbirth: evidence and debate*. London: Churchill Livingstone.

Myles, T. D., Santolaya, J. (2003) Maternal and neonatal outcomes in patients with a prolonged second stage of labor. *Obstetrics and Gynecology* 102, 52–8. www.greenjournal.org/cgi/content/full/102/1/52

Nasir, A., Korejo, R., Noorani, K. J. (2007) Childbirth in the squatting position. *Journal of the Pakistan Medical Association* 57(1), 19–22.

Neal, J. L., Lowe, N. K., Patrick, T. E., Cabbage, L. A., Corwin, E. J. (2010) What is the slowest-yet-normal cervical dilation rate among nulliparous women with spontaneous labor onset? *Journal of Obstetrics Gynaecology and Neonatal Nursing* 39(4), 361–9.

NICE (National Institute for Health and Clinical Excellence) (2007) *Clinical Guideline 55: Intrapartum Care*. London, NICE. www.nice.org.uk

Nolan, M. (2011) What is women's experience of being at home in early labour? *NCT New Digest*. Research. Jan.

Ockenden, J. (2001) The hormonal dance of labour. *The Practising Midwife* 4(6), 16–17.

Odent, M. (1998) Use of water during labour – updated recommendations. *MIDIRS* 8(1), 68–9.

Parry, D. (2003) Reversing the Chi. *Midwifery Matters*. Issue 98: www.radmid.demon.co.uk/Chi.htm

Rahnama, P., Ziaei, S., Faghihzadeh, S. (2006) Impact of early admission in labour on method of delivery. *International Journal of Gynaecology and Obstetrics*, 92(3), 217–20.

Roberts, C. L., Torvaldsen, S., Cameron, C. A., Olive, E. (2004) Delayed versus early pushing in women with epidural analgesia: a systematic review and met-analysis. *British Journal of Obstetrics and Gynaecology* 111(12), 1333–40.

Roberts, C. L., Algert, C. S., Cameron, C. A., Tovaldsen, S. (2005) A meta-analysis of upright positions in the second stage to reduce instrumental deliveries in women with epidural analgesia. *Acta Obstetricia et Gynecologica Scandinavica* 84(8), 794–8.

RCM (Royal College of Midwives) (2005) *Campaign for Normal Birth*. www.rcmnormalbirth.org.uk

RCM (2010) *The RCM Survey of Positions Used in Labour and Birth*. London, RCM.

Russell, J. G. B. (1982) The rationale of primitive delivery positions. *British Journal of Obstetrics and Gynaecology* 89, 712–5.

Simkin, P., Ancheta, R. (2005) *The Labour Progress Handbook*. Oxford, Blackwell Publishing.

Sleep, J., Roberts, J., Chalmers, I. (2000) The second stage of labor. In Enkin, M., Keirse, M. J. N. C., Neilson, J., Crowther, C., Duley, L., Hodnett, E., Hofmeyr, J. (eds) *A Guide to Effective Care in Pregnancy and Childbirth*, pp. 289–99. Oxford, Oxford University Press.

Smyth, R. M. D., Allderd, S. K., Markham, C. (2007) Amniotomy for shortening spontaneous labour. *Cochrane Database of Systematic Reviews*, Issue 4.

Spiby, H., Green, J., Renfrew, M. *et al.* (2008) Improving care at the primary/secondary interface: a trial of community-based support in early labour. *The ELSA trial*. York: Mother and Infant Research Unit, Department of Health Sciences, University of York. www.york.ac.uk/

Walsh, D., Downe, S. (2010) *Labour Rythms. Essential Midwifery Practice Intrapartum Care*, pp. 64–5. Oxford, Wiley-Blackwell.

Walsh, D. (2000a) Evidence-based care. Part 3: assessing women's progress in labour. *British Journal of Midwifery* 8(7), 449–57.

Walsh, D. (2000b) Evidence-based care. Part 6: limits on pushing and time in the second stage. *British Journal of Midwifery* 8(10), 604–8.

Walsh, D. (2007) *Rhythms in the First Stage of Labour. Evidence based care for normal labour – a guide for miwives*, pp. 29–43. London, Routledge.

Walsh, D. (2010) Labour rhythms vs labour progress: one final update. *BJM* 18, 482.

Wang, F., Shen, X., Guo, X., Peng, Y., Gu, X. (2009) Epidural analgesia in the latent phase of labor and the risk of cesarean delivery: a five-year randomized controlled trial. *Anesthesiology* 111(4), 871–80.

WHO (2003) *Managing Complications in Pregnancy and Childbirth: A Guide for Midwives and Doctor*, pp. 61–2. Publication Dept of Reproductive Health and Research. Geneva, WHO.

Winter, C., Duff, M. (2010) The progress of labour; oderly chaos. In McCourt, C. (ed.) *Childbirth, Midwifery and Concepts of Time*. London, Berghahn Books.

Zhang, J., Troendle, J., Yancey, M. (2002) Reassessing the labour curve. *American Journal of Obstetrics and Gynecology* 187, 824–8.

Zhang, J., Troendle, J., Mikolajczyk, R. (2010) The natural history of the first stage of labour. *Obstetrics and Gynaecology* 115(4), 705–10.

10 Assisted birth: ventouse and forceps

Cathy Charles

Introduction

With good labour support, most women will experience a spontaneous vaginal delivery. Some women, however, for a variety of reasons, will not. For those women the options are either an instrumental delivery or a caesarean section (CS). An instrumental delivery carried out competently, in a supportive atmosphere, can still be a triumph for a woman, and a source of celebration. However, there is an increased risk of morbidity and reduced maternal satisfaction with assisted delivery. Many women may feel they have failed, and the experience may leave physical and/or emotional scars. Others may be relieved to have avoided a CS and move quickly on to enjoy their baby. Clinical competence is vital, and emotional support through the experience is equally important.

Incidence and facts

- 12–14% of UK births were instrumental in 2010, with 16.7% in Northern Ireland (BirthChoiceUK; Bragg *et al.*, 2010; ESRI, 2011).

The Midwife's Labour and Birth Handbook, Third Edition. Edited by Vicky Chapman and Cathy Charles.
© 2013 John Wiley & Sons, Ltd. Published 2013 by John Wiley & Sons, Ltd.

- In the USA the rising caesarean section (CS) rate has reduced instrumental deliveries to <5% (Werner *et al.*, 2011).
- Forceps are used for around 50% of instrumental births in England and Wales in 2010, but in >75% of all instrumental births in Scotland (BirthChoiceUK).
- There are significant morbidity risks following instrumental delivery, but CS in second stage also carries high morbidity risk and has implications for subsequent births (RCOG, 2005; O'Mahony *et al.*, 2010).
- A Chinese study (Li *et al.*, 2011) suggests babies born by instrumental rather than spontaneous vaginal/CS delivery may be more likely to develop psychological problems, possibly due to high cortisol levels. More research is needed, but if this is so, it is particularly important to minimise the stress of an instrumental birth.
- The skill of the practitioner in both choosing the appropriate method for the particular circumstances, and in applying the instrument correctly, may well be the key factors in success.

Avoiding an instrumental delivery

The incidence of a forceps/ventouse delivery varies widely in different settings. Women who start labour at home or in a midwifery unit have 'a substantially lower incidence of assisted deliveries' compared with an obstetric unit (BECG, 2011). Good labour practice in all settings is likely to reduce the incidence of instrumental delivery and will include the following:

- Continuous support in labour especially by a non-staff carer (Hodnett *et al.*, 2011).
- Encouraging mobilisation/upright position (Gupta *et al.*, 2012; Lawrence *et al.*, 2009).
- Avoidance of epidural (Hodnett *et al.*, 2011), although if instrumental delivery is performed, this is the most effective analgesia.
- Avoidance of continuous cardiotocograph (CTG) monitoring for low-risk women (NICE, 2007).
- Avoidance of arbitrary second-stage time limits if progress is being made (Sleep *et al.*, 2000). There is some evidence that maternal and fetal morbidity increases after 3 hours in the second stage (Cheung *et al.*, 2004; Allen *et al.*, 2009), but there is known maternal morbidity with instrumental delivery (Sleep *et al.*, 2000; Dupuis *et al.*, 2004).
- Use of intravenous (IV) oxytocin in a slow second stage, particularly for primigravidae with poor contractions (NICE, 2007).
- Delaying pushing for women with epidurals for 1–2 hours reduces mid-cavity or rotational deliveries (Roberts *et al.*, 2004), and allowing up to 4 hours for second stage (NICE, 2007) and non-supine position increases the spontaneous delivery rate (Downe *et al.*, 2004). There is no evidence that discontinuing an epidural for the pushing stage speeds delivery and it increases pain (Torvaldsen *et al.*, 2004).

Indications for an instrumental delivery

- Failure to progress/maternal exhaustion in second stage. NICE (2007) suggests primigravidae should deliver within 3 hours of start of active phase, and nulliparas within 2 hours.

- Fetal heart rate concerns (and/or fetal blood sample pH <7.20).
- Elective shortening of the second stage for fetal/maternal benefit, e.g. epileptic mother – however, there are few absolute indications as obstetricians differ in their views.

In some parts of the world CS is not an option, and an instrumental birth, even if the criteria are not ideal, may be the only chance of delivery and/or to protect the life of the mother and baby. Also in some cultures avoiding CS has particular importance, as it may allow a woman to have a greater number of future babies.

Types of instrument

Forceps vary depending on whether traction alone or fetal head rotation is required. There are two basic designs:

- Straight forceps (e.g. Kjelland's) used for rotational births.
- Curved forceps (e.g. Neville Barnes or Wrigley's) which align with the curve of the pelvis so cannot be rotated. Also known as outlet or 'lift-out' forceps.

'Soft' forceps may have the fetal sides padded with pliable polyurethane pads with self-adhesive backing or a permanent soft rubber coating.

Ventouse cups may be metal, plastic or silicone. Both posterior and anterior cups exist. Traditionally ventouse cups attach to a suction pump, but more recently a single-use complete hand-held (e.g. 'Kiwi', see Figure 10.1) system is available which does not require a separate vacuum machine and is operated by only one person. This frees up other staff to concentrate on the woman, rather than a machine. Its small size may make it less intimidating to the woman.

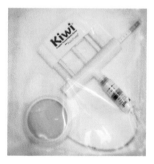

Fig. 10.1 Kiwi ventouse omnicup. *Photo by Debbie Gagliano-Withers.*

Both forceps and ventouse can be used for rotational manoeuvres: forceps can exert greater traction force (20 kg) than ventouse (10 kg) (WHO HRL). There is, however, a UK trend away from difficult rotational deliveries and towards CS, particularly if the head is well above the spines. A well-performed rotational delivery is an amazing thing to behold, but the risks are not to be dismissed, and there are fewer obstetricians with the confidence and skills to undertake them.

Choice of instrument

Neither method has a dramatically different effect on long-term neonatal outcomes, despite hot debate and sometimes prejudiced discussion. NICE (2007) concludes that the decision should be made according to the clinical situation and the experience of the practitioner. The skill of the practitioner may well be the key factor in instrumental delivery success.

- Ventouse is a relatively simple technique to learn, and is less dependant than forceps on accurate assessment of the fetal head position.
- Ventouse allows spontaneous head rotation: forceps rely on the user to manually rotate the blades as required.
- Ventouse may be used to help flex a deflexed head (Hofmeyr, 2004) but forceps can be used for face presentation or aftercoming head of a breech baby.
- Forceps are more likely to achieve vaginal delivery than ventouse, but preceed more CSs, third/fourth-degree tears with/without episiotomy, vaginal trauma, general anaesthesia, flatus incontinence or altered continence and neonatal facial injuries (O'Mahony *et al.*, 2010). Often there is sequential use (i.e. ventouse tried first, followed by forceps) which can complicate the analysis for each individual method.
- Cephalhaematoma and retinal haemorrhage is more likely in ventouse births (O'Mahony *et al.*, 2010). Werner *et al.* (2011) suggest that ventouse increases the risk of neurological complications (neonatal seizures, intraventricular hemorrhage, and subdural haemorrhage: these are the most likely determinants of long-term developmental problems), although Cochrane review does not support this (O'Mahony *et al.*, 2010).
- Ventouse may be difficult if there is marked caput, or the baby has lots of hair, as suction is hard to maintain.
- Ventouse may be inadvisable after repeated fetal blood sampling, as it risks further scalp trauma.
- Ventouse requires maternal effort. Forceps do not, so may be more suitable if the woman has a dense epidural.
- Forceps are more painful, so may be less preferable if the woman does not have an epidural.
- Soft cups are more likely to fail than metal cups but less likely to cause scalp injury (O'Mahony *et al.*, 2010).
- Hand-held ventouse cups (e.g. Kiwi) are possibly slightly more successful than silastic cups, but marginally less than metal cups (Attilakos *et al.*, 2005; O'Mahony *et al.*, 2010).
- Ventouse is particularly inadvisable for preterm birth due to the soft fetal skull.

Much research fails to specify exactly which type of forceps/ventouse was used, and this makes comparison of methods difficult, as there are clear differences between different instruments, e.g. soft versus metal ventouse cups, or rotational versus outlet forceps.

Care of a woman undergoing instrumental delivery

A calm, sensitive approach is crucial. Explanations need to be clear and informative, with plenty of support given to the woman and her birth partner(s), for whom such an experience may be a frightening ordeal.

Communication

Debating options at this stage of labour is not always easy. Some women may be feeling very much in control. Others may be exhausted, in extreme pain, and not receptive to discussion. If there are concerns about the condition of the baby, staff may feel under pressure to press on with an assisted delivery and limit debate. It is easy to talk glibly of 'informed choice'; many distressed women in labour will consent to almost anything that offers them a way out.

Birth partners can feel extremely stressed and tired; they may display anger or aggression, as they try to cope with their own and their partner's distress. It may be the partner, rather than the woman, who asks questions at this point. Conversely they may block discussion, saying 'Just get on with it; she's been through enough'.

The woman should be aware of the possibility of CS, should the instrumental attempt fail. Increasingly these days obstetricians incline towards a 'trial of ventouse/forceps' in theatre, for anything other than the most simple 'lift-out' birth. This reduces the time taken for CS if the instrumental delivery fails, but a theatre is a cold clinical environment in which to give birth.

Reducing fear

Instrumental deliveries can be frightening for women – and sometimes staff too.

> '*As fluorescent lights go on, the room fills with people, she hears the metallic clang of lithotomy poles, the sound of tearing paper as instrument packs are opened, the loud voices of people issuing instructions. She may feel disorientated, as the bed is pumped higher, she is tilted back, moved down the bed, legs uncomfortably suspended. As well as these sounds and sensations, she senses the anxiety levels of her attendants (– there is something very dramatic about to happen here, so no matter how much pain I'm in now, it is about to get a whole lot worse –)*'* (Charles, 2002).

Ideally one staff member should focus solely on the emotional needs of the woman and her birth partner(s). If another midwife is not available, this might be a maternity auxiliary/care assistant.

Resist the urge to put all the lights on: a sudden flood of fluorescent light is frightening, increases the atmosphere of drama and may make a woman feel naked and vulnerable. Perineal illumination and 'spot' areas of lighting, where necessary, are quite sufficient.

Analgesia

NICE (2007) recommends that instrumental birth should have tested effective analgesia. This is the woman's decision, guided by professional advice. Some women want to get the birth over with quickly, rather than wait for further analgesia. Sometimes a situation of clinical urgency reduces the options.

Theoretically, ventouse delivery pain is not significantly greater than from spontaneous birth, since the cup, unlike forceps, takes up no space alongside the head. Pain mainly results from initial cup insertion (unless epidural/spinal in situ), and subsequent checking of the instrument's position, followed by the usual delivery sensations.

However, fear may increase pain perception. Ensure that someone is there to prepare and support her through these moments.

- Epidural analgesia may be advisable for a forceps delivery. Ensure that it is adequately 'topped up' prior to delivery. Some doctors may instead administer a pudendal block.
- Entonox may be helpful +/– other methods of analgesia.
- Perineal infiltration of lignocaine may help; there may also be some placebo effect.
- Explain to a woman undergoing ventouse delivery that her urge to push is important, as this birth will be a joint effort. There is no evidence, however, that it is helpful to switching off an epidural infusion for the pushing phase or for instrumental delivery (see Chapter 1): it tends to increase distress rather than help the woman push.

Use of IV oxytocin

If contractions are weak, then oxytocin augmentation may be considered. NICE (2007) cautions against oxytocin for the second stage, but does not give any rationale. It will be an individual clinical decision and local guidelines may apply. Oxytocin for other stages of labour is normally started low and increased gradually; but if used for instrumental delivery a fairly high dose of oxytocin is usually started immediately. This prevents time being wasted in gradually increasing the dose, and since the delivery is now imminent, any adverse effects are likely to be transitory.

Positioning

- Following explanations and consent, the woman's legs should be gently and symmetrically lifted and supported in an adducted hip position. Lithotomy is not essential although some women may be comfortable in this position, particularly if staff experiment with pole height and adjust the position of the woman's buttocks relative to the poles.
- An instrumental delivery is perfectly possible with two helpers supporting the heels (Charles, 2002).
- For ventouse, other positions such as left lateral or squatting have been suggested (Johanson, 2001). Most professionals prefer to apply the cup with the woman in a semi-recumbent position. Once applied, there is no reason why she should not take up a lateral or squatting position. Squatting is known to increase the pelvic outlet diameter. Having said this, many professionals are more comfortable working with the method they are accustomed to and may resist alternative suggestions.
- Think aortocaval occlusion. Often this is forgotten during instrumental delivery. Create a small lateral tilt from a wedge or pillow if the woman is lying flat.

Bladder care

Most women produce little urine in the second stage and/or have difficulty micturating. Catheterisation was once routine prior to instrumental delivery. Vacca (1997) however states: 'A catheter need only be passed if the woman is unable to void or if the bladder is visibly or palpably distended'. In the absence of substantial research, professionals should use clinical judgement or adhere to local protocol. An indwelling catheter should be removed, or the balloon deflated, before delivery (RCOG, 2005).

Episiotomy

This should *not* be a routine intervention performed with every instrumental delivery (Vacca, 1997; AAFP, 2012) or done simply to prevent a tear. An episiotomy is usually only indicated for severe fetal distress (Sleep *et al.*, 2000; Hartmann *et al.*, 2005), although as forceps take up space alongside the head, there may be an increased indication during a forceps delivery for access to apply forceps. A mediolateral rather than midline episiotomy appears to reduce third/fourth-degree tears following forceps deliveries (Riskin-Mashiah *et al.*, 2002; Viswanathan *et al.*, 2005).

If indicated it should only be performed when the perineum has been stretched thin by the descending head. Use your clinical judgement, taking into account the flexibility of the perineum. Early episiotomy increases maternal morbidity, blood loss and haematoma formation, extension to the anal sphincter or rectum, and postpartum pain (Sleep *et al.*, 2000).

Consent for instrumental delivery should not imply that consent is given for episiotomy without further discussion.

Assisting at an instrumental delivery

Mutual staff support

Instrumental deliveries are stressful for everyone. Staff are often intimidated by the 'medicalised' atmosphere, but should try to avoid appearing rushed. Usually there is reasonable time to prepare. Even if the intervention is for fetal distress, remember that if this were a CS the 'decision to delivery time' would be longer.

The doctor/midwife delivering the baby may appear calm but will be under pressure. Rudeness and roughness towards the woman, however, should not be tolerated. Positive attitudes and efficiency in opening packs, preparing equipment and communicating information will help ensure a safe birth and give the mother confidence in her helpers.

Interestingly, when asked who delivered their baby, 11% of women delivered by a doctor using forceps and 40% by ventouse reported that both the doctor and midwife delivered the baby: surely an example of teamwork (Redshaw *et al.*, 2007).

Equipment preparation

To an extent, this will depend on local practice:

- Cleanse and possibly drape (not really necessary!) the vaginal area.
- Open sterile instrument packs and assist the delivering professional as requested.
- For ventouse, an assistant may need to attach the suction tubing to the machine and control the pressure. Leaks are usually due to poor tubing attachment or the release pedal having been left depressed following a previous delivery.

Instrumental procedure

Once packs are opened, the clinician normally performs a forceps delivery without further direct help.

For a ventouse delivery using a suction machine, the delivering professional gives instructions. Normally pressure starts at 0.2 kg/cm^2 and then increases to 0.8 kg/cm^2 in one step. There is no evidence that slowly increased pressure is of any benefit (Vacca, 1997).

The head should descend with each pull. The procedure should be abandoned if there is no evidence of progressive descent with each pull, if a ventouse cup detaches two/three times and/or if delivery is not imminent after three pulls by an experienced clinician (RCOG, 2005; AAFP, 2012). Experienced midwives and doctors often recognise when a head will not deliver after just one pull, and abandon the attempt immediately. Conversion to forceps delivery may be appropriate, e.g. for extensive caput or poor maternal effort. This is a critical moment for decision-making however, and failed forceps delivery may compound the problem. CS may eventually be indicated.

The incidence of shoulder dystocia and postpartum haemorrhage increases with instrumental delivery. Anticipate and be prepared.

Advocacy/accountability

Whilst the delivering professional is responsible for their own practice, midwives continue to have a duty of care towards their client and are still accountable for their practice. If a midwife feels that further analgesia is required, or that the delivering professional is having difficulties, they must speak out, acting as an advocate for the client. This is not always easy.

Post-procedure care

- A midwife should record any aspects of the birth, for example, start of procedure and fetal heart auscultation.
- Following birth, if all is well, events should follow just as if the woman had delivered unaided; skin-to-skin contact and early breastfeeding should be encouraged in the normal way. Parents should be aware that the baby's head may appear marked or moulded, but that this should disappear within hours.
- Diclofenac 100 mg rectally (PR) following delivery/suturing is the anti-inflammatory drug of choice (Dodd *et al.*, 2004). There is no evidence that prophylactic antibiotics reduce post-instrumental delivery infections (Liabsuetrakul *et al.*, 2004).

Midwife instrumental delivery

Some UK midwives now carry out instrumental deliveries, following formal training and assessment, under specified criteria. Academic supporting courses exist, e.g. at Bradford University http://www.bradford.ac.uk/postgraduate/midwifery/ (masters level) and Bournemouth University (Alexander *et al.*, 2002).

Currently midwife instrumental practitioners undergo a more rigorous training and assessment process than most obstetricians. A high rate of inappropriate placement of the vacuum cup by obstetricians has been cited as a reason for re-addressing obstetrician training needs (Sau *et al.*, 2004) and obstetric training packages exist, e.g. the Management of Emergency Obstetrics and Trauma (MOET) and also the American Academy of Family Physicians (AAFP); also some developed specifically for low-income countries. The World Health Organization Reproductive Health Library (WHO RHL) has a teaching video programme on vacuum extraction.

Many midwives may be uncomfortable with the idea of midwife ventouse/forceps practitioners, feeling that it is just a cost-saving measure and erodes the concept of a midwife's involvement in normal birth (Davies and Iredale, 2006; Scotsman, 2006). Others suggest that a woman may get better care from a midwife (Charles, 1999; Alexander *et al.*, 2002). The debate continues, but midwife ventouse practitioners have been successfully practising low-risk ventouse deliveries for over ten years in the UK with good maternal and neonatal outcomes (Awala *et al.*, 2006).

Do midwife practitioners bring anything special to instrumental birth?

- Midwives have a philosophy of promoting normal birth, which means they may not always rush to perform instrumental birth when asked, but make other practical suggestions to facilitate spontaneous birth.
- They may be more aware of the importance of a relaxed birth environment, e.g. calm atmosphere, low lighting and minimal noise.
- They may use their awareness of a woman's fear and loss of control to make the experience less stressful.
- They may be more likely to consider slow delivery of the head and selective (rather than routine) episiotomy, thus reducing perineal trauma.
- They may be more receptive than other clinicians to ideas such as ventouse in lateral or squatting positions.

Of course, none of the above will be true if the wrong kind of midwives become instrumental practitioners. Midwives are not mini-obstetricians. They should be recruited for training by midwives and selected for attitude as much as clinical skills. We do not need midwives who are by nature interventionist or drama queens (or kings).

Criteria for a midwife instrumental delivery

The criteria may vary according to local protocol.

- Fully dilated cervix
- Occipitoanterior (OA) position (but not necessarily direct OA), well flexed
- No asynclitism
- Head no longer palpable (i.e. fully engaged) abdominally
- Head below the level of the ischial spines
- Minimal caput/moulding
- Good contractions
- Verbal maternal consent obtained.

If fetal distress occurs in a stand-alone midwife-only unit and a ventouse/forceps midwife is called in, it is sensible to call an ambulance as well. If the circumstances are inappropriate for instrumental delivery, or the attempt fails immediate transfer is necessary.

Preparation

History

Review the antenatal and labour history, note parity; length of labour and fetal position during labour. Beware of a slow 7–10 cm cervical dilatation interval. Slow second-stage progress, particularly in multigravidae, may indicate disproportion and/or malpresentation.

Assessment

A midwife instrumental delivery should not normally be attempted unless the criteria given above are met. It is important to remain focused and analytical throughout, and not be swayed by the enthusiasm of other staff, or parents, to achieve delivery. It is particularly hard in stand-alone midwife-led units to decline an instrumental delivery, because this means transfer to another unit. However, transfer following failed instrumental delivery, sometimes with an episiotomy and a stressed mother and baby, is worse. See Box 10.1 for an ethical dilemma.

Perform an abdominal palpation and vaginal examination, with consent. Do not rely on the opinion of others, even if several staff reassure you: 'It's definitely OA … '. Check for yourself.

Monitor the contractions; if poor strength and/or frequency, then IV oxytocin may be advisable.

Box 10.1   Ethical dilemma for a ventouse midwife.

Imagine you are working in a stand-alone midwife unit. You are called for a sustained fetal bradycardia. The baby is OP, the head slightly deflexed, slightly asynclitic but below the spines. The head does not feel particularly large, and you think it would probably deliver with a ventouse cup. However, your criteria specify that the head must be OA, well flexed with no asynclitism.

The bradycardia is not recovering. An ambulance has been called but has not yet arrived and the obstetric unit is thirty minutes away. Do you decline to assist, because the case does not fit your midwife ventouse criteria, even though you believe ventouse delivery is possible and may save a baby's life? Or do you risk a failed ventouse, perhaps contributing to further fetal distress, and criticism for working outside your normal role?

This is a difficult situation. There are no answers, and each midwife must come to their own conclusion. It is to be hoped the midwife would be supported in choosing either option. Good supervisory and risk management review should take into account the skills and intentions of the midwife, in trying to weigh up all the pros and cons of attempted ventouse. Whatever you choose to do, accurate record-keeping is essential, showing you have understood the situation and thought through the possible options and outcomes. Anyone judging the case will want to see that the midwife was not simply being reckless but was acting in a considered and responsible way.

This author encountered exactly this dilemma and chose to perform an OP ventouse delivery. The outcome was good and she was supported in her decision. It is interesting to speculate whether she would have been so well supported if the outcome had been adverse.

Communication

Prior to physical examination, the midwife should introduce him/herself to the woman and partner. Attitude at this time is extremely important, and gaining a woman's confidence is crucial. In cases of presumed fetal distress, this discussion may have to be brief, but most people understand and under such circumstances will want actions rather than words.

It is important to acknowledge the woman's hard work so far. Explain the situation and confirm the woman's (and her partner's) understanding. Try to present options, if possible, e.g. 'If I confirm that the baby is in the right position for ventouse delivery, then we can either do it now, or see how your pushing goes over the next fifteen minutes . . . ', giving the woman the choice. Some women, however, may be too distressed to make such choices, or may perceive this as indecision. Midwifery judgement should be used, as with all women in labour, to decide the level of information given.

Remember that most post-birth emotional trauma appears to be associated with poor information giving and perceived loss of control (Green, 1990). Never underestimate a woman's capacity to make choices, however distraught she may appear.

Please read the preceding section entitled 'Care of a woman undergoing instrumental delivery' for general comments on instrumental delivery, including *analgesia, positioning* and *bladder care*. The following section describes aspects specific to midwife ventouse or forceps delivery.

Midwifery ventouse delivery

Midwife ventouse deliveries are normally performed using silc cups or single operator hand-held plastic cups. Check the suction by applying the cup to your hand. (See also 'Assisting at an instrumental delivery' above.)

- Cup insertion is often painful, but with increasing experience, it can be performed smoothly and gently. Entonox may help.
- Immediately following a contraction (warn the woman what is about to happen), insert the squeezed, externally lubricated cup by gently slipping two fingers of the other hand into the vagina, retracting the perineum and sliding the cup into the space created. Avoid pressing the clitoris or urethra.
- Manouvre the cup into the optimal position (see Figure 10.2). The centre of the cup should lie over the 'flexion point' which, in a well-flexed OA position, is typically 3 cm from the posterior fontanelle (Vacca, 1997).
- If the cup is correctly applied so that its centrepoint lies over the flexion point, with the sagittal suture running centrally down, then traction will result in the smallest

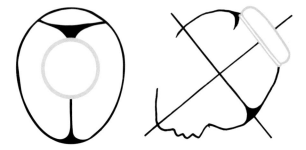

Fig. 10.2 Application of the ventouse cup. The cup is manoeuvred into the optimal position. In an occipitoanterior position the flexion point is typically around 3 cm from the posterior fontanelle with the sagittal suture running centrally down.

diameters of the fetal head (the suboccipitobregmatic and biparietal) being drawn through the birth canal (see also page 45, Chapter 2, for fetal skull diameters). This minimises traction, increasing the likelihood of a successful birth, reducing maternal/fetal trauma. In practice maternal tissue often inhibits cup positioning, so then the cup is simply placed as near as possible to the posterior fontanelle.

- The woman is often distressed following cup application, so reassure and congratulate her that the cup is now in place, and she has got through an unpleasant moment.
- Apply 0.2 kg/cm^2 pressure, and then check the position and ensure no maternal tissue is trapped in the cup. The process of feeling round the cup is another painful moment, especially anteriorly where space is tight, so warn the woman and proceed gently. If satisfactory, increase to 0.8 kg/cm^2 in one step.
- Await the next contraction. Encourage the woman to get her breath back and focus on the coming need to push. Sometimes it helps to smile, get eye contact, and encourage an atmosphere of controlled excitement: 'It really won't be long now ... '. This may recharge the atmosphere, giving the woman more energy. Beware though: a 'high adrenaline' environment may scare some women.
- Some practitioners like to place a forefinger on the cup edge and a second alongside on the baby's head, so any cup separation is detected quickly
- With the contraction, encourage the woman to push and apply steady traction perpendicular to the cup, initially downwards. As the head comes under the symphysis and extends, the cup will move, and the traction needs to follow the curve of the birth canal round and upwards.
- Very gentle steady traction *slightly* to one side, then another, may help dislodge a stuck head. This must be done with great caution. Avoid the temptation to repeatedly 'rock' the head: this may cause scalp trauma.
- As already discussed, it is not essential to perform an episiotomy for a ventouse delivery (Vacca, 1997; AAFP, 2012); use clinical judgement and obtain consent, as with any birth.
- Overexcited staff may be tempted to deliver the head quickly. Unless there is good reason to hurry, resist this urge. Remember how slowly a primigravid woman normally delivers; fast perineal stretching will cause increased pain and tissue trauma. Once the head is guided to the perineum, the woman's expulsive urge may do most of the rest of the work. Some midwives will hardly pull at all, as the perineum slowly distends.
- Do not remove the cup until the head has fully delivered: tempting though it is to discard the cup and return to a nice normal birth, if things suddenly slow down it is traumatic for both woman and baby to endure cup reapplication.

Gentle skilled ventouse births can be true collaborations between midwife and mother. There are reports of women who believe they had only minimal help and deny they have had an instrumental delivery (Charles, 1999).

Midwife forceps delivery

- Ensure that the woman has adequate analgesia: forceps are usually more painful than ventouse.
- Check the blades lock before using them (they may not be a matching pair).

- Lubricate the blades well.
- Immediately after a contraction (warn the woman first!) insert the left blade with the shank initially vertical, protecting the left vaginal wall with two fingers of the right hand.
- The blade should slide fairly easily in to lie parallel to the fetal head axis. If not, abandon the procedure.
- The second blade should be similarly inserted, and the blades locked. Depressing the handles slightly can help lock the blades.
- Check for correct application (see Figure 10.3):
  - The posterior fontanelle should be midway between the shanks and 1 cm above them.
  - The sagittal suture should be in the midline: try to palpate the lambdoidal sutures to confirm this (see Fig 8.1 page 131).
- With a contraction encourage the woman to push: perform traction by pulling on the blades with one hand and pressing down on the shanks.
- The traction axis will change as the head descends along the J-shape of the birth canal.
- Consider episiotomy, especially for primigravidae, as forceps take up space alongside the head.
- As the head crowns traction becomes vertical. Remove the blades before the head is completely out to decrease perineal tension. Think about slow delivery of the head (see Ventouse delivery above).

Advocacy/accountability

See also the earlier section 'Care of a woman undergoing instrumental delivery'. Remember: you are a midwife, not an obstetrician. Do not be drawn into making decisions outside your remit.

Post-birth discussion and care

Most ventouse/forceps midwives discuss the birth with the parents afterwards, congratulating the mother on her courage and endurance, and giving an opportunity for questions and explanations. Sometimes this is practicable only immediately following the birth. It is helpful to inform a woman that any subsequent birth is unlikely to require another assisted delivery. Some women and partners may find discussion supportive and reassuring. Others may be too shocked by events to be ready to 'revisit' them, or too preoccupied by their new baby to care. Be sensitive to this.

Postnatal exercises have been shown to improve urinary continence at 3 months postpartum in women who had instrumental deliveries and/or babies >4000 g (Ciarelli and Cockburn, 2002).

Records

Indications and assessment for instrumental delivery, details of procedure and outcome should be recorded. Instrumental midwives may wish to keep a logbook of

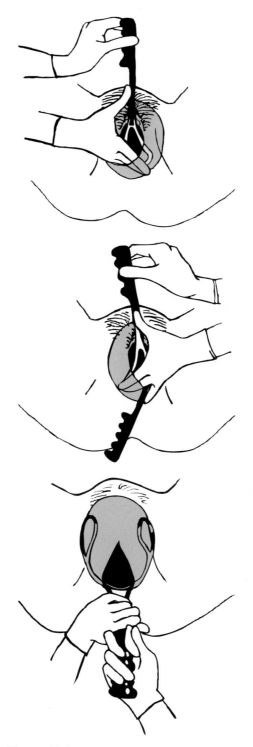

Fig. 10.3   Application of forceps blades.

deliveries (see Appendix 10.1) and periodically review their practice, e.g. numbers of failed deliveries.

It is helpful to log any instrumental deliveries that, after assessment, the midwife decides not to perform, and the subsequent outcome. These 'declined deliveries' may indicate a ventouse/forceps midwife's skill as much as the successful births achieved (see Appendix 10.2).

Logbooks may form part of an overall audit of ventouse/forceps midwife deliveries in some locations.

Summary

- Instrumental deliveries are stressful for women, partners and staff. Sensitivity is vital.
- Consent should always be sought before any intervention.
- Warn a woman of the possibility of CS if instrumental delivery fails.
- Midwives are accountable for their own practice, even when another professional has taken over the delivery. Although difficult, voice any concerns about suboptimal care.
- Midwife ventouse/forceps deliveries may be carried out under specified criteria.
  - Ensure adequate analgesia.
  - Avoid aortocaval occlusion.
  - Routine catheterisation/episiotomy is unsupported by evidence.
  - Prepare a woman for the pain of ventouse cup/forceps insertion.
  - Encourage slow head delivery to minimise perineal trauma.
  - Anticipate shoulder dystocia and PPH.
  - Midwife ventouse/forceps practitioners are not obstetricians.
- Give post-delivery analgesia (e.g. diclofenac 100 mg PR).
- A post-birth discussion may be helpful for a woman and her partner.
- Encourage postnatal exercises.

References

AAFP (American Academy of Family Physicians) (2012) *Advanced Life Support in Obstetrics (ALSO) Course Syllabus Manual*. Leawood, Kansas, AAFP.

Alexander, J., Anderson, T., Cunningham, S. (2002) An evaluation by focus group and survey of a course for midwifery ventouse practitioners. *Midwifery* 18, 165–72. Abstract: http://eprints.bournemouth.ac.uk/3948/

Allen, V. M., Baskett, C. M., O'Connell, C. M. *et al.* (2009) Maternal and perinatal outcomes with increasing duration of the second stage of labor. *Obstetrics and Gynecology* 113(6), 1248–58.

Attilakos, G., Sibanda, T., Winter, C., Johnson, N., Draycott, T. (2005) A randomised controlled trial of a new handheld vaccum extraction device. *International Journal of Obstetrics and Gynecology* 112(11), 1510–15.

Awala, A., Nethra, S., Walker, D., Charles, C. (2006) The midwife ventouse: a safe practice. *MIDIRS* 16(2), 181–3.

BECG (Birthplace in England Collaborative Group) (2011) Perinatal and maternal outcomes by planned place of birth for healthy women with low risk pregnancies: the

Birthplace in England national prospective cohort study. *British Medical Journal* 343. http://www.bmj.com/content/343/bmj.d7400. or www.npeu.ox.ac.uk/birthplace BirthChoiceUK *website www.birthchoiceuk.com*

Bragg, F., Cromwell, D., Edozien, L., Gurol-Urganci, I., Mahmood, T., Templeton, A., van der Meulen, J. (2010) Variation in rates of caesarean section among English NHS trusts after accounting for maternal and clinical risk: cross sectional study. *British Medical Journal* 341, 5065. http://www.bmj.com/content/341/bmj.c5065.full

Charles, C. (1999) How it feels to be a midwife ventouse practitioner. *British Journal of Midwifery* 7(6), 380–2.

Charles, C. (2002) Practising as a midwife ventouse practitioner in an isolated midwife-led unit setting. *MIDIRS Midwifery Digest* 12(1), 75–7.

Cheung, Y., Hopkins, I., Caughey, A. (2004) How long is too long: does a prolonged second stage of labour in nulliparous women affect maternal and neonatal morbidity? *American Journal of Obstetrics and Gynaecology* 191, 933–8.

Ciarelli, P., Cockburn, J. (2002) Promoting urinary continence in women after delivery: randomised controlled trial. *British Medical Journal* 324(378), 1241–7.

Davies, J., Iredale, R. (2006) An exploration of midwives' perceptions about their role. *MIDIRS Midwifery Digest* 16(4), 455–60.

Dodd, J., Hedayati, H., Pearce, E., Hotham, N., Crowther, C. A. (2004) Rectal analgesia for the relief of perineal pain after childbirth: a randomised controlled trial of diclofenac suppositories. *An International Journal of Obstetrics and Gynaecology* 111(10), 1059–64.

Downe, S., Gerrett, D., Renfrew, M. J. (2004) A prospective randomised trial on the effect of position in the passive second stage of labour on birth outcome in nulliparous women using epidural analgesia. *Midwifery* 20(2): 157–68.

Dupuis, O., Madelenat, P., Rudigoz, R. (2004) Faecal and urinary incontinence and delivery: risk factors and prevention. *Gynaecology, Obstetrics and Fertility* 32, 540–8.

ESRI (The Economic and Social Research Institute) (2011) *Perinatal Statistics Report 2009.* Health Research and Information Division, The Economic and Social Research Institute. http://www.esri.ie/news_events/latest_press_releases/perinatal_statistics_repo_3/index.xml

Green, J. M. (1990) Expectations, experiences and psychological outcomes of childbirth: a prospective study of 825 women. *Birth* 17(1), 15–23.

Gupta, J., Hofmeyr, G., Shehmar, M. (2012) Position in the second stage of labour for women without epidural anaesthesia. *Cochrane database of systematic reviews*, Issue 5.

Hofmeyr, G. J. (2004) Obstructed labor: using better technologies to reduce mortality. *International Journal of Gynecology and Obstetrics* 85 (1 Suppl. 1), S62–S72.

Lawrence, A., Lewis, L., Hofmeyr, G., Dowswell, T., Styles, C. (2009) Maternal positions and mobility during first stage labour. Cochrane Database of Systematic Reviews, Issue 2.

Li, H.-T., Ye, R., Achenbach, T., Ren, A., Pei, L., Zheng, X., Liu, J.-M. (2011) Caesarean delivery on maternal request and childhood psychopathology: a retrospective cohort study in China. *British Journal of Obstetrics and Gynaecology* 118, 42–8.

Hartmann, K., Viswanathan, M., Palmieri, R., Gartlehner, G., Thorp, J., Lohr, K. (2005) Outcomes of routine episiotomy: a systematic review. *JAMA* 293, 2141–8.

Hodnett, E. D., Hofmeyr, G. J., Sakala, C., Weston, J. (2011) Continuous support for women during childbirth (Cochrane Review). *Cochrane database of systematic reviews*, Issue 2. http://library.nhs.uk/evidence/

Johanson, R. (2001) The baby lifeline B.I.R.T.H. series. Interactive educational video series. Baby Lifeline Trading, Coventry. Reviewed by V. Tinsley. *MIDIRS* 11(2), 284–5.

Johnson, C., Keirse, M. J. N. C., Enkin, M., Chalmers, I. (2000) Hospital practices – nutrition and hydration in labor. In Enkin, M., Keirse, M. J. N. C., Neilson, J. (eds) *A Guide to Effective Care in Pregnancy and Childbirth*, 3rd edn, pp. 255–66. Oxford, Oxford University Press.

Liabsuetrakul, T., Choobun, T., Peeyananjarassri, K., Islam, M. (2004) Antibiotic prophylaxis for operative vaginal delivery. *Cochrane Database of Systematic Reviews*, Issue 3.

MOET (Management of Emergency Obstetrics and Trauma) (2007) *Course Manual* (revised 2009). London, RCOG Press. http://www.rcog.org.uk/catalog/book/moet_manual

NICE (National Institute for Health and Clinical Excellence) (2007) *Clinical Guideline 55: Intrapartum Care*. London, NICE.

O'Mahony, F., Hofmeyr, G. J., Menon, V. (2010) Choice of instruments for assisted vaginal delivery. *Cochrane Database of Systematic Reviews*, Issue 11.

Redshaw, M., Rowe, R., Hockley, C., Brocklehurst, P. (2007) *Recorded Delivery: The Findings from a National Survey of Women's Experience of Maternity Care*. NPEU. www.npeu.org.uk

Riskin-Mashiah, S., O'Brien, Smith, E., Wilkins, I. (2002) Risk factors for perineal tear: can we do better? *American Journal of Perinatology* 19, 225–34; reprinted in September 2007 *MIDIRS* 384.

Roberts, C. L., Torvaldsen, S., Cameron, C. A., Olive, E. (2004) Delayed versus early pushing in women with epidural analgesia: a systematic review and met-analysis. *British Journal of Obstetrics and Gynaecology* 111(12), 1333–40.

Royal College of Obstetricians and Gynaecologists (RCOG) (2005) *Operative Vaginal Delivery: Clinical Guideline 26*. www.rcog.org.uk

Sau, A., Sau, M., Ahmed, H., Brown, R. (2004) Vacuum extraction: is there any need to improve the current training in the UK? *Acta Obstetricia et Gynecologica Scandinavica* 83, 466–70.

Scotsman (2006) Midwives to perform risky forceps births. Online newspaper: 14 May http://www.scotsman.com/news/health/midwives-to-perform-risky-forceps-births-1-1411767).

Sleep, J., Roberts, J., Chalmers, I. (2000) The second stage of labor. In Enkin, M., Keirse, M. J. N. C., Neilson, J., *et al.* (eds) *A Guide to Effective Care in Pregnancy and Childbirth*, 3rd edn, pp. 289–99. Oxford, Oxford University Press.

Torvaldsen, S., Roberts, C. L., Bell, J. C., Raynes-Greenow, C. H. (2004) Discontinuation of epidural in labour for reducing the adverse delivery outcomes associated with epidural analgesia. *Cochrane Database of Systematic Reviews*, Issue 4.

Vacca, A. (1997) *Handbook of Vacuum Extraction in Obstetric Practice*. Albion, Queensland, Australia, Vacca Research.

Viswanathan, M., Hartmann, K., Palmieri, R., Lux, L., Swinson, T., Lohr, K., Gartlehner, G., Thorp, J. (2005) The use of episiotomy in obstetrical care: a systematic review. *Evidence Report/Technology Assessment* 112, 1–8.

WHO RHL (World Health Organization Reproductive Health Library) *Vacuum extraction*. http://apps.who.int/rhl/videos/en/index.html

Werner, E. F., Janevic, T. M., Illuzzi, J., Funai, E. F., Savitz, D. A., Lipkind, H. S. (2011) Mode of delivery in nulliparous women and neonatal intracranial injury. *Obstetrics and Gynecology* 118(6), 1239–46.

Appendix 10.1   Midwife ventouse practitioner log book record

Midwife ventouse practitioner log book record
Ventouse Practitioner name .... Unit ....
Case no ....   Date.................   Time of delivery ....
Client name.................................. Reg no .... Age.............
Address ....
Gestation .... Gravida/Para ....
Induction: Yes/No   Method...............
Augmentation: 1st stage .... 2nd stage ....
INDICATION FOR VENTOUSE ....
Abdo palpation .... Fifths palpable per abdo ....
Contractions ....
Vaginal examination: Dilatation.......... Station .... Caput .... Moulding ....

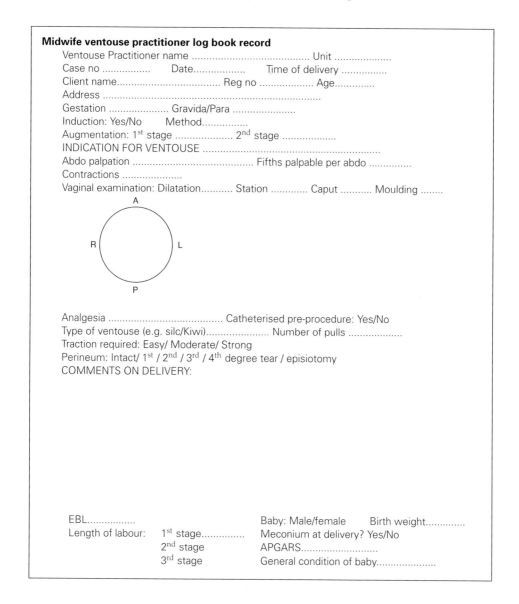

Analgesia .... Catheterised pre-procedure: Yes/No
Type of ventouse (e.g. silc/Kiwi)...................... Number of pulls ....
Traction required: Easy/ Moderate/ Strong
Perineum: Intact/ 1st / 2nd / 3rd / 4th degree tear / episiotomy
COMMENTS ON DELIVERY:

EBL.................   Baby: Male/female   Birth weight.............
Length of labour: 1st stage...............   Meconium at delivery? Yes/No
                      2nd stage   APGARS...........................
                      3rd stage   General condition of baby....................

Appendix 10.2   Decision to decline midwife ventouse delivery

It is recognised that midwife ventouse practitioner (MVP) skill may be determined not just by successful ventouse deliveries achieved, but also by declining to attempt ventouse extraction on unsuitable cases. MVPs should complete this form whenever asked to do a delivery which, following assessment, they decide not to perform.

An MVP may decide against a ventouse delivery for any reason. It is understood that decision making, particularly in an isolated community unit, is not always easy.

This form merely aims to monitor MVP decision making. It should in no way inhibit midwives from calling in an MVP for an opinion.

Please note: if an MVP *actually starts* a ventouse delivery, which is then abandoned, s/he should not complete this form, but fill in the existing MVP log book form, and complete a risk-management form, in the usual way.

Do not file this form in client's maternity notes. Please retain a copy for your ventouse practitioner log book.

MVP name:................................... **Maternity Unit:** ....
Date:...............................
Client name: .... **Hospital no:** .... **Age:** ....
Address: .... **Gravida/Para:** .... **Gestation:** ....

History/reason for ventouse request:...

Abdo palpation:... **Contractions:**..
Cervical dilatation:....................... **Station:**..................... **Moulding:**............... **Caput:**.................
Position:..

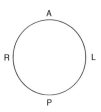

Reason for declining ventouse and action taken:

Outcome:

11 Caesarean section

Cathy Charles

Introduction

Some women readily choose caesarean section (CS); some are reluctantly persuaded to undergo CS, and some have CS thrust suddenly upon them with little chance to make any truly informed choice.

CS can save the life of a mother and/or baby. The problem is that it is often performed unnecessarily. This largely lies in the domain of obstetric decision making, outside the power of the midwife. However, the midwife still has some degree of influence, in supporting a woman's right to choose, and on occasions in challenging the rationale behind the decision.

Incidence and facts

- The overall CS rate in England rose from 9% in 1980 to 25% in 2010. In the wider UK it is now 26–30% (BirthChoice, UK).
- CS rates elsewhere in Europe vary widely: the lowest (<20%) are in Sweden, Norway, Finland, Lithuania, Slovenia, Flanders, Brussels and the Czech Republic. The highest (30%) are in Italy and Portugal (Euro-Peristat Group, 2008).
- Elective CS accounts for 9% of **all** UK births (Bragg *et al.*, 2010).

The Midwife's Labour and Birth Handbook, Third Edition. Edited by Vicky Chapman and Cathy Charles.
© 2013 John Wiley & Sons, Ltd. Published 2013 by John Wiley & Sons, Ltd.

- The last major CS survey found that 22% CSs were for fetal distress and 20% for failure to progress (Thomas and Paranjothy, 2001).
- 72% CSs are for previous CS or breech presentation (elective or emergency) (Bragg *et al.*, 2010).
- In one study 90% of breech presentations were delivered by CS; 57% of which were elective (Bragg *et al.*, 2010).
- This rising CS rate has not improved neonatal outcomes and increases maternal morbidity/mortality risk (NCCWCH, 2004).
- Regional anaesthesia is recommended for CS. Direct anaesthetic death accounts for 3% of all maternal deaths in the UK (CMACE, 2011); all deaths were under general anaesthetic (GA).

Risks and benefits of CS

Benefits

The subject of the benefits of CS can be contentious: there are multitudinous beliefs frequently cited by the public (Bewley and Cockburn, 2002), and unfortunately also by health professionals, which vary in their accuracy.

The overwhelming reason for CS is obviously to prevent mortality and morbidity in mothers and babies. NICE (2011) do not offer an opinion on an optimal CS rate, but the World Health Organization states that a CS rate of 10–15% reflects appropriate intervention, and a higher rate confers no health benefits (WHO, 1985).

- CS may be the only means of delivering a baby in truly obstructed labour. The alternative is fetal, and ultimately maternal, death.
- CS *may* play a minimal role in reducing cerebral palsy (brain injury due to oxygen deprivation) in babies. However, only around 10% cerebral palsy appears to be birth related, and CS appears to make no difference (NICE, 2004).
- CS may improve outcomes in breech presentation, although many challenge this (see Chapter 14). Research into vaginal breech outcomes is often measuring the adverse result of poorly managed supine breech extractions with interventionist manoeuvres.
- CS may reduce some, but not all, urinary incontinence and uterovaginal prolapse. It makes no difference to faecal incontinence (NICE, 2004).
- CS reduces the likelihood of 'obstetric shock' (NICE, 2011).
- Prevention of perineal injury (NICE, 2011) unless of course the woman has a CS following failed vaginal/instrumental birth with an episiotomy. Abdominal scar pain is of course unavoidable, although NICE rather bizarrely suggests that CS reduces intrapartum and 3 day postpartum abdominal pain compared with vaginal birth.
- Some women have a morbid fear of childbirth (tocophobia), which counselling may not dispel. CS may give them a sense of control and reduce fears.
- Elective CS offers some women a sanitised birth experience. Witness the 'celebrity cult' of elective CS; these women may be labelled in the popular press as 'too posh to push'.
- A small number of women with pelvic problems, e.g. congenital hip dislocation, may benefit from CS, although most can be helped to have a normal birth.

- Elective CS is convenient: the parents know and/or can plan in advance the date of their baby's birth. This may be relevant for parents wishing to avoid a baby being born on the anniversary of a previous stillbirth.
- A Chinese study (Li *et al.*, 2011) suggests babies born by elective CS develop fewer psychological problems than following instrumental delivery, possibly due to reduced cortisol levels, although more research is needed. Studies from other cultures should be treated with caution as they may reflect a different approach to delivery.
- CS can assist in the resuscitation of a woman with cardiac arrest (see Chapter 18).
- Perceived protection from litigation ('action bias'): clinicians may believe they will be judged to have done their best if a CS is performed, even if the outcome is no better, or even worse (see Chapter 22).

Risks

CS carries morbidity and mortality risks for mothers, and some neonatal risk, particularly in the second stage of labour. CS is more likely than vaginal birth to result in:

- Longer hospital stay (average 3–4 days CS, 1–2 days vaginal birth) (NICE 2011).
- Abdominal scar pain.
- Postpartum haemorrhage (PPH) leading to hysterectomy (NICE, 2011).
- Future pregnancy risk, e.g. placenta praevia, uterine rupture, antepartum stillbirth and repeat CS (NICE, 2004). *'Attempts to increase the VBAC rate make little sense without addressing the reason for the problem in the first place. Reducing the number of primary cesareans deals with the problem where it originates. Unless measures are instituted to reverse the rapidly rising cesarean rate, catastrophic complications from placenta accreta and percreta associated with multiple repeat cesareans soon may be a greater problem than uterine rupture'* (Scott, 2010).
- Reduced likelihood of having another baby (NICE, 2004).
- Thromboembolic disease, heart attack, cardiac arrest and ITU admission (NICE, 2011).
- Maternal death. *'Further research is needed to estimate more robustly what, if any, is the increased risk of maternal deaths associated with CS, particularly those undertaken without a clinical indication'* (CEMACH, 2004).
- Neonatal morbidity: increased adverse respiratory outcomes, particularly after elective CS, low blood sugar and poor temperature regulation (NICE, 2004; Kolas *et al.*, 2006). Babies of mothers undergoing elective CS are up to twice as likely to be admitted to neonatal intensive care unit than following vaginal delivery (Kolas *et al.*, 2006; NICE, 2011).
- Low mood: elective CS in particular may result in lower maternal hormone levels (oxytocin, endorphins, catecholamines and prolactin) which can affect postnatal mood, self-esteem and breastfeeding (Buckley, 2005) although NICE (2011) suggests breastfeeding rates are unaffected.
- Post-traumatic stress disorder: this can result from any birth (Kitzinger and Kitzinger, 2007), but there are many accounts of post-traumatic stress disorder following emergency CS (BTA website). This 'anecdotal' evidence may be dismissed by some clinicians. It may not be so much the CS itself, but the sense of

loss of control and poor support that causes psychological trauma. This is a complex area, as conversely some vaginal birth PTSD victims subsequently choose elective CS.

- CS (including postnatal stay) costs double that of instrumental delivery and 2–3 times more than spontaneous vaginal birth (Henderson *et al.*, 2001). For every 1% rise in CS the NHS spends an extra £5 million per year (NHSIII website).

Stemming the flow

There is a wide-ranging debate about the reasons for the current steep rise in the CS rate (Odent, 2004; NHSIII, 2007). Numerous birth initiatives aim to stem this epidemic including the RCM campaign for normal birth (RCM, 2007) and the National Service Framework (DoH, 2004). The NHS Institute has published *Pathways to success – a self-improvement toolkit* (NHSIII, 2007) aimed at enabling trusts to assess their performance and make practice changes to reduce CS rates and offer better care to those women who have CS.

CS may be reduced by the following:

- Home birth (NICE, 2011).
- Birthing centre: both instrumental birth and CS are reduced for women who start labour in a birthing centre (BECG, 2011).
- Supporting women who choose vaginal birth after caesarean (VBAC) (NICE, 2011): giving these women unbiased, factual information improves VBAC uptake (see Chapter 12). Inform them that women who attempt VBAC after ≤4 CSs have no increased risk of fever or bladder/surgical injuries, and the risk of uterine rupture, although higher for planned VBAC, is rare (NICE, 2011).
- Offering continuous support in labour (Hodnett *et al.*, 2011; NICE, 2011).
- Offering induction of labour after 41 weeks gestation (NICE, 2011) (see Chapter 19).
- Avoidance of continuous cardiotocograph (CTG) monitoring for low-risk women (NICE, 2007; NICE, 2011). Some even question its value in high-risk women, since Cochrane review can find no evidence that it improves outcomes (Alfirevic *et al.*, 2006).
- Performing fetal blood sampling (FBS) prior to CS for abnormal CTG, according to NICE (2011). However, Cochrane review found no evidence of higher CS rates when FBS was not available (Alfirevic *et al.*, 2006).
- Offering external cephalic version for breech presentation (NICE, 2011).
- Revisiting the so-called evidence which suggests CS is automatically the safer mode of delivery for breech (see breech chapter).
- Considering resting the uterus if labour is slow, to allow lactic acid levels to recover, rather than tiring it further with oxytocin (Wray, 2010).
- Involving consultants in the CS decision (NICE, 2011).
- Performing high quality instrumental deliveries by experienced clinicians.
- Addressing doctors' influence on women's decision-making. Studies show the obstetrician's experience, gender, workplace practices and whether working privately or NHS affects their advice on mode of delivery (Thomas and Paranjothy, 2001).

Indications for elective CS

NICE (2011) lists the following:

- **A term singleton breech (if external cephalic version is contraindicated or has failed)** – however, see Chapter 14 for further discussion. It is surprising that NICE still persists in promoting CS for breech despite questionable research.
- **A twin pregnancy with first twin breech** although NICE can offer no research to support this, but instead say it is 'common practice' (see Chapters 14 and 15).
- **Primary genital herpes in third trimester** as this decreases neonatal infection.
- **Placenta praevia**, i.e. a placenta that partly ('minor') or completely (major') covers the internal cervical os.
- **Morbidly adherent placenta** proven by doppler ultrasound and possibly MRI scan.

NICE (2011) states that CS should not be routinely offered to women with the following:

- **Twin pregnancy when the first twin is cephalic at term.**
- **Preterm birth.** There is no evidence that CS improves the already high morbidity for this group.
- **Small for gestational age babies** for the above reason.
- **High body mass index (BMI).**
- **HIV positive women** on highly active anti-retroviral therapy with a viral load of <400 copies per ml or women on any anti-retroviral therapy with a viral load of <50 copies per ml. In these circumstances the risk of HIV transmission is the same for CS and vaginal birth (NICE, 2011).
- **Hepatitis B or hepatitis C.**
- **Genital herpes recurrence.** As long as this is not a primary outbreak, there is no evidence of high risk of transmission.

Maternal request

The issue of elective CS for maternal request creates hot debate, with one lobby stating that a woman has the right to choose the birth of her choice while others feel that no one should have the right to choose unnecessary major abdominal surgery which absorbs scarce resources (Dimond, 1999; Dodwell, 2002).

In 2004 NICE stated that maternal request alone was not an indication for CS and that further clarification should be sought and counselling offered. In 2011 NICE changed its advice, suggesting that a woman requesting CS due to anxiety about childbirth, should be offered referral to a healthcare professional with expertise in providing perinatal mental health support, but if the woman continued to request CS after discussion then a planned CS should be offered. This is a controversial view, and has generated much press discussion, and at times misprepresentation, with the popular press reporting that all women are now entitled to a CS on demand.

The experience of CS

CS may come as a blessed relief to a woman after an arduous pregnancy and/or labour. Conversely, she may feel deeply disappointed that she has been unable to give birth naturally. If the CS is an emergency she may be frightened and apprehensive as her birth plans fall apart and events move out of her control. Choice can disappear as the quiet birthing room is invaded suddenly by noise, light and unknown people. She and her partner may even believe that she or their baby might die. Good care and support are critical in helping the woman achieve a positive experience whatever the circumstances and greet her baby with joy.

The principles of care are broadly the same whether a woman is undergoing elective or emergency CS, although the urgency of emergency CS will increase stress levels for everyone. Even if an elective CS, the woman's decision may not have been easy, and she may have the same fears as anyone else undergoing CS.

Elective CS birth plan

It is interesting to speculate why so few women undergoing elective CS write a birth plan. Perhaps they do not feel they have any control over this highly medicalised procedure. Although it is not common practice, it is perfectly possible for a woman to write down her preferences (Lowdon and Chippington Derrick, 2007). The process of enquiring/imagining what may happen may help her and her partner prepare for the event. A written birth plan may also be harder for staff to disregard. Responding to individual preferences may take some staff out of their comfort zone and remind them that there is a person at the centre of the proceedings, not a series of formulaic actions to be performed.

> 'Women's preferences for the birth, such as music playing in theatre, lowering the screen to see the baby born, or silence so that the mother's voice is the first the baby hears, should be accommodated where possible' (NICE, 2004).

The only slight concern for some midwives is that the pseudo-normalisation of the procedure by use of birth plans, low lights and music may give the impression that CS is a normal way for a baby to be born. Walsh (2010) describes the prettification of hospital labour rooms (not theatres as such, but the description applies) as 'faking domesticity and homeliness when beneath the surface technology and professional hegemony are lurking with intent'.

Midwifery care for CS

Consent: (see www.dh.gov.uk/en/DH_103643) Whilst some might question the quality and objectivity of CS information given to many women, in practical terms consent for elective CS is comparatively straightforward. An emergency situation, however, may be quite different. A 'competent' woman has the right to refuse CS even if she or her baby's health would clearly benefit, and the woman should be made aware of this (DoH, 2001; NICE, 2011). The midwife may have to support a woman's right to refuse in the face of strong opposition, occasionally even that of her partner.

Written consent is advisable, but in an emergency not essential, as long as the mother has verbally consented, or is not well enough to consent. Consent is *not* 'informed' when a distressed, frightened woman is forced to sign a piece of paper she can barely focus on, while a doctor gabbles out the risks of a CS which the woman may believe is now essential to save her baby's life. Such 'consent' will have little validity in a court of law under questioning by any competent lawyer.

Question the obstetrician politely and calmly if you feel there is not a good indication for CS. If there is an abnormal fetal heart rate pattern in the first stage, FBS is recommended first, if technically possible and not contraindicated (NICE, 2004), although disappointingly FBS does not appear to affect CS rates (Alfirevic *et al.*, 2006) or neonatal outcomes (NICE, 2007). Junior/middle grade doctors should not be making the final decision. A consultant obstetrician should be involved in any decision to offer a CS which will, in theory, depend on evidence of clinical benefit to mother and baby (NICE, 2011). In practice this 'consultation' may consist of a quick phone call to a consultant with a scenario explained in such a way that s/he can hardly disagree. Be sensitive to the difficult position the obstetricians may be in. Pressure from parents (and sometimes midwives) to perform a CS, along with fears of an adverse outcome, criticism and litigation, can make their job very hard.

Give emotional support. If CS is elective, or occurs for slow labour progress, women usually have time to prepare emotionally. The woman may feel relieved that things are finally drawing to an end and/or distressed that she has been unable to have a vaginal birth. All women need support, but an emergency CS for 'fetal compromise' can be particularly frightening. Hold the woman's hand, give her eye contact and show her warmth: let her know that her baby will be here soon, that she is doing her very best in difficult circumstances, and that the birth will be a triumph no matter what. Birth partners can be tired and emotional too – don't forget to support them. Partners may appear angry. Sometimes they say 'I knew this was going to happen'; following vaginal birth they may forget these transient negative thoughts, but when emergency CS occurs, they feel the bad experience was almost foreseeable.

Accept your own feelings. Midwives may feel disappointment in realising their care has not been enough to achieve a vaginal birth. You are no longer the lead caregiver and may feel disempowered and frustrated, perhaps especially so if you do not agree with the decision for CS. Do not let this affect your behaviour towards the woman. It is not her fault, and she needs your support now more than ever.

Physical preparation

- **Haemoglobin result.** It is sensible to have this prior to any birth, but particularly CS, as 4–8% women lose >1000 ml at CS (NICE, 2011). It is not necessary to routinely perform group and save, crossmatch or clotting screen prior to CS according to (NICE, 2011) although many believe it is wise practice to check platelets at least.
- **Site intravenous cannula.** A preload of crystalloid/colloid is recommended if CS under regional anaesthesia (NICE, 2011).
- **Clarify the level of urgency:** NICE (2011) define four levels of urgency:
    (1) Immediate threat to the life of the woman or fetus.
    (2) Maternal or fetal compromise which is not immediately life-threatening.
    (3) No maternal or fetal compromise but needs early delivery.
    (4) Delivery timed to suit woman or staff.
    A safe decision-to-delivery interval for emergency (NICE say 'unplanned') CS for presumed fetal distress is not definable, as it will, of course, vary with individual circumstances, but NICE suggest as an audit standard:

- ○ 30 min for category 1: 'immediate perceived threat to life of mother/baby'.
- ○ 75 mins for category 2: 'maternal or fetal compromise which is not immediately life-threatening'.

This is ONLY to be used for measuring a unit's general performance through audit, and 'not to judge multidisciplinary team performance for any individual CS' (NICE, 2011). NICE suggest, perfectly logically, that a category 1 CS should be performed as quickly as possible once the decision has been made, whilst acknowledging that rapid delivery has risks too.

- **Give antacids** or similar drugs pre-CS to reduce gastric volume and acidity and **antiemetics** reduce risk of vomiting during CS (NICE, 2011).
- A **catheter** is normally sited for a regional block due to potential bladder dysfunction and over-distension (NICE, 2011), and possibly to ensure a full bladder does not obstruct surgery/risk bladder damage, although the routine use of catheters for CS has been questioned (Ghoreishi, 2003). 4% of women develop a urinary tract infection following CS with an indwelling Foley catheter despite antibiotic prophylaxis (Horowitz *et al.*, 2004). If there is time, ask the woman if she would prefer to have the catheter sited in theatre or in her room first.
- **Shave.** A lower segment CS will often be at/below the pubic hair line, so a shave is normally performed. Again this can be done in theatre or the woman's room. An electric shaver with disposable head is probably the most comfortable option. Disposable single-use razors are uncomfortable if used dry; soap and water or shaving foam is considerate.

  'Advise the woman to shave 3 cm of pubic hair herself. She then feels in control and prepared' (Victoria, elective CS mother).
- RCOG (2009) suggests steroids should be given to reduce the risk of respiratory morbidity in all babies born by elective caesarian section (ELLSCS) prior to 38 weeks.

In theatre

Table tilt: the operating table should be tilted at 15 degrees (NICE, 2011).

Anaesthesia: The Royal College of Anaesthetists and NICE (2011) recommend that CS should usually be performed under regional anaesthesia (e.g. spinal/epidural). CMACE (2011) reports a maternal death under anaesthesia: see Box 11.1.
Paradoxically the rare event of a CS under GA may make staff less proficient in dealing with failed intubation (CMACE, 2011).

If the mother is having a GA, her birth partner may not be allowed in the theatre. It is not clear why this is often the case, and this archaic practice is being challenged in more progressive hospitals where staff recognise that it should be up to the couple to decide what is best for them and their baby. Whether the partner is present or absent for the birth, he or she may wish to cuddle the baby at the earliest opportunity and perhaps offer skin-to-skin contact (SSC) until the mother is awake.

Environment. Do not be intimidated by the number of other staff in theatre and avoid picking up on anyone else's negativity. Sometimes when the team is stressed individuals may appear irritable, withdrawn or cold. Do not let this become infectious. Keep a relaxed and warm manner towards the woman, even if yours is the only

Box 11.1   Maternal death under GA: CMACE (2011) Case study.

A woman had a working epidural in labour when it was decided to perform a Category 2 CS. Subsequently there was a sustained fetal bradycardia, which escalated the urgency to Category 1. The woman died after failed tracheal intubation. The epidural had not been topped up for surgical anaesthesia because the anaesthetist planned to top the epidural up in theatre. If the epidural had been topped up when it was decided she was to have a CS, general anaesthesia may not have been required.

Epidural anaesthesia for operative delivery: learning points

'Epidural analgesia that has been working well in labour should be topped up to provide full surgical anaesthesia without delay once the decision for operational delivery has been made. If the woman cannot be immediately transferred to an operating theatre and full epidural anaesthesia is established on the labour ward, the anaesthetist and full resuscitation equipment should be immediately available and full "epidural monitoring" provided.' (CMACE, 2011)

smiling face in the room. She may like to have music playing, a running commentary, or silence so her voice is the first her baby hears. She may want the lights dimmed briefly for the moment of birth and/or photographs taken. These things are easier to plan and implement for an elective CS, but even in an emergency many choices can still be fulfilled. Blithely ignore any staff who cast their eyes to heaven at your strange requests: the mother is the centre of events and the staff are there for her, not the other way around.

Temperature. Make sure the theatre is warm. CS babies are more prone to hypothermia (NICE, 2004). Staff often notice theatres are cold: they are large rooms with a constant airflow (Ellis, 2005). Put on the resuscitaire as soon as possible (its heater will also help warm the room), although hopefully it will not be needed, as SSC is advised, and a well baby will not need to be separated from its parents.

A screen may protect the mother and partner from seeing too much, but some parents wish to watch their baby being born. Always ask: never assume.

Scrubbing to assist. Some hospitals require midwives to scrub to assist the obstetrician, but others have theatre staff to do this. Midwives may have views on this, feeling they are there to be 'with women', not 'with obstetrician'; if scrubbing is necessary, try to ensure that there is someone free to be with the woman. Anaesthetists are, however, usually very good at connecting with women and their partners. It is not so much the *quantity* of staff, but the *quality* of care that is important.

Use of forceps: NICE (2011) recommends forceps only used if the head is difficult to deliver, also that the effect on neonatal morbidity from the *routine* use of forceps at CS is unclear.

Uterotonics: NICE (2011) recommend oxytocin 5 IU by slow intravenous injection following CS birth to reduce PPH.

Prophylactic antibiotics are recommended before skin incision, as 8% of CS women develop endometritis, urinary tract and wound infection: this reduces maternal infection better than post-incision with no apparent neonatal effects (NICE, 2011).

Delayed cord clamping (DCC): unless there are serious neonatal concerns DCC of at least three minutes is perfectly possible and likely to be beneficial to the baby: the baby could lie on the woman's chest (preferably) or legs – see page 28 for DCC benefits.

Alternatively the cord could be milked towards the baby (see page 28). It may fall to the midwife to try to change the mindset of resistent staff who think this is an extreme idea.

Cord blood analysis. An arterial sample is required following emergency CS (see Chapter 23) (NICE, 2011).

Resuscitation. If fetal compromise is suspected, or following general anaesthesia, a practitioner trained in advanced newborn resuscitation should be present (NICE, 2011) (see Chapter 18).

Scrubbing up to take the baby: a midwife normally scrubs up to receive the baby from the obstetrician. Time pressure may mean that the midwife feels that the baby must be immediately 'processed' (weighed, given vitamin K, wrapped and labelled) prior to being given to – often – the partner. Ideally, however, the midwife should try to facilitate **skin-to-skin contact (SSC)** (see pages 25 and 212 for benefits). The baby can be placed almost immediately onto the mother's chest. It can be technically tricky, as the baby often needs to be placed high up to avoid encroaching on the 'sterile field' of the abdomen. Enlightened anaesthetists are increasingly helpful in assisting with SSC. If the mother is unwell or declines it, consider the partner; babies given SSC with their fathers following CS cry less and appear calmer (Erlandsson *et al.*, 2007). There should, in an ideal world, be no rush to weigh and measure the baby: this special time is important. Erlandsson concludes:

> *'The father can facilitate the development of the infant's prefeeding behaviour in this important period of the newborn infant's life and should be regarded as the primary caregiver ... during the separation of mother and baby.'*

Postnatal care

Recovery room. Women should be observed on a one-to-one basis by trained recovery staff until they are stable, have regained airway control and can communicate (NICE, 2011).

Breastfeeding can be started in the recovery room. CS mothers are less likely to start breastfeeding in early hours after birth, for obvious reasons. Delayed mother–baby contact can result in lower postnatal mood for up to 8 months (Rowe-Murray and Fisher, 2001). Make sure the mother is not drowsy: theatre recovery staff are usually helpful at ensuring the safety and comfort of mothers and babies, with cot sides and pillows.

Observations. Regular observations identify problems early. Check half-hourly for the first 2 hours then 'hourly thereafter' (NICE, 2011): usually around 2 hours if all is well. Local guidelines may apply. Report problems to an obstetrician.

- **Pulse, BP, respiratory rate.**
- **Pain and sedation.** Ensure the woman is comfortable. Opioid analgesia can over-sedate some women.
- **Observe lochia and wound site.**
- **Check urine output.** Ensure the catheter is free draining and the tubing not kinked.

Analgesia. Women may vary greatly in their needs. Opioid drugs and non-steroidal anti-inflammatories (NSAIDs) (check for contraindications) give good pain relief following CS (NICE, 2011), with paracetamol for milder pain. NSAIDs reduce the need for opioids, so should be used as an adjunct to any analgesia unless contraindicated (NICE, 2011).

Check analgesia has been prescribed and given. Advise the woman to ask for further analgesia early, as pain is easier to control before it has built up; regular analgesia is usually sensible for the first few days as pain can be debilitating for a new mother with a baby to care for.

Check any patient-controlled analgesia (PCA) functions correctly: CMACE (2011) reports a postnatal ward death from PCA overdose.

Beware of drugs written on *anaesthetic charts* but not transferred to prescription sheets: this may result in drug errors.

Thromboprophylaxis. Thromboembolism is a leading cause of direct maternal death. Ensure thromboembolic stockings and/or low-molecular-weight heparin LMWH) have been prescribed for post-CS women, particularly if emergency CS and/or other risk factors exist. LMWH should be given 4 hours after spinal/epidural is established or after epidural catheter removal (RCOG, 2009; NICE, 2011; CMACE, 2011).

Eating and drinking can be resumed when the woman wishes if she is recovering well with no complications (NICE, 2011).

General support. Women need lots of assistance, particularly in the first few hours. Make sure that she is comfortable with plenty of supportive pillows and a drink and the call bell is accessible. Reassure her that she can ring at any time for help. Tuck the baby in with her if she wishes, and is awake enough and not sedated: ensure the baby is safe. Try to anticipate her needs as well as respond to them.

Postnatal discussion. Following emergency CS women should be offered the opportunity to discuss the reasons for it and the implications for future pregnancies with a knowledgeable professional, backed up by printed information (Murphy *et al.*, 2005: NICE, 2011) (see Chapter 12). She may wish to tell her story endlessly at first, particularly if the CS was an emergency; give her space to do this. Referral to a support group may help.

Tell a woman that she has been very brave to undergo major abdominal surgery for the sake of her baby.

Summary

- The steep rise in CS has not improved maternal or neonatal health.
- Good midwifery care and avoiding unnecessary interventions reduce CS.
- Women requesting elective CS should have a full discussion of risks and benefits.
- Consider a birth plan for elective CS.
- Politely challenge a CS which you believe is unnecessary.
- Give maximum emotional support to the woman and birth partner.
- Ignore negativity: from other staff make the woman the centre of attention.
- Physical care:
  - Site IV cannula; obtain Hb result
  - Give antacids
  - Insert catheter (usually) and shave
  - Ensure warm theatre
  - Check if she wants a screen in situ
  - Prophylactic antibiotics are recommended

○ Take arterial cord bloods if emergency CS
○ Call an advanced newborn clinician if fetal compromise suspected
- Try to enable SSC with mother: if not, suggest father.

Postnatally:

- Breastfeed in recovery room ASAP.
- Observe vital signs, lochia, wound and urine output.
- Ensure that analgesia and thromboprophylaxis prescribed, given and *recorded on drug chart* (not just anaesthetic sheet).
- She can eat and drink when she wishes.
- Give lots of support and help her get comfortable.
- Postnatal review for emergency CS is helpful.

Support groups for women following CS

Birth Trauma Association (BTA) www.birthtraumaassociation.org.uk
Caesarean birth and VBAC information www.caesarean.org.uk
National Childbirth Trust www.nct.org.uk

Further reading

Gallagher-Mundy, C. (2004) *Caesarean Recovery*. London, Carroll and Brown.
National Childbirth Trust (1999) *Caesarean Sections*. London, NCT.
NHS Institute for Innovation and Improvement website *Pathways to Success: A Self-Improvement Toolkit Guidelines to Reduce CS*. www.institute.nhs.uk
RCOG (2007) *Green-top Guideline No. 45: Birth after Previous Caesarean Birth*. www.rcog.org.uk

References

Alfirevic, Z., Devane, D., Gyte, G. (2006) Continuous cardiotocography (CTG) as a form of electronic fetal monitoring (EFM) for fetal assessment in labour. *Cochrane Database of Systemic Reviews*, Issue 3.
Bewley, S., Cockburn, J. (2002) The unfacts of 'request' caesarean section. *BJOG: an International Journal of Obstetrics and Gynaecology* 109(6), 597–605.
BirthChoice UK. *www.birthchoiceuk.com*
(Birthplace in England Collaborative Group (BECG) (2011) Perinatal and maternal outcomes by planned place of birth for healthy women with low risk pregnancies: the Birthplace in England national prospective cohort study. *British Medical Journal* 343:d7400.
Bragg, F., Cromwell, D., Edozien, L., Gurol-Urganci, I., Mahmood, T., Templeton, A., van der Meulen, J. (2010) Variation in rates of caesarean section among English NHS trusts after accounting for maternal and clinical risk: cross sectional study *British Medical Journal* 341: 5065. http://www.bmj.com/content/341/bmj.c5065.full
Buckley, S. (2005) *Gentle Birth, Gentle Mothering*. Brisbane, Queensland, One World Press.
CMACE (Centre for Maternal and Child Enquiries) (2011) *Saving mothers' lives: reviewing maternal deaths to make motherhood safer: 2006–2008*. The Eighth Report of the Confidential

Enquiries into Maternal Deaths in the United Kingdom *BJOG 118*, (suppl.1), 1–203. http://onlinelibrary.wiley.com/doi/10.1111/j.1471-0528.2010.02847.x/pdf

CEMACH (Confidential Enquiry into Maternal and Child Health) (2004) *Why Mothers Die 2000–2002. The Sixth Report of Confidential Enquiries into Maternal Deaths in the United Kingdom*. London, RCOG Press. http://cemach.interface-test.com/Publications/CEMACH-Publications/Maternal-and-Perinatal-Health.aspx

Dimond, B. (1999) Is there a legal right to choose a caesarean? *British Journal of Midwifery* 7(8), 515–8.

Dodwell, M. (2002) Should women have the right to a clinically unnecessary CS? *MIDIRS Midwifery Digest* 12(2), 274–7.

DoH (Department of Health) (2001) *Good Practice in Consent Implementation Guide: Consent to Examination or Treatment*. London, DoH.

DoH (2004) *National Service Framework for Children, Young People and Maternity Services: Executive Summary 40496*. www.dh.go.uk

Ellis, J. (2005) Neonatal hypothermia. *Journal of Neonatal Nursing* 11, 76–82.

Erlandsson, K., Dsilna, A., Fagerberg, I., Christensson, K. (2007) Skin-to-skin care with the father after caesarean birth and its effect on newborn crying and prefeeding behaviour. *Birth* 34(2), 105–13.

Euro-Peristat Group (2008) *European Perinatal Health Report. Better statistics for better health for pregnant women and their babies*. Paris, EURO-PERISTAT Group. www.europeristat.com/publications/european-perinatal-health-report.shtml

Ghoreishi, J. (2003) Indwelling urinary catheters in caesarean delivery. *International Journal of Gynaecology and Obstetrics* 83(3), 267–70.

Henderson, J., McCandlish, R., Kumiega, L., Petrou, S. (2001) Systematic review of economic aspects of alternative modes of delivery. *British Journal of Obstetrics and Gynaecology* 108, 149–57.

Hodnett, E. D., Gates, S., Hofmeyr, G. J. and Sakala, C., Weston, J. (2011) Continuous support for women during childbirth. *The Cochrane Database of Systematic Reviews*, Issue 2.

Horowitz, E., Yogev, Y. and Ben-Haroush, A. (2004) Urine culture after catheterisation. *International Journal of Gynaecology and Obstetrics* 85, 276–8.

Kitzinger, C., Kitzinger, S. (2007) Birth trauma: talking to women and the value of conversation analysis. *British Journal of Midwifery* 15(5), 256–64.

Kolas, O., Saugstad, A., Dalveit, A., Nilsen, S., Oian, P. (2006) Planned caesarean vs planned vaginal delivery at term: comparison of newborn infant outcomes. *American Journal of Obstetrics and Gynaecology* 195(6), 1538–43.

Li, H.-T., Ye, R., Achenbach, T., Ren, A., Pei, L., Zheng, X., Liu, J.-M. (2011) Caesarean delivery on maternal request and childhood psychopathology: a retrospective cohort study in China. *British Journal of Obstetrics and Gynaecology* 118: 42–8.

Lowdon, D., Chippington Derrick, D. (2007) *CS and VBAC Information*. www.caesarean.org.uk

Murphy, D., Pope, C., Frost, J., Liebling, R. (2005) Women's views on the impact of operative delivery in the second stage of labour: qualitative interview study. *British Medical Journal* 327(7427), 1132–5.

NCCWCH (National Collaborating Centre for Women's and Children's Health) (2004) *Caesarean Section: Clinical Guideline*. London, RCOG Press.

NICE (National Institute for Health and Clinical Excellence) (2001) *Clinical Guideline D – Induction of Labour*. London, NICE. www.nice.org.uk

NICE (2004) *Clinical Guideline 13: Caesarean Section*. London, NICE. www.nice.org.uk

NICE (2007) *Clinical Guideline 55: Intrapartum Care.* London, NICE. www.nice.org.uk

NICE (2011) *Clinical Guideline 132: Caesarean Section.* London, NICE. www.nice.org.uk

NHS (2007) *NHS Maternity Statistics, England.* London, Information Centre for Health and Social Care. www.ic.nhs.uk/webfiles/publications/maternity0506/NHSMaternity StatsEngland200506.pdf

NHSIII (NHS Institute for Innovation and Improvement) (2007) *Delivering Quality and Value. Pathways to Success Toolkit.* London, NHSIII. www.institute.nhs.uk

Odent, M. (2004) *The Caesarean.* London, Free Association Books.

RCM (Royal College of Midwives) (2007) *Campaign for Normal Birth.* www.rcmnormalbirth .org.uk

RCOG (2009) Thromboprophylaxis during pregnancy, labour and after vaginal delivery. *RCOG Green Top Guidelines.* www.rcog.org.uk

Rowe-Murray, H. J., Fisher, J. R. W. (2001) Operative intervention in delivery is associated with compromised early mother-infant interaction. *BJOG International Journal of Obstetrics and Gynaecology* 108(10), 1068–75.

Scott, J. R. (2010) Solving the vaginal birth after cesarean dilemma. *Obstetrics and Gynecology* 115(6), 1112–3.

Thomas, J., Paranjothy, S. (2001) *National Sentinel Caesarean Section Audit Report.* London, RCOG Press.

Walsh, D. (2010) Birth environment. In Downe, S., Walsh, D. (eds) *Intrapartum Care*, p. 45. Oxford, Wiley Blackwell.

Wray, S. (2010) *Scientists say 25% of caesareans could be avoided.* http://www.liv.ac.uk/2004 website/newsroom/press_releases/2004/05/uteri.htm

WHO (1985) Appropriate technology for birth. *Lancet* 2, 436–7.

12 Vaginal birth after caesarean section

Vicky Chapman

'There is something in the act of giving birth, especially if the environment is supportive, that you can't experience if you have a cesarean. We're starting to understand it with the help of science (how hormones are at play during a birth and how they work), and research is beginning to show the possible impact of giving birth on personal growth' (Vadeboncoeur, 2011).

Introduction

Women who have had a previous caesarean section (CS) often want to try for a vaginal birth in subsequent pregnancies, commonly referred to as *vaginal birth after caesarean* or VBAC. For some women, fear of repeating past negative labour experiences and the unpredictability of birth means that labour can be a daunting prospect (Lowdon and Chippington Derrick, 2007). However, others choose VBAC because they fear another CS, they are influenced by the shorter recovery time and/or they want the experience and satisfaction of a normal birth (Emmett *et al.*, 2006).

Incidence and facts

In 1985 the World Health Organization issued a consensus statement suggesting there were no additional health benefits associated with a CSR above 10–15%.

- The CS rate (CSR) was 24.8% (162 512) in England in 2010–11 (NHS Maternity Statistics England, 2011) and 14% of these were repeat elective CS.
- CS is more expensive: for every 800 births conducted as normal deliveries instead of CS, the NHS would save £1 million (OHE, 2007).
- There is emerging evidence of serious harm relating to multiple CS (Guise *et al.*, 2010) including significant placenta percreta/accreta risk, prelabour stillbirth and reduced fertility.
- The 2001 National CS Audit recommended 'a trial of labour should be considered in women who have had a previous CS' (RCOG, 2001).
- VBAC is a reasonable and safe choice for the majority of women with prior CS; the UK VBAC success rate is 72–76% (RCOG, 2007).
- NICE (2011) suggest that for birth following one previous CS:
  - Planned repeat CS marginally increases maternal mortality
  - Planned VBAC marginally increases neonatal mortality
  - Perinatal mortality is not statistically different between the two groups
- Uterine rupture is very rare, but is increased in women attempting VBAC: 22–74:10 000 (RCOG, 2007)

The influence and opinions of professionals

The RCOG found most obstetricians failed to recognise the degree of their influence over women's CS/VBAC decision (RCOG, 2001; Emmett, 2006).

- CS is recommended more frequently by obstetricians who are male, junior in experience or working in the private health sector (RCOG, 2001).
- When asked about themselves 25% of obstetricians would choose elective CS over vaginal birth *in a straightforward pregnancy* (RCOG, 2001). Fewer female obstetricians than male would choose a CS (Groom *et al.*, 2002; MacDonald *et al.*, 2002). These rates are higher than reported in other women surveyed (RCOG, 2001), and in contrast to personal preferences of midwives, 96% of whom would prefer a vaginal delivery (Dickson and Willett, 1999).
- A large study found that 8–90% (average 44%) of CS women were offered a trial of labour in subsequent pregnancies (RCOG, 2001).
- Most obstetricians surveyed believed that elective CS was not the safest option for the mother, although 50% thought it was the safest option for the baby (RCOG, 2001).
- To address a high CS rate, some UK hospitals have introduced midwifery-led clinics for VBAC women with strict criteria, resulting in around 95% VBAC attempt rates.

VBAC or elective CS

'In women having had a previous CS there are risks associated with both a trial of labour and with repeat CS. The greatest risk of adverse maternal outcomes occurs in a failed trial of labour. However, successful VBAC has the fewest complications and therefore the failure rate

for trial of labour is likely to be an important determinant of the overall comparative risks of a trial of labour and repeat CS' (NICE, 2011:13.4).

Women do not make decisions based on the same perceived statistical risks and safety concerns as professionals: women's decisions tend to be based on their previous delivery experience(s), ease of recovery and family responsibilities, rather than primarily for their own safety or that of their infant (Eden *et al.*, 2004). When asked, 45% of women preferred VBAC, 27% had their choice determined by medical factors, 20% would opt for a repeat elective CS; the remaining 6.2% had no clear preference (RCOG, 2001).

Considerations and risks associated with VBAC

- NICE (2011) report the intrapartum fetal death for planned VBAC is similar to a primigravid labour at 10 in 10 000, which is small but higher than for planned repeat CS at 1 in 10 000. In contrast to this, Menacker *et al.* (2010) found no differences in neonatal mortality risk between VBAC and repeat CS.
- Uterine rupture is a rare but serious risk for women with previous CS.
- Vaginal delivery is associated with postnatal perineal pain and trauma, increased risk of urinary incontinence and uterovaginal prolapse (NICE, 2011).
- Attempted VBAC has an unknown outcome: there is unpredictability as to whether birth will be normal, assisted or emergency CS. An emergency CS can be a huge disappointment and may reignite past frightening experiences.
- Labour is more likely to be monitored and medicalised; caregivers may be preoccupied with risk and not provide the level of emotional support a woman needs. This type of labour experience can create feelings of powerlessness, inadequacy and anxiety in women.

Risks associated with CS

- Operative risks include bladder/ureter injury (1:1000); it is rare for women to need intensive care following childbirth but more likely after CS (9:1000) (NICE, 2011).
- Neonatal risks include neonatal respiratory morbidity, especially <39/40, NICU/ SCBU admission and longer length of hospital stay (Morrison *et al.*, 1995; Kamath *et al.*, 2009).
- Primigravid women who undergo CS are at increased risk in their subsequent pregnancy for anaemia, placental abruption, uterine rupture and hysterectomy (Jackson *et al.*, 2012). Multiple CS increases risks of placenta accreta (Langdana *et al.*, 2001), antepartum stillbirth and reduced future fertility (NICE, 2011).
- The rate of placenta praevia in a second pregnancy for women with vaginal first births is 4.4:1000 births, compared to 8.7:1000 births for women with CS first birth (Gurol-Urganci *et al.*, 2011). Previous CS women with placenta praevia had more adverse events than if they had had previous vaginal birth: blood transfusion (15% versus 32%), hysterectomy (0.7–4% versus 10%), and maternal morbidity (15% versus 23–30%) (Guise *et al.*, 2010).
- Postnatal recovery is slower after CS: with more abdominal pain, longer hospital stay and increased postnatal readmission. Postoperative infections (e.g. endometritis, urinary tract/wound infection) occur in 8% of CS and reduced mobility increases risk of venous thromboembolism (NICE, 2011).

- The risk of serious complications increases significantly relative to increasing number of repeated caesareans: NICE (2011) therefore stipulate that knowledge of the woman's intended number of future pregnancies is an important factor to consider during the decision-making process for either planned VBAC or repeat CS.

What improves the success rate in VBAC?

The VBAC success rate is 72–76% (RCOG, 2007) which is similar to a primigravida. More recent data suggest that women with three or more prior CSs who attempt VBAC have similar rates of success and risk for maternal morbidity as those with one or two prior CSs. (Cahill *et al.*, 2010). A previous successful vaginal delivery is the best indicator of potential VBAC success. See Table 12.1 for related risk factors.

Table 12.1   Related risk factors for VBAC.

	Increased possibility of successful VBAC	Reduced likelihood of VBAC
Maternal factors	<35 years old Body mass index <30	Short stature Body mass index >30 Non-white ethnicity (RCOG, 2007)
Previous obstetric history	One previous vaginal birth (success rate 87–90%)	Previous preterm CS delivery (RCOG, 2007)
	Previous CS for breech	Previous CS for 'cephalopelvic disproportion' (CPD)
		Oxytocin use in previous labour (NICE, 2011)
		Previous baby >4000 g (RCOG, 2007)
Midwifery/ obstetric care	Involvement of a consultant obstetrician in CS decision-making	Continuous electronic fetal monitoring
	Intermittent auscultation (IA)	Induction of labour (RCOG, 2007)
	Female companion/support during labour (Hodnett, 2007)	Cervical dilatation <4 cm on admission
	Planned home birth	(RCOG, 2007)
	Mobilisation/upright postures (RCM, 2010)	

Induction of labour for VBAC

The VBAC rate following IOL is slightly lower than in spontaneous labour VBAC rate, at around 75% (Vause and Macintosh, 1999). A large Norwegian study reported 94 uterine ruptures (5:1000) in previous CS women having IOL. The highest risk was after IOL, especially using prostaglandin, where the risk was up to 13 times higher. The authors recommended 'induction should be discouraged in mothers with previous caesarean section, as it carries the highest risk, and most catastrophic consequences, of uterine rupture for both mother and neonate. If needed, mechanical induction should be used instead of medical induction by prostaglandins' (Al-Zirqi *et al.*, 2010). Risk of uterine rupture in VBAC is 8:1000 for IOL with non-prostaglandin agents; 24:1000 with prostaglandin IOL (NICE, 2011).

NICE (2011) suggest that during IOL previous CS women should be monitored closely, with access to electronic fetal monitoring and with immediate access to CS, because they are at increased risk of uterine rupture. IOL should also take place on the labour ward.

Place of birth

A woman who has had a previous CS is considered 'high risk' and NICE (2011) advise that planned VBAC should be conducted in a suitably staffed and equipped delivery suite, with continuous intrapartum care and monitoring and available resources for immediate CS and advanced neonatal resuscitation.

Women who feel pressured, obstructed or unsupported sometimes opt out of the acute hospital system. Most birthing centres do not encourage VBAC, but women may still choose to give birth there, or even at home. Some NHS midwives are uncomfortable supporting home birth VBAC and women may turn to independent midwives (Lowdon and Chippington Derrick, 2007). However, as discussed in Chapter 6 (home birth), all midwives have a duty to provide care and support at home, even if the pregnancy is not considered low risk. Planned home birth reduces women's CS risk (NICE, 2011). Women wanting a home birth are usually highly motivated, labour is physiologically spontaneous, and labour not 'interfered with'.

Preparing for birth at home/birthing centre

See also Chapter 6.

- **Care as per normal labour.** The midwife must instil confidence in the woman and strike a balance between maintaining a caring, reassuring presence while also being unobtrusively vigilant for signs of possible rupture.
- **Ruptured uterus.** While there are no reported cases of this occurring at a home birth in the UK (Lowdon and Chippington Derrick, 2007), the midwife should be well supported by colleagues, her supervisor of midwives and be up to date on VBAC issues (for signs and symptoms of rupture see Box 17.1, page 276).
- **Transfer.** The transfer rate for a woman attempting home VBAC is thought to be higher, possibly as midwives and mothers tend to be cautious and transfer at the first sign of trouble. One small study reported a 28% VBAC transfer rate although none was for a ruptured uterus (Chamberlain *et al.*, 1994).

Midwifery care for VBAC labour

Women should not be pressured to consent to any particular aspect of care. Since a ruptured uterus is rare, many women undergo 'routine' interventions which involve iatrogenic risk and subsequent morbidity.

First stage

One-to-one midwifery care. Continuous intrapartum care is vital for the provision of quality emotional support and important for the recognition and management of uterine scar rupture.

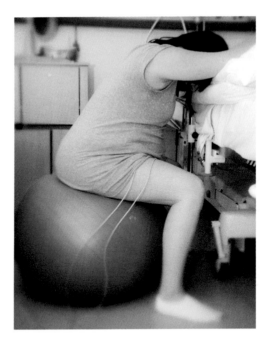

Some women may approach labour with trepidation, affected by memories of a previously stressful labour, perhaps ending in a frightening emergency situation (Horn, 2007). Particular reassurance may be required at the point in labour when the previous CS occurred. Knowing the reason for the previous CS may help midwives prevent a recurrence.

Consultant opinion. Consultant obstetricians should be involved in any decision making for CS, because evidence suggets this reduces the likelihood of unecessary CS (NICE, 2011).

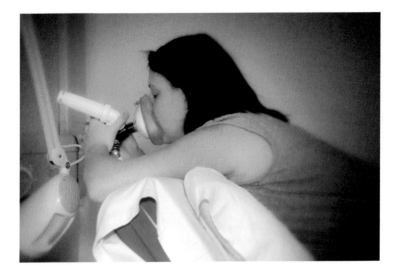

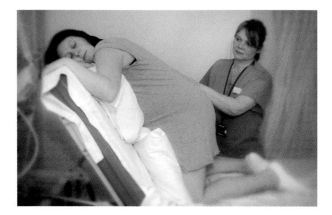

Monitoring the fetal heart rate (FHR). Electonic fetal monitoring (EFM) in high-risk women increases labour interventions, including CS, without reducing the perinatal mortality rate (Alfirevic *et al.*, 2007). One study showed VBAC women undergoing EFM had a higher non-reassuring fetal heart rate (FHR) and CS rate than women receiving intermittent monitoring (IA) without any improvement in outcome (Madaan and Trivedi, 2006).

Despite a lack of evidence to support CTG the RCOG (2007) recommend continuous fetal monitoring for VBAC women. In retrospective reviews in 55–87% cases of ruptured uterus the CTG was abnormal (Guise *et al.*, 2004); pathological features include variable and/or late decelerations followed by fetal bradycardia (Menihan, 1999). Farmer *et al.*, 1991 found that 'the most common manifestation of a scar separation was a prolonged fetal heart rate deceleration (70%)'. Abnormal fetal heart rate patterns have high false positives and are an unreliable diagnostic tool for fetal compromise: any gross FHR abnormalities are likely to be picked up whatever the form of monitoring.

Some VBAC support groups criticise routine CTG for VBAC (Beech Lawrence, 2001) and describe staff acting unprofessionally or threateningly, exaggerating risks and coercing women into CTG monitoring.

Scrupulous IA is a valid alternative, and any woman declining CTG needs to be supported in labour and her choices respected.

Epidural. VBAC is not a contraindication to an epidural (RCOG, 2007). Some clinicians recommend epidurals 'just in case' a CS is needed while others suggest it could mask uterine rupture pain. Women should be aware that epidurals carry a risk of complications and interventions which may complicate an otherwise straightforward labour.

Intravenous (IV) access and bloods (for FBC/crossmatching). A timely cannula saves time in a later possible emergency, but it is uncomfortable and restricts movement. If the woman accepts, cap it, enabling freer movement, and flush regularly. If she declines it can be sited later, just as for any other emergency CS. Label and store blood ready or send off if required.

Warm water immersion. Some hospitals actively support VBAC women to labour in water because it improves the spontaneous birth rate. Monitoring is possible with EFM telemetry or by IA. Note: a cannula is contraindicated in water as it constitutes an infection risk to the woman.

Nutrition and regular antacids. There is no strong evidence that antacids in labour prevent aspiration under anaesthesia (Gyte and Richens, 2006); however, these are often recommended for high risk/VBAC women. NICE highlights uncertainty over eating in labour versus risk of aspiration under anaesthesia, stating that isotonic drinks during labour prevent ketosis without increasing gastric volume (NICE, 2011).

Slow labour. More likely with a large baby, postmaturity, cephalopelvic disproportion (CPD) or malposition, all of which make successful vaginal delivery less likely. Midwives should aim to negate iatrogenic slow progress by avoiding opiates or epidurals; encouraging mobility and upright postures and maintain continuous, supportive one-to-one care. Enkin (2000) suggests slow progress should not always result in CS: careful oxytocin use, avoiding hyperstimulation, following consultant opinion and maternal discussion (RCOG, 2007) may be effective (see Chapter 19). Serial vaginal examination, preferably by the same person, may help assess progress (RCOG, 2007).

Second stage of labour

Many VBACs are forceps or ventouse assisted as fear of uterine rupture and lack of confidence in the birth process leads to a desire to conclude VBAC as quickly as possible. If progress is slow, upright maternal birthing positions, non-active pushing and avoiding arbitrary second stage time limits improve the spontaneous vaginal birth rate (Walsh, 2000). While studies on second stage duration are not VBAC-specific, 'allowing' a longer second stage increases vaginal delivery rate, reduces CS and has no adverse effect on neonatal morbidity, although there is a small increased risk of shoulder dystocia (Myles and Santolaya, 2003). There is some evidence that second stage >4 hours increases the risk of more severe perineal trauma, PPH and infection (Myles and Santolaya, 2003).

- Restricting the duration of the second stage due to fear of uterine rupture is not evidence-based and increases trauma / morbidity.
- Active pushing (valsalva) is potentially dangerous for VBAC women as it includes prolonged breath holding and forced bearing down which carries multiple risks including raised intrauterine pressure.

Third stage

- A scar on the uterus is not a contraindication to a physiological third stage.
- If the placenta appears retained, be cautious: it may have adhered to the myometrium of the previous scar (placenta accreta or morbidly adherent placenta) and may require hysterectomy to control haemorrhage (Langdana *et al.*, 2001) although if not bleeding conservative management is sometimes tried where the cord is cut short and placenta left in situ to be reabsorbed by the body. Inform the doctor early if the placenta appears retained; be aware bleeding may be concealed.

Uterine scar rupture

Uterine rupture is rare and has relatively weak risk factors (Landon, 2010).

- Previous vaginal delivery/ VBAC reduces the risk of rupture.
- Short interpregnancy interval, prior preterm CS, single layer uterine closure, IOL and augmentation increase the risk of rupture (Landon, 2010).

While no unique clinical feature indicates uterine rupture (RCOG, 2007), many women and midwives report a woman's *unease* or *distress* as a common feature (Lowdon and Chippington Derrick, 2002). Farmer *et al.* (1991) found that bleeding and pain were unlikely findings (3.4% and 7.6% respectively). The most common manifestation of scar separation was prolonged fetal heart rate deceleration. For more on uterine rupture see Chapter 17, pages 276–277.

Summary

In hospital

- Give plenty of extra reassurance, positive support and maintain one-to-one midwifery care.
- Possible precautions:
  - Cannula and bloods (test only in an emergency)
  - Eating and drinking is not contraindicated but be cautious – consider antacids.
- Observe unobtrusively for signs of uterine rupture: listen to the woman.
- Serious FHR changes are the most common sign of uterine rupture.
- Prostaglandin/artificial rupture of the membranes/oxytocics should be used with caution.
- Epidural is not contraindicated.

At home/birthing centre

- Ensure you have support and in turn offer reassurance and positive care.
- Be unobtrusive monitoring for signs of uterine rupture.
- Be prepared for transfer if necessary.

Acknowledgement: photos in this chapter by Debbie Gagliano-Withers.

References

Alfirevic, Z., Devane, D., Gyte, G. M. (2007) Continuous cardiotocography (CTG) as a form of electronic fetal monitoring (EFM) for fetal assessment during labour (Review). *Cochrane Library*, Issue 3.

Al-Zirqi, I., Stray-Pedersen, B., Forsén, L., Vangen, S. (2010) Uterine rupture after previous caesarean section. *BJOG: An International Journal of Obstetrics and Gynaecology* 117, 809–20.

Beech Lawrence, B. (2001) Electronic fetal monitoring: do NICE's new guidelines owe too much to the medical model of childbirth? *The Practising Midwife* 4(7), 31–3.

Cahill, A., Tuuli, M., Odibo, A., Stamilio, D., Macones, G. (2010) Vaginal birth after caesarean for women with three or more prior caesareans: assessing safety and success. *British Journal of Obstetrics and Gynaecology* 117, 422–7.

Chamberlain, G., Wraight, A., Crowley, P. (1994) *National Birthday Trust Report – Report of the Confidential Enquiry into Home Births*. London, Parthenon Publishing.

Dickson, M. J., Willett, M. (1999) Midwives would prefer a vaginal delivery. *British Medical Journal* 319, 1008.

Eden, K. B., Hashima, J. N., Osterwell, P., Nygren, P., Guise, J. M. (2004) Childbirth preferences after cesarean birth: a review of the evidence. *Birth* 31, 49.

Emmett, C., Shaw, A., Montgomery, A., Murphy, D. (DiAMOND study group) (2006) Women's experience of decision making about mode of delivery after a previous caesarean section: the role of health professionals and information about health risks. *An International Journal of Obstetrics and Gynaecology* 113(12), 1438–45.

Enkin, M. (2000) Labour and birth after a previous caesarean section. In Enkin, M., Keirse, M. J. N. C., Neilson, J. *et al.* (eds) *A Guide to Effective Care in Pregnancy and Childbirth*, 3rd edn, pp. 359–71. Oxford, Oxford University Press.

Farmer, R. M., Kirschbaum, T., Potter, D., Strong, T. H., Medearis, A. L. (1991) Uterine rupture during trial of labor after previous cesarean section. *American Journal of Obstetrics and Gynecology* 165, 996–1001.

Groom, K. M., Patterson-Brown, S., Fisk, N. M. (2002) Temporal and geographical variation in UK obstetricians' personal preference regarding mode of delivery. *European Journal of Obstetrics, Gynecology, and Reproductive Biology* 100, 185–8.

Guise, J. M., McDonagh, M. S., Osterweil, P., Nygren, P., Chan, B. K., Helfand, M. (2004) Systematic review of the incidence and consequences of uterine rupture in women with previous caesarean section. *British Medical Journal* 329, 19–25.

Guise, J. M., Eden, K., Emeris, C., Denman, M. A., Marshall, N., Fu, R. R., Janik, R., Nygen, P., Walker, M. (2010) Vaginal birth after cesarean: new insights. *Evid Rep Technol Assess (Full Rep)* 191(1), 397.

Gurol-Urganci, I., Cromwell, D. A., Edozien, L. C., Smith, G. C., Onwere, C., Mahmood, T. A., Templeton, A., van der Meulen, J. H. (2011) Risk of placenta previa in second birth after first birth cesarean section: a population-based study and meta-analysis. *BMC Pregnancy Childbirth* Nov 21:11:95.

Gyte, G. M. L., Richens, Y. (2006) Routine prophylactic drugs in normal labour for reducing gastric aspiration and its effects. *Cochrane Database of Systematic Reviews*, Issue 3.

Hodnett, E. D., Gates, S., Hofmeyr, G. J., Sakala, C. (2007) Continuous support for women during childbirth. *Cochrane Database of Systematic Reviews*, Issue 3.

Horn, A. (2007) VBAC at Home. *www.homebirth.org.uk*

Jackson, S., Fleege, L., Fridman, M., Gregory, K., Zelop, C., Olsen, J. (2012) Morbidity following primary cesarean delivery in the Danish National Birth Cohort. *American Journal of Obstetrics and Gynecology*. 206, 139.e1–5.

Kamath, B. D., Todd, J., Glazner, J. E., Lezotte, D., Lynch, A. M. (2009) Neonatal outcomes after elective cesarean delivery. *Obstetrics and Gynecology* 113(6), 1231–8.

Landon, M. B. (2010) Predicting uterine rupture in women undergoing trial of labour after prior cesarean delivery. *Semin Perinatology* 34(4), 267–71.

Langdana, F., Geary, M., Haw, W., Keane, D. (2001) Peripartum hysterectomy in the 1990s: any new lessons? *Journal of Obstetrics and Gynaecology* 21, 121–3.

Lowdon, D., Chippington Derrick, D. (2002) VBAC on whose terms. *AIMS Journal* 14, 1.

Lowdon, D., Chippington Derrick, D. (2007) CS and VBAC Information *www.caesarean.org.uk*

Madaan, M., Trivedi, S. (2006) Intrapartum electronic fetal monitoring vs intermittent auscultation in post-caesarean pregnancies. *International Journal of Obstetrics and Gynaecology*, 94, 123–5.

MacDonald, C., Pinion, S., McCleod, U. (2002) Scottish female obstetricians' views on elective caesarean section and personal choice for delivery. *Journal of Obstetrics and Gynaecology* 22, 586–9.

Menacker, F., MacDorman, M. F., Declercq, E. (2010) Neonatal mortality risk for repeat cesarean compared to vaginal birth after cesarean (VBAC) deliveries in the United States, 1998–2002 birth cohorts. *Maternal and Child Health Journal* 14(2), 147–54.

Menihan, C. A. (1999) The effect of uterine rupture on fetal heart rate patterns. *Journal of Nurse-Midwifery* 44(1), 40–6.

Morrison, J. J., Rennie, J. M., Milton, P. J. (1995) Neonatal respiratory morbidity and mode of delivery at term: of timing of elective caesarean section. *British Journal of Obstetrics and Gynaecology* 102, 101–6.

Myles, T. D., Santolaya, J. (2003) Maternal and neonatal outcomes in patients with a prolonged second stage of labor. *Obstetrics and Gynecology* 102, 52–8.

NICE (2008) *Clinical Guideline D – Induction of Labour*. London, NICE.

NICE (2011) *Full Clinical Guideline 132 Caesarean Section*. London, NICE.

NHS Maternity Statistics England (2011) *HES Online Hospital Episode Statistics. The information centre for health and social care: Maternity Data* 2010–11. www.hesonline.nhs.uk

RCM (2010) *The RCM's Survey of Positions used in Labour and Birth*. London: RCM.

RCOG (2001) Royal College of Obstetricians and Gynaecologists Clinical Effectiveness Support Unit. *National Sentinel Caesarean Section Audit Report* (Thomas, J., Paranjothy, S., eds). London, RCOG Press.

RCOG (2007) *Green-top Guideline No. 45: Birth After Previous Caesarean Birth*. London, RCOG Press. www.rcog.org.uk

Vause, S., Macintosh, M. (1999) Evidence based case report: use of prostaglandins to induce labour in women with a caesarean section scar. *British Medical Journal* 318, 1056–8.

Walsh, D. (2000) Evidence-based care: Part 6: limits on pushing and time in the second stage. *British Journal of Midwifery* 8(10), 604–8.

Vadeboncoeur, H. (2011) Making the case for VBAC. An interview by Kimmelin Hull. A research blog about healthy pregnancy, birth and beyond. *Science and Sensibility*. www.scienceandsensibility.org/?tag + how-to-achieve-a-vbac

13 Preterm birth

Charlise Adams

Introduction

'The birth of a baby should be one of the most special and joyful experiences a family can have and yet every year thousands of families experience the pain of . . . seeing a tiny child fight for life' (Briley *et al.*, 2002).

Preterm birth (PTB) is defined as the delivery of a baby before 37 completed weeks gestation. It is the single most important cause of death or morbidity for newborn babies (Saigal and Doyle, 2008). The lower the gestational age, the greater the problems, although outcomes have dramatically improved in recent years, particularly for babies between 27–28 weeks (EPIcure, 2008). A woman in unexpected preterm labour may be very stressed and midwifery care needs to be skilled and compassionate. Good multidisciplinary teamwork is essential. Although labour is likely to be more closely scrutinised and susceptible to increased intervention, with good care it is still possible for many mothers to achieve a safe and satisfying birth.

The Midwife's Labour and Birth Handbook, Third Edition. Edited by Vicky Chapman and Cathy Charles.
© 2013 John Wiley & Sons, Ltd. Published 2013 by John Wiley & Sons, Ltd.

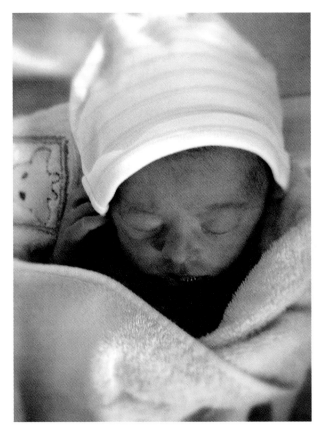

Fig. 13.1   Preterm babies are vulnerable to heat loss: always put on a hat.

Incidence and facts

- Worldwide 5–10% of all live births are preterm with around 28% neonatal deaths (out of 4 million per year) directly attributable to preterm birth PTB (Lawn *et al.*, 2005).
- In England and Wales, the PTB rate is 8.6%, i.e. one live baby in twelve:
  - 93% of preterm births occur after 28 weeks
  - 6% of preterm births occur between 22 and 27 weeks.
- Almost 50% of UK PTBs are by caesarean section (CS), often elective prelabour CS (RCOG, 2006a).
- Preterm babies are more prone to hypothermia, hypoglycaemia, jaundice, infection and respiratory distress. More serious risks are intraventricular haemorrhage, deafness, retinopathy of prematurity, blindness, necrotising enterocolitis (NEC), cerebral palsy and death (Kenyon *et al.*, 2001).
- A preterm baby is more likely to survive if it is a singleton, not small for dates and experiences a cephalic vaginal birth (Tyson *et al.*, 2008). Girls have a higher survival rate than boys (Kent *et al.*, 2011). Gestational age is the single most important predictor of survival (Lucey *et al.*, 2004).

Causes and associated factors of preterm birth

PTB is often unpredictable, although numerous risk factors exist, including poor economic status, pre-existing medical conditions and previous PTB (Tucker and McGuire, 2004). Causes are often unknown or multifactorial.

'Both preterm labour and PPROM are now considered a syndrome initiated by multiple mechanisms including infection/inflammation, uteroplacental ischemia/haemorrhage, uterine overdistension, stress, and other immunologically mediated processes. However, a precise mechanism cannot be established in most cases' (Goldenberg and McLure, 2010).

The two most common risk factors for PTB are multiple pregnancy – up to 30% of UK PTBs (ONS, 2007) – and infection, particularly intrauterine. Up to 80% of CS PTBs with intact membranes have shown bacteria and inflammatory response in the amniotic fluid so infection is probably a key cause of PTB (Goldenberg *et al.*, 2000). Preterm babies born with an infection have a four times higher mortality rate than other preterm babies (RCOG, 2006b).

Identifying women at risk of preterm labour is imprecise; also prediction does not yet mean prevention. Several prediction methods are available, e.g. infection screening, cervical scanning and biochemical markers (fetal fibronectin, salivary oestriols and interleukins), but no single reliable method of predicting preterm delivery exists (Briley *et al.*, 2002).

Place of delivery

Ideally all preterm babies should be born in a hospital with a neonatal intensive care unit (NICU) although babies over 35 weeks may well be cared for on a normal ward within that hospital. Transfer to a NICU-equipped hospital is advisable for women with threatened preterm labour, however, transfer may be unwise if the birth is imminent or the woman's condition is unstable; e.g. bleeding or severe pre-eclampsia.

If transfer is required, decide whether a midwife escort is needed. Any escorting staff must be trained to assist in transfer/unexpected PTB (CESDI, 2003).

With increasing pressure on NICU cots, a woman may have to transfer in labour or postnatally a long distance away, sometimes hundreds of miles from her home, particularly if the baby is very preterm or has particular problems requiring specialist support. Occasionally mothers and babies may be separated for hours or days, as it is not always possible to accommodate the mother, or she may be too ill to travel. This is an unsatisfactory but sometimes unavoidable situation.

Preterm prelabour rupture of membranes (PPROM)

PPROM complicates only 2% of pregnancies but is associated with 40% of preterm deliveries (RCOG, 2006b).

Possible complications of PPROM

- Oligohydramnios
- Abruption

- Cord prolapse/compression
- Ascending infection
- Preterm birth with associated morbidity
- Intrapartum fetal compromise
- Stillbirth/neonatal death

(RCOG, 2006b; Walkinshaw, 2001)

If PPROM occurs at 24–34 weeks gestation 50% of women will deliver within 4 days and 70–80% within 1 week (Walkinshaw, 2001). Primary causes of neonatal death following PPROM are sepsis (leading to a four times increased mortality rate compared with other preterm babies) and prematurity/pulmonary hypoplasia (RCOG, 2006b).

Diagnosis of PPROM

Listen closely to the woman's story and offer a sterile speculum examination to observe pooled liquor. **Do not perform a digital vaginal examination if the woman is not in labour** – sepsis is a particular risk for preterm babies. Nitrazine tests and microscopic examination of liquor (ferning test) have high false positive results (17% nitrazine, 6% ferning) so are not recommended; ultrasound to detect oligohydramnios may be helpful (RCOG, 2006b).

Management of PPROM

- **Observe for signs of clinical chorioamnionitis** (RCOG, 2006b):
  - Maternal temperature, pulse and fetal heart rate – report pyrexia or maternal/fetal tachycardia. RCOG recommend 4–8 hourly monitoring but since many women go home if labour does not start, this is not always practicable.
  - Uterine tenderness or offensive smelling discharge.
- **Antibiotics**: erythromycin for 10 days is recommended (RCOG, 2006b). Studies show reduced neonatal and maternal morbidity, including chorioamnionitis, neonatal infection and abnormal cerebral ultrasound. Antibiotics may delay delivery so steroids can be given (Kenyon *et al.*, 2001; RCOG, 2006b).
- **A high vaginal swab (HVS)** is often requested although there is a high false positive rate of 25% which can lead to unnecessary intervention (RCOG, 2006b).
- **Give corticosteroids** as prescribed, to mature fetal lungs.

Interventions which are felt to be of little or no use in PPROM are (RCOG, 2006b):

- **Tocolysis** following PPROM: labour may be starting for a reason, e.g. sepsis, in which case the baby needs to be delivered
- Routine weekly investigations, e.g. high vaginal swabs (HVS), full blood count (FBC), and C-reactive protein (CRP) are poor indicators of maternal infection (RCOG, 2006b).

Corticosteroids for threatened preterm birth

Administration of corticosteroids to the mother prior to preterm birth has been demonstrated (Shah, *et al.*, 2012) to reduce

- neonatal death by 31%
- respiratory distress syndrome (RDS) by 44%
- intraventricular haemorrhage by 46%
- necrotising enterocolitis (NEC)
- systemic infections
- NICU admission and ventilatory support.

Corticosteroids are normally given from 24–34 weeks: see Table 13.1. A senior paediatrician should be consulted for earlier preterm babies. There is little research into multiple pregnancy but corticosteroids are probably helpful as with singleton babies.

Table 13.1   Betamethasone/dexamethasone.

Indications:	Threatened preterm delivery 24–34/40 gestation (Roberts & Dalziel, 2007) to reduce risk of RDS, IVH and NEC. Betamethasone appears better at reducing RDS.
Dosage and frequency:	Total dose of 24 mg in 24–48 hours: precise frequency unimportant (RCOG, 2006b): EITHER two doses of 12 mg (12–24 hours apart) OR four doses of 6 mg (4–12 hours apart). Outcomes are best if the birth occurs between 24 hours and 7 days after administration. RCOG (2006b) states insufficient evidence on longer-term benefits/risks to recommend routine repeat courses.
Route:	Ideally IM. Oral less effective (RCOG, 2006b).
Contraindications:	Caution if maternal systemic infection, including TB /sepsis (RCOG 2006b; JFC, 2012).
Side effects:	No negative short/long-term effects noted in mother or baby (RCOG, 2006b) as most steroid side effects are associated with long term use (JFC, 2012).
Cautions:	Diabetes not a contraindication to antenatal corticosteroids, but give additional insulin according to an agreed protocol and closely monitor women (RCOG, 2006b).

Tocolysis in threatened preterm labour

Tocolysis is not associated with prevention of PTB and has no clear effect on perinatal or neonatal morbidity (RCOG, 2002). It is not normally recommended in the presence of PPROM, but may gain time for a course of corticosteroids or in utero transfer. Atosiban and nifedipine appear effective in delaying birth for up to 7 days; ritodrine is another option (RCOG, 2002). Nifedipine is unlicensed for oral use but appears to have fewer side effects. Magnesium sulphate does not delay birth, but appears to reduce the risk of cerebral palsy, so RCOG (2002) recommend it is used alongside other tocolytic drugs at least 24 hours prior to delivery.

The use of tocolytics should be avoided if:

- the baby has already died or has an abnormality incompatible with life
- the fetal or maternal condition requires urgent delivery
- the woman has active vaginal bleeding – as tocolytics relax the uterus
- PPROM and/or infection is present.

Monitoring the fetal heart in preterm labour

Continuous electronic fetal monitoring (EFM) may be considered when in labour, particularly if there are other fetal concerns, e.g. IUGR. NICE (2007) recommends preterm labour as one indication for EFM. However, Cochrane review found that EFM in preterm labour appears to have no advantage over intermittent auscultation (IA) and increases maternal morbidity, CS and possibly cerebral palsy (Alfirevic *et al.*, 2007). It also restricts the woman's mobility.

EFM is likely to be more easily interpretable in older preterm babies than very early ones. Very premature small babies can be difficult to monitor continuously, and preterm cardiotocographs (CTGs) may be difficult to interpret as they differ from those at term. Preterm (particularly very preterm) CTGs tend to have a higher baseline, sometimes 170 bpm, and decelerations which are not necessarily truly pathological: Atalla *et al.* (2000) suggest that most preterm babies with unsatisfactory CTG traces will not be acidotic. EFM is also an unreliable tool for predicting future neurodevelopmental impairment of premature infants of very low birth weight (Nisenblat *et al.*, 2006).

Once a CTG is performed clinicians are likely to have a low threshold for action in a preterm labour, although as stated earlier this may not improve the outcome.

Ultimately the method of monitoring is the woman's choice. Many women may be very willing to have continuous monitoring in the belief that it is the safest option, but midwives should be aware that if the woman declines, or monitoring is impracticable, IA is a perfectly acceptable alternative. If it is decided to perform IA, it should be carried out scrupulously (see Chapter 3).

Midwifery care

Most care and support will be the same as for any labour (see Chapter 1) but women in preterm labour may be particularly anxious.

- **Continuous, supportive, one-to-one midwifery care** is proved to reduce interventions and improves maternal and fetal outcomes (Hodnett *et al.*, 2011).
- **Discuss with the parents** what may occur at/after the birth: i.e. who will be present, anticipated resuscitation, ventilatory support and the likelihood of NICU care.
- **Minimise environmental stress.** Try to reduce external stressful stimuli of bright lights, noise, interruptions and lack of privacy. PTBs may attract more staff: ask yourself: does this person really need to be in the room?
- **Multidisciplinary communication is essential.** Inform labour ward coordinator, obstetrician, NICU staff and paediatric team. Delegate someone else to do this if the woman needs your full attention.
- **Transfer.** If transferring in from home or midwife-led unit, ensure the acute unit is informed in advance so they can prepare for the woman's arrival.
- **Position.** Encourage mobility and upright postures if possible to aid optimal fetal positioning, progress and descent. As with any labour, avoid the supine position as it may cause FHR abnormalities, increased duration of second stage, episiotomy and instrumental delivery (Gupta *et al.*, 2012). A non-supine position also improves outcomes in women with epidurals (Roberts *et al.*, 2005).
- **Monitor the FHR.** See earlier discussion on EFM versus IA.
- **Minimise digital VEs.** Always consider what is to be gained by VE, which may lead to ascending infection, especially with PPROM.

- **Observe for infection.** Since preterm labour is often due to infection, be vigilant for maternal pyrexia, fetal/maternal tachycardia or offensive smelling liquor. Discuss with obstetrician re need for blood cultures or bacteriological specimens/swabs.
- **Eating and drinking is not contraindicated**, and while there is no good evidence for antacids like ranitidine or cimetidine in normal labour (Gyte and Richens, 2006) some preterm labours may be considered high enough risk to justify 4-hourly antacids. *If nifedipine is being used for tocolysis be aware that ranitidine and cimetidine may interact with it, causing profound hypotension* (Johnson, 2010).
- **Avoid narcotic analgesia**, e.g. pethidine: may cause neonatal respiratory depression, drowsiness and depressed reflexes, including the suck reflex (NICE, 2007) which is often poor anyway in a preterm baby.
- **Artificial rupture of the membranes (ARM) is not recommended** since any potential cord compression may be particularly serious for a preterm baby and there is a risk of exacerbating ascending infection/chorioamnionitis.
- **Fetal blood sampling (FBS) is contraindicated** <34 weeks (NICE, 2007) and has not been shown to hold an advantage over EFM without fetal blood sampling (Alfirevic *et al.*, 2007).
- **Prepare the resuscitaire.** Check equipment. Provide baby clothes, hat and warm towels, plastic/bubble wrap. Have small laryngoscope, endotracheal tubes (ETTs) and masks available. Preterm labours can progress rapidly, so be prepared. If the baby is very preterm a specialist resuscitaire with additional equipment may be used. If using a standard resuscitaire, reduce pressures to 20–25 cm water (normally 30–40 cm water for term birth).

Second stage of labour

- **Keep the room warm.** Shut windows and switch off fans when birth is close.
- **Avoid forced pushing.** Prolonged breath holding and closed glottis pushing is associated with fetal compromise, forceps delivery and lower Apgars (Keirse, 2000) which can have more serious consequences for a preterm infant. Let the woman push at her own pace.
- **Avoid episiotomy.** The only indications are acute fetal compromise and, if absolutely necessary, an unyielding perineum (Keirse, 2000). Episiotomy does not protect the preterm fetal head.
- **Summon relevant staff.** Whilst it may not always be necessary for an obstetrician to be present, they are more likely to be there if the baby is very preterm, and should be quickly available if problems arise in any PTB. A practitioner experienced in preterm resuscitation should be present for most PTBs, although this may be unnecessary for older preterm babies >35 weeks.
- **Always expect the unexpected**. Preterm babies can arrive very quickly before all relevant staff are present, so be prepared for the best laid plans to go awry. All midwives should be aware of the basic principles of resuscitation and initial management of preterm babies.

Mode of delivery

Vaginal delivery is preferable for singleton cephalic babies (Figueroa and Rouse, 2010). Ventouse delivery is not recommended <34 weeks due to the baby's soft skull (Keirse,

2000). Forceps delivery may damage the fetal head (Keirse, 2000) and the old practice of preterm elective forceps delivery has been abandoned.

Almost 50% of preterm infants are delivered by CS (RCOG, 2006a) despite no clear evidence of automatic advantage over a vaginal birth (NICE, 2011). CS can be lifesaving for severely compromised babies but involves risks to the fetus: a very small preterm baby can be difficult to deliver by CS; care must be taken to avoid trauma to the fragile skin and tissues. NICE (2011) also states that 10% of CSs performed at 27–28 weeks require a classical (upper segment) uterine incision which may affect a woman's future pregnancies. Many preterm CSs are performed, for fetal or maternal concerns, on women who are not in labour, which skews the statistics: if a woman actually goes into preterm labour she has a more than 50% likelihood of a vaginal birth.

Care immediately after birth

Care will vary depending on the gestation, size and condition of the baby. The main immediate risks are:

- **Heat loss** due to high surface area relative to mass, and less insulating fat.
- **Respiratory difficulty** due to immature lung formation and a reduced ability to endure hypoxia during labour. The more preterm a baby is, the more unlikely it is to establish adequate breathing.

Delayed cord clamping (DCC)

NICE (2007) disappointingly recommends early cord clamping for all actively managed third stages. This advice is being challenged and NICE is reviewing it (see Chapter 1, page 28). Delayed cord clamping is likely to be particularly beneficial for preterm babies. Benefits are likely to outweigh the risks.

The UK Resuscitation Council (UKRC) accepts a possible jaundice risk, but states that DCC for vigorous preterm babies improves blood pressure during stabilisation, reduces intraventricular haemorrhage (IVH) and need for blood transfusion (Rabe *et al.*, 2012; Richmond and Wyllie, 2010). Late-onset sepsis may also be reduced (Mercer *et al.*, 2006). DCC does not pose an immediate threat to the preterm baby in the immediate post-partum adaptation period (Rabe *et al.*, 2012).

There is no consensus over how long to delay clamping. The UKRC suggests that while there is no research to guide DCC for non-vigorous preterm babies, those born in apparently good condition will benefit from DCC of at least one minute or until the cord stops pulsating (Richmond and Wyllie, 2010), and up to 3 minutes gives greater benefits. In fact the UKRC suggests that preterm babies should actually have a longer period with the cord unclamped than term babies, as they will benefit more (Richmond and Wyllie, 2010).

It is possible and beneficial to perform DCC following CS (Cernadas *et al.*, 2006). The baby could be put on the mother's legs or preferably skin-to-skin on her chest.

Having said all this, it may be hard in practice to facilitate DCC for a preterm baby, since the midwife is usually not the only practitioner in control at the point of birth. For only slightly preterm babies one minute or more of DCC may be easier to achieve. However, significantly preterm babies that will require extensive resuscitation – ironically those that probably will benefit from DCC the most! – tend to be whisked off quickly to the resuscitaire. While Rabe *et al.* (2012) suggest that 30–45 seconds of DCC is feasible in preterm infants below 33 weeks, staff may feel anxious about these fragile babies. In theory, initial resuscitation could be carried out on the bed with the baby still attached to the cord between the mother's legs, but in practice there are few paediatricians or neonatal practitioners who would be happy to go along with this. There is likely to be an understandable urgency to get a very preterm and/or floppy baby onto a resuscitaire in a good light. However, as a compromise, it may be possible to 'milk the cord' towards the baby to give an extra transfusion of blood in a short time.

All studies on DCC involve active management of the third stage. It is unlikely that a true physiological third stage (leaving baby attached to the placenta until delivery) would be achieved with a preterm delivery but especially if the baby will require ventilatory support. If the cord is not clamped until the delivery of the placenta, materno-fetal blood transfer will happen naturally.

DCC will reduce the pH of the arterial blood, so if cord blood sampling is performed it is advisable to note the period of delay prior to clamping, to avoid unnecessary concerns and adverse medicolegal implications.

Whenever the cord is cut, leave the baby's end long in case umbilical catheterisation is required later: this is an excellent intravenous access site provided by nature, and can save time and trauma, as IV access can be difficult, especially in very preterm babies.

Skin-to-skin contact

There is good evidence that skin-to-skin contact should be considered the gold standard of care for most preterm babies as there are many physiological and psychological benefits for both mother and baby (see Box 13.1).

It has even been suggested that preterm or LBW infants could be regarded as external fetuses needing skin-to-skin contact to promote maturation (Nyqvis *et al.*, 2010).

If the mother is unable to provide skin-to-skin contact but the baby is in good condition then partners can also provide it.

Box 13.1   Skin-to-skin contact (SSC) at birth in preterm infants.

- **Improves clinical outcomes** in both term and preterm infants (Moore *et al.*, 2007) stabilising the heart rate, respiratory response/rate and oxygen requirements (Bergman *et al.*, 2004; Christenson *et al.*, 1992).
- **Provides better warmth** compared to radiant overhead heaters or incubators (Bergman, 2004) protecting even infants <1500 g (Christenson *et al.*, 1998) against hypothermia.
- **Reduces cardiorespiratory instability:** separated preterm infants weighing 1200–2200 g demonstrate hyperarousal and separation anxiety response patterns (Bergman *et al.*, 2004) many hours following birth, affecting heart rate and respiration. SSC relaxes the baby and normalises breathing and heart rate.
- **Promotes maternal–infant attachment and pleasure** of the mother and her baby, also significantly improves breastfeeding uptake and duration (De Chateau & Wilbert, 1997, Moore *et al.*, 2007) which is particularly beneficial for preterm infants.
- **Promotes earlier positive feelings in fathers** (Sullivan, 1999).
- **Seems to have no side effects** making it the most obvious and sensitive form of care for preterm infants.

SSC should not be pursued, however, if the baby is born in poor condition requiring intensive intervention, e.g. urgent need for intubation and ventilation.

Aim to deliver the baby onto the mother's chest immediately, or as soon as possible. Dry the baby, cover the outer part of the baby with a pre-warmed blanket or space blanket (but do not put it between baby and mother) and put on a hat on the baby (Moore *et al.*, 2012).

Skin-to-skin care may lead into a more prolonged pattern of close contact between mothers and babies, known as kangaroo mother care, i.e. a low birth weight baby kept close to the mother's body (in a similar way to marsupials), placed between her breasts, covered and held in position by her clothes (WHO, 2003).

Kangaroo care has been shown to be exceptionally successful when used in developing countries in place of incubators. If a baby is born unexpectedly at home the mother's body may act as a perfect natural incubator whilst awaiting further assistance.

It must be remembered, however, that there may be times when the urgent clinical needs of the baby outweigh the benefits of skin-to-skin contact, particularly if the baby has significant respiratory difficulty and/or is very preterm.

Resuscitation

Ideally PTBs will take place with an experienced paediatrician or neonatal practitioner in attendance. Midwives should be aware of the principles of preterm resuscitation so that they can assist, or lead the resuscitation if birth occurs unexpectedly, e.g. at home.

Chapter 18 covers neonatal resuscitation in detail, but preterm babies have some specific needs.

Immediate action following birth for babies needing resuscitation

- **Call for help** if experienced assistance is not already present.
- **Assess the baby** visually quickly: pale and floppy or pink and alert?
- **Place** baby between the mother's legs, with the cord still attached and unclamped so the baby can benefit from extra blood and oxygen. Bag and mask ventilation may be carried out with the baby in this position, although if the baby is in very poor condition a resuscitaire may allow better access.
- **If further resuscitation needed** (or paediatrician/neonatal practitioner requests) then clamp and cut the cord (consider milking the cord several times towards the baby first if DCC is not possible) and move baby to a heated resuscitaire.
- When the cord is cut, **leave it long** for possible IV access.
- **Think warmth:** either dry the baby OR place the wet baby in a plastic bag/sheet (e.g. bubble wrap) up to the neck.
- Put a **hat** on the baby.
- **Intubation only by experienced professionals**! Remember it is better to perform good bag and mask ventilation than for an inexperienced intubator to waste time and risk injury to the baby. Most midwives are not trained to intubate as this is a skill which needs to be practised regularly.
- **Ensure equipment is size appropriate:** the mask should make a good seal over nose and mouth with no leaks. Prepare equipment for intubation by an experienced professional: small laryngoscope, endotracheal tubes ≤ 3.0 depending on size of baby.
- **Check the pressure:** ensure that any method of lung inflation has a pressure of 20–25 cm water (normally 30–40 cm for term babies): i.e. 500 ml self-inflating bag with

a blow-off valve set at 20–25 cm, and/or compressed air/oxygen on a resuscitaire with pressure set at 20–25 cm. If heart rate does not improve consider increasing up to 30 cm water but no higher.

- **Avoid excessive chest movement** during inflation especially in <30 week babies as this may cause lung overdistension.
- **Surfactant** is recommended to reduce alveolar surface tension to prevent RDS: administered via an ETT by a specialist health professional (Sinha *et al.*, 2008).
- If chest compressions are required **do them gently** – don't panic; stay calm, stay focused.
- **Handle the baby very gently** as preterm skin is often fragile: dragging towels across the skin may cause damage.

Care related to specific types of preterm labour

Very preterm infants (22–26 weeks)

A very preterm baby is much more likely to die, either at or shortly after birth. EPICure (2008) reports that in England and Wales:

- 7% of UK babies born at 22 weeks survive
- 42% born at 24 weeks survive
- 78% born at 26 weeks survive.

Also in 10–15% PTBs the baby has died before labour starts or has lethal malformations incompatible with life. These very sad situations will come as a shock to the parents and this can be an extremely distressing time. See Chapter 21 for more information on stillbirth and neonatal death.

The increasingly high survival rates of very preterm infants are compounded by corresponding levels of disability, although morbidity is improving due to technical advances such as ventilatory support, administration of corticosteroids and surfactant therapy (Larson *et al.*, 2010). Around 30–50% of live babies born <25 weeks (or weighing <750g at birth) have a moderate or severe disability (Costeloe *et al.*, 2000; Tyson *et al.*, 2008).

Care for very preterm labour should include:

- An ultrasound scan to confirm fetal presentation, and possibly serious abnormalities (Keirse, 2000).
- Staff trained in neonatal resuscitation and thermal care of neonates and at least one clinician experienced in tracheal intubation should attend the birth of any baby <28 weeks (CESDI, 2003).
- Prior to the birth the parents should be able to discuss with an experienced paediatrician the prognosis and likely events following the birth, and whether or not to commence treatment or resuscitation in a very preterm or extremely ill baby. This discussion should be documented.
- Due to heightened emotions and anxiety many parents find it difficult to process information. Staff must be prepared to repeat explanations and talk in sensitive, understandable terms about the possible outcome, however bleak, for the baby.

Breech presentation

Breech presentation is more common in preterm infants and is associated with an increased incidence of congenital abnormality, stillbirth and neonatal mortality than cephalic preterm infants (Keirse, 2000). Preterm breech infants are also more likely to present with incomplete presentations, e.g. footling, with associated risks of umbilical cord prolapse and a premature urge to push. The optimal mode of delivery for preterm breech has not been fully evaluated in clinical trials and the relative risks for the preterm infant and mother remain unclear. RCOG (2006a) advise against routine CS for preterm breech, and advise discussion on an individual basis with the woman and her partner. A CS would be more likely to be recommended for a complicated breech presentation, e.g. footling.

See Chapter 14 for more information on breech birth.

Multiple pregnancies

Around 50% of multiple pregnancies deliver preterm, making up 12% of all PTBs (Ananth and Vintzileos, 2006) and women expecting multiples are usually aware of this possibility. The risks are greater than for singleton PTB. A second-born twin has a higher risk of a poor perinatal outcome than the first-born, although again optimal mode of delivery is unclear and likely to depend on individual circumstances (Hofmeyr *et al.*, 2011). See Chapter 15 for more information on multiple births.

Preterm birth at home

Unplanned, quick birth at home is usually very straightforward, in itself, but can occasionally present the midwife with a compromised preterm baby. Sometimes the mother too is unwell; indeed this may have caused her preterm labour.

Hypothermia is extremely serious in preterm babies (CESDI, 2003) and is the primary risk for babies 'born before arrival' (BBA) (Loughney *et al.*, 2006). Dry the baby thoroughly at birth, and give skin-to-skin contact promptly with the mother (see Box 13.1 for benefits). In addition, put a hat on the baby and cover well. Keep the room warm. If you decide to use a plastic bag (e.g. if the baby has to be separated from the mother for resuscitation), do not dry the baby. A food grade bag, e.g. roasting bag, is perfectly suitable, although there may be raised eyebrows at your request.

Hospital transfer is advisable for any baby <35–36 weeks; many preterm babies appear well at delivery but can develop respiratory and other difficulties in the hours following birth.

Unless the baby requires active resuscitation, consider skin-to-skin 'kangaroo care' for transfer. Ambulance staff may be reluctant to transfer an 'unsecured' baby but may relent when the benefits are explained.

See Chapter 6 for more information on home birth and BBA.

Postnatal care

This book is not the forum for a detailed account of postnatal care of a preterm baby. However, the midwife has a key role in promoting the importance of a preterm baby

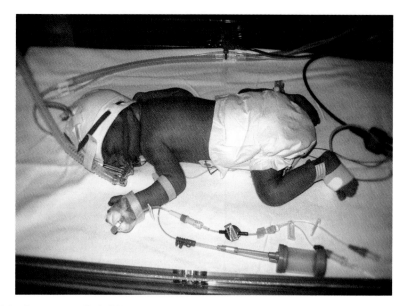

Fig. 13.2   Parents may find NICU technology intimidating.

having breastmilk. Preterm babies are those who benefit the most from natural milk, and who are most damaged by artificial milk. Early hand/pump expressing, freezing breast milk if necessary for future use, should be encouraged. Even if the mother has no intention of ultimately breastfeeding, she may agree to give at least one or two first feeds of colostrum to help protect her fragile baby.

Much psychological support is need for families with preterm babies. It is important to monitor women postnatally for PND. Wherever possible attempt to see the woman and her family at home following discharge of the baby from hospital, and give her time to talk through the experience.

Summary

- Communicate clearly with parents and be prepared to repeat information.
- Main risks of PTB are hypothermia and respiratory difficulty.
- Ideally specialist staff should be available, but PTB can happen anywhere, any time: be prepared to take control.
- Keep the room warm.
- Always put a hat on the baby.
- Encourage DCC or try to milk the cord towards the baby if separation is necessary.
- Encourage mother-baby skin-to-skin contact unless the baby needs immediate and intensive attention.
- If baby has to be separated either dry it well OR put it wet into a plastic bag with face exposed: ALWAYS keep warm even during resuscitation.
- Remember basic principles of resuscitation; use size appropriate equipment.
- Good bag and mask ventilation should be adequate until specialist help arrives.
- Drop ventilator equipment pressures to 20–25 cm water (term: 30–40 cm water).

Evidence supports:

- Antenatal corticosteroid administration 24–34 weeks
- Maternal antibiotic administration if PPROM or suspected maternal infection.

Evidence supports *avoiding*:

- ARM or 'routine' VE
- Narcotic analgesia
- Active pushing
- Supine maternal position
- FBS
- Ventouse/forceps
- Non-indicated episiotomy
- Early clamping of the umbilical cord.

Useful contacts

BLISS, The Premature Baby Charity www.bliss.org.uk
Tommy's the Baby Charity Research, education and information for parents and professionals. www.tommys-campaign.org

References

Alfirevic, Z., Devane, D., Gyte, G. M. (2007) Continuous cardiotocography (CTG) as a form of electronic fetal monitoring (EFM) for fetal assessment during labour (Review). *Cochrane Library*. Issue 3.

Ananth, C. V., Vintzileos, A. M. (2006) Epidemiology of preterm birth and its clinical subtypes. *Journal of Maternal Fetal and Neonatal Medicine* 19(12), 773–82.

Briley, A., Crawshaw, S., Hughes, J. (2002) *Premature Labour – Information for Parents*. London, Tommy's the Baby Charity.

Cernadas, J. M. C., Carroli, G., Lardizabal, J. (2006) Effect of timing of cord clamping on neonatal venous hematocrit values and clinical outcome at term: a randomized, controlled trial *Pediatrics* 118(3), 1318–9.

CESDI (2003) *Project 27/28: An Enquiry into Quality and Care and its Effect on Survival of Babies Born at 27/28 Weeks*. London, The Stationery Office.

Costeloe, K., Hennessy, E., Gibson, A. (2000) EPICure study: outcomes to discharge from hospitals for infants born at the threshold of viability *Pediatrics* 106, 659–71.

EPIcure (2008) *Survival after Birth before 27 Weeks of Gestation*. http://www.epicure.ac.uk/overview

Figueroa, D., Rouse, D. J. (2010) Location, mode of delivery and intrapartum issues for the preterm gestation. In Berghella, V. (ed.) *Preterm Birth: Prevention and Management*. Chichester, Wiley Blackwell.

Goldenberg, R. L., McLure, E. M. (2010) The epidemiology of preterm birth. In Berghella, V. (ed.) *Preterm Birth: Prevention and Management*. Chichester, Wiley Blackwell.

Goldenberg, R. L., Hauth, J. C., Andrews, W. W. (2000) Intrauterine infection and preterm delivery. *New England Journal of Medicine* 342, 1500–7.

Gupta, J., Hofmeyr, G., Shehmar, M. (2012) Position in the second stage of labour for women without epidural anaesthesia. *Cochrane database of systematic reviews*, Issue 5.

Hodnett, E. D., Hofmeyr, G. J., Sakala, C., Weston, J. (2011) Continuous support for women during childbirth. *Cochrane database of systematic reviews*, Issue 2. http://library.nhs.uk/evidence/

Hofmeyr, G., Barrett, J., Crowther, C. (2011) Planned caesarean section for women with a twin pregnancy. *Cochrane database of systematic reviews*. http://summaries.cochrane.org/CD006553/planned-caesarean-section-for-women-with-a-twin-pregnancy

JFC (Joint Formulary Committee) (2012) *British National Formulary*, 63rd ed. London: BMJ Group and Pharmaceutical Press.

Kent, A., Wright, I., Abdel-Latif, M., The New South Wales and Australian Capital Territory Neonatal Intensive Care Units Audit Group (2011) Mortality and adverse neurologic outcomes are greater in preterm male infants. *Pediatrics* (10), 1542–78.

Kenyon, S., Taylor, D., Tarnow-Mordi, W. (2001) Broad spectrum antibiotics for spontaneous preterm labour: the ORACLE I randomised trial. *Lancet* 375, 979–88.

Keirse, M. (2000) In Enkin, M., Keirse, M., Neilson, J. (eds) *A Guide to Effective Care in Pregnancy and Childbirth* 3rd edn. Oxford, Oxford University Press.

Larson, J. E., Desai, S. A., McNett, W. (2010) Perinatal care and long-term implications. In Berghella, V. (ed.) *Preterm Birth: Prevention and Management*. Chichester, Wiley-Blackwell.

Lawn, J. E., Cousens, S., Zupan, J. for the Neonatal Survival Steering Team (2005) Four million neonatal deaths: When? Where? Why? *Lancet* 365, 891–900.

Lucey, J. F., Rowan, C. A., Shiono, P., Wilkinson, A. R., Kilpatrick, S., Payne, N. R., Horbar, J. D., Carpenter, J., Rogowski, J., Soll, R. F. (2004) Fetal infants: the fate of 4172 infants with birthweights of 401 to 500 grams – the Vermont Oxford Network experience (1996–2000). *Pediatrics* 113, 1559–66.

Loughney, A., Collis, R., Dastgir, S. (2006) Birth before arrival at delivery suite: Associations and consequences. *British Journal of Midwifery* 14(4), 204–8.

Mercer, J. S., Vohr, B. R., McGrath, M. M., Padbury, J. F., Wallach, M., Oh, W. (2006) Delayed cord clamping in very preterm infants reduces the incidence of intraventricular hemorrhage and late-onset sepsis: a randomized, controlled trial. *Pediatrics* 117(4), 1235–42.

Moore, E. R., Anderson, G. C., Bergman, N., Dowswell, T. (2012) Early skin-to-skin contact for mothers and their healthy newborn infants. *Cochrane Database of Systematic Reviews*, Issue 5.

NICE (2007) *Clinical Guideline 55: Intrapartum Care*. London, National Institute for Health and Clinical Excellence. http://guidance.nice.org.uk/CG55/Guidance

NICE (2011) *Clinical Guideline 132: Caesarean Section*. London, NICE. www.nice.org.uk

Nyqvis, K. H., Anderson, G. C., Bergman, N., Cattaneo, A., Charpak, N., Davanzo, R., Ewald, U., Ibe, O., Ludington-Hoe, S., Mendoza, S., Pallás-Allonso, C., Ruiz Peláez, J. G., Sizun, J., Widström, A.-M. (2010) Towards universal Kangaroo Mother Care: recommendations and report from the First European conference and Seventh International Workshop on Kangaroo Mother Care. *Acta Pædiatrica* 99, 820–6.

ONS (Office for National Statistics) (2007) *Preterm Births, Preterm births data*. http://www.ons.gov.uk/ons/publications/re-reference-tables.html?edition=tcm%3A77-50818

Rabe, H., Diaz-Rossello, J., Duley, L., Dowswell, T. (2012) Effect of timing of umbilical cord clamping and other strategies to influence placental transfusion at preterm birth on maternal and infant outcomes. *Cochrane Database of Systematic Reviews*, Issue 8.

RCOG (Royal College of Obstetricians and Gynaecologists) (2006a) *The Management of Breech Presentation. Guideline No. 20b*. London, RCOG. http://www.rcog.org.uk/womens-health/clinical-guidance/management-breech-presentation-green-top-20b

RCOG (2006b, revised 2010) *Preterm, Prelabour Rupture of Membranes. Green Top Guideline 44.* London, RCOG *http://www.rcog.org.uk/womens-health/clinical-guidance/preterm-prelabour-rupture-membranes-green-top-44*

RCOG (2002, revised 2011) *Tocolytic Drugs for Women in Preterm Labour. Green Top Guideline 1b.* London, RCOG. http://www.rcog.org.uk/womens-health/clinical-guidance/tocolytic-drugs-women-preterm-labour-green-top-1b

Richmond, S., Wyllie, J. (2010) *Newborn Life Support.* Resuscitation Council (UK). http://www.resus.org.uk/pages/nls.pdf

Roberts, D., Dalziel, S. (2007) Antenatal corticosteroids for accelerating fetal lung maturation for women at risk of preterm birth. *Cochrane Database of Systematic Reviews,* Issue 4.

Saigal, S., Doyle, L. W. (2008) An overview of mortality and sequelae of preterm birth from infancy to adulthood. *Lancet* 371, 261–9.

Shah, V. S., Ohlsson, A., Halliday, H. L., Dunn, M. (2012) Early administration of inhaled corticosteroids for preventing chronic lung disease in ventilated very low birth weight preterm neonates. *Cochrane Database of Systematic Reviews,* Issue 5.

Sinha, S. K., Gupta, S., Donn, S. M. (2008) Immediate respiratory management of the preterm infant (2008) *Seminars in Fetal and Neonatal Medicine* 13(1), 24–9.

Tucker, J., McGuire, W. (2004) Epidemiology of preterm birth. *British Medical Journal* 329, 675–8.

Tyson, J., Parikh, N., Langer, J., Green, C., Higgins, R. (2008) Intensive care for extreme prematurity: moving beyond gestational age. *New England Journal of Medicine* 358, 1672–81.

Walkinshaw, S. (2001) In Chamberlin, G., Steer, P. (2001) (eds) *Turnbull's Obstetrics,* 3rd edn. London, Churchill Livingstone.

World Health Organization (WHO) (2003) *Kangaroo Mother Care: A Practical Guide.* WHO. http://www.who.int/maternal_child_adolescent/documents/9241590351/en/

14 Breech birth

Lesley Shuttler

Introduction

Breech presentation is where the lie of the baby is longitudinal and the baby's buttocks are in the lower segment of the mother's uterus.

Following the term breech trial (TBT) (Hannah *et al.*, 2000), midwives today may have limited experience of seeing, or being involved in caring for, a woman having a vaginal breech birth. They may approach a vaginal breech birth with the same lack of confidence and fear observed in inexperienced obstetricians. However, midwives need to remember that in carefully selected/assessed women, vaginal breech birth can be a safe and fulfilling birth option (Alarab *et al.*, 2004; RCOG, 2006a; Glezerman, 2006; Maier *et al.*, 2011; Michel *et al.*, 2011). Midwives should have the skills to assist a planned spontaneous breech birth where the labour is progressing well, and recognise when it is not.

Approximately one third of all breech presentations are undiagnosed at onset of labour (Evans, 2012a). It is, therefore, important that midwives are prepared to deal with this eventuality and that they have the training, knowledge and skills to assist the woman and her baby (CMACE, 2011; Robinson, 2000). There is no research to support caesarean section (CS) as the optimum method of delivery in these cases.

The Midwife's Labour and Birth Handbook, Third Edition. Edited by Vicky Chapman and Cathy Charles.
© 2013 John Wiley & Sons, Ltd. Published 2013 by John Wiley & Sons, Ltd.

Incidence

- 25% of babies adopt a breech position at some time in pregnancy; 3–4% remain breech at term (RCOG, 2006a).
- The TBT (Hannah *et al.*, 2000) has increased breech caesarean rates. The UK CS rate for breech was 69% in 1993 (RCOG, 2001). In England now it is 90%, with 57% elective CS (Bragg *et al.*, 2010), and in Ireland 92.3% (Fitzpatrick *et al.*, 2011): other countries have had similar increases.
- 20% of UK stillbirths and 28% of neonatal deaths are breech presentation; of these 88% of stillbirths and 73% of neonatal deaths are delivered vaginally. However, presentation is unlikely to be causally related to death (CMACE, 2011). Many vaginal breech births are unexpected preterm births, which in themselves carry a higher risk of mortality.

Facts

- Many babies appear to adopt a breech presentation for no particular reason. However, a minority will adopt a breech position because of problems such as short or entangled cord, prematurity, placenta praevia, uterine or fetal abnormalities.
- Irrespective of mode of delivery, breech presentation is associated with increased subsequent disability; in a few cases failure to adopt a cephalic presentation may be a marker for fetal impairment (RCOG, 2006a).
- For a woman with predisposing factors like diabetes, fetopelvic disproportion, a previous macrosomic baby, or a suspected large baby and poor labour progress, a CS is usually advisable (RCOG, 2006a).
- Evidence suggests that external cephalic version (ECV) should be offered to all women with an uncomplicated breech baby at term (37–42 weeks) (NICE, 2003; RCOG, 2006b).
- Following TBT, the RCOG (2006a) advises, 'Women should be advised that planned (breech) CS carries a reduced perinatal mortality and early neonatal morbidity … compared with planned vaginal birth', but the TBT trial has been criticised for clinical and methodological flaws. Later follow-up of TBT babies showed that while initial perinatal deaths for planned CS were lower, more babies died later: by two years old infant death rates and neurodevelopmental delay were the same for CS and vaginal delivery groups (Whyte *et al.*, 2004).
- Women should be facilitated to make an informed choice about their birth options and should not be coerced into one particular mode of delivery. These discussions should include the possible differences between a 'managed' vaginal breech birth and one 'facilitated' by a skilled practitioner.
- Breech babies usually have a good heart rate at birth but may be slower to breathe spontaneously than cephalic babies, and may require bag-and-mask ventilation to establish breathing.

Types of breech presentation

The baby in a breech presentation will adopt a variety of positions, similar to a cephalic baby, with the sacrum being the denominator. Table 14.1 illustrates different breech presentations.

Table 14.1   Types of breech presentation.

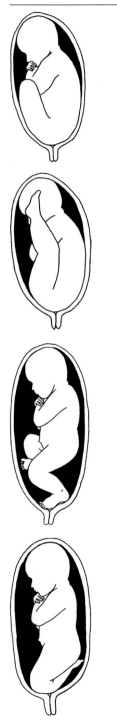

Complete (flexed or full breech)
Incidence: 10% of term and preterm breeches (Frye, 2010)

The baby sits cross-legged with flexed knees and hips: feet are tucked up against its bottom

This position is most common in multigravidae

Extended (incomplete or frank breech)
Incidence: 45–50% (AAFP, 2012) or 60–70% (Frye, 2010) of term breeches

The baby's legs are flexed at the hip but with straight knees: the legs lie alongside the trunk

This position is most common in primigravidae near term as knee flexion is restricted by firm uterine and abdominal muscles

Footling
Incidence: 20–25% of preterm breeches and 10–20% (Frye, 2010) or 35–45% (AAFP, 2012) of term breeches

One or both knees and/or hips are extended with one or more feet below the buttocks

Knee/kneeling
Incidence: <5% of term breeches (Frye, 2010)

One or both hips are extended and the knees are flexed: the knees are at the height of or below the buttocks

This is the rarest presentation

Others
Occasionally a presentation may be compound, e.g. one leg footling, the other extended

Women's options and the provision of care

Midwives need to explore their own feelings and prejudices and remain unbiased and non-judgemental, acting in a manner that will facilitate both informed choice and decision-making as well as enabling the woman to access appropriate care.

- Explore the options: ECV, managed vaginal delivery, physiological breech birth, CS; home or hospital.
- Women can choose who assists at the birth: an NHS/independent midwife, or an obstetrician.
- Discuss the possible difference between a vaginal breech birth that is 'managed' and one that is 'facilitated' by a skilled practitioner/midwife. Managed/medicalised breech birth tends to include a package of epidural anaesthesia, routine episiotomy and lithotomy position for the delivery. A facilitated birth encourages the breech baby to birth through supporting the woman in upright postures and only inter-vening should a direct indication arise.
- Choice may be restricted due to 'local policy' or a lack of suitably skilled practition-ers.
- Where a hospital is unable to safely offer the woman the option of a vaginal breech birth, she should be referred to another practitioner or hospital where this choice is available (RCOG, 2006a).

Self-help measures

A woman may wish to try self-help measures to turn a breech antenatally, promoting a feeling of active involvement. Methods include postural management, e.g. knee-chest position and pelvic rocking, visualisation, swimming, massage, talking to her baby and complementary therapies such as hypnotherapy, homeopathy, acupuncture, acupres-sure, moxibustion, chiropractic or osteopathic intervention. There is little hard evidence for any of these methods. Only acupuncture and moxibustion have undergone ran-domised controlled trials (RCTs) (Neri *et al.*, 2004; Coyle *et al.*, 2005). Whilst results look promising, the evidence base is incomplete for these and all self-help/complementary measures. Do *et al.* (2011) plan to undertake another RCT into moxibustion for cephalic version, concluding that it is an acceptable option for both women and clincians, and could increase choice or women if it proves effective.

External cephalic version

All women should be offered information about the safety and benefits of ECV at term. When it is undertaken by a trained operator, the success rate is around 50%. This rate, however, may vary from 30 to 80% depending on several factors including engagement of the breech, liquor volume, uterine tone, race and parity (RCOG, 2006b).

- The success rate of ECV may be increased by the use of tocolysis (RCOG, 2006b).
- Following successful ECV, spontaneous reversion to breech presentation is quoted as <5% (Impey and Lissoni, 1999).
- Hofmeyr (2000) suggests that even during labour, if the membranes remain intact ECV with tocolysis appears to have a reasonable success rate.

- Rhesus negative women who have ECV performed should be offered anti-D prophylaxis (NICE, 2002).

The use of ECV before term (i.e. 34–35 weeks), whilst increasing the likelihood of cephalic presentation at birth, does not appear to reduce the CS rate and may increase the rate of preterm birth (Hutton and Hofmeyr, 2006; Hutton *et al.*, 2011).

Caesarean section

Many obstetricians now recommend CS for breech presentation regardless of individual circumstances. This is primarily due to the TBT (Hannah *et al.*, 2000), which reported an increased 1% mortality risk and 2.4% early neonatal morbidity risk in breech vaginal delivery over CS. Hannah *et al.* concluded: 'planned caesarean section is better than planned vaginal birth for the term fetus in the breech presentation'. Whilst this recommendation has been largely accepted and implemented by obstetricians, others have challenged it (Robinson, 2000/2001; Banks, 2001; Gyte, 2001; Lancet Correspondence, 2001). One criticism is that the 'vaginal' breech deliveries in the TBT were dorsal 'managed' breech extractions, and women were not allowed to labour in upright positions. Some women also moved from their randomised groups, potentially confounding the result. Glezerman (2006, 2012) concludes that in the light of serious methodological and clinical flaws 'the original term breech trial recommendations should be withdrawn'. Alarab *et al.* (2004) state that with strict selection criteria, adherence to a careful intrapartum protocol and an experienced obstetrician in attendance a vaginal breech delivery at term can be achieved safely.

In a 2-year follow-up study to the TBT (Whyte *et al.*, 2004), an unexpectedly high number of babies born by breech CS showed later neurodevelopmental delay, which balanced the smaller numbers of perinatal deaths in that group. It was concluded that 'planned cesarean delivery is not associated with a reduction in risk of death or neurodevelopmental delay in children at 2 years of age'. Another observational prospective study with an intent-to-treat analysis demonstrated a lower mortality and morbidity than the TBT (Goffinet *et al.*, 2006), and this is replicated in other studies (Maier *et al.*, 2011; Michel *et al.*, 2011).

Cochrane review of three studies (including Hannah) also found that planned caesarean section compared with planned vaginal birth reduced perinatal or neonatal death (i.e. mortality at or soon after birth) but that since at two years there were no differences in the outcome 'death or neurodevelopmenatal delay': any neonatal benefits came 'at the expense of somewhat increased maternal morbidity' (Hofmeyr *et al.*, 2003).

The practice of CS for breech babies in the belief that it is safer may become a self-fulfilling prophecy as attendants become less skilled in vaginal breech birth. With a rising breech CS rate too, few clinicians have vaginal breech experience (RCOG, 2006a). It is to be hoped that in the next few years, the debate following the TBT will lead to a better understanding of breech issues, and that women will not be pressured into CS without proper consideration of the relative risks.

RCOG (2006a) Guidelines for the Management of Breech Presentation state:

- Women should be fully informed on all aspects relating to breech birth both for current and future pregnancies and have careful assessment before selection for vaginal breech birth.

- Induction of labour may be considered if individual circumstances are favourable.
- Augmentation in labour is not advisable. Slow progress at any stage should be considered as possible fetopelvic disproportion, and a CS may then be indicated.
- Routine CS for a preterm breech baby should not be advised.
- Diagnosis of breech presentation during labour should not be a contraindication for vaginal breech birth.
- In a twin pregnancy where the first baby is breech, it is suggested that the data relating to a singleton breech can be used to aid decision-making. Where the second twin is breech, the RCOG (2006a) states that routine CS should not be performed. (For more information on twins see Chapter 15.)

Midwives are strongly advised to read and evaluate all the literature for themselves. It may also fall to them to inform colleagues, managers and obstetricians of current national guidelines.

Concerns and possible complications with a breech birth

Hypoxia

Hypoxia has been identified as the commonest cause of death in breech babies. CESDI (2000) suggests that lack of recognition and inaction are major factors. Causes include cord compression and head entrapment. These risks may be largely due to the lack of an experienced birth attendant.

Umbilical cord prolapse

Incidence: 3.7% in breech presentation (primigravidae 6%, multigravidae 3%) (Confino *et al.*, 1985).

Umbilical cord prolapse is more common in preterm labour and incomplete presentations (e.g. footling), and following artificial rupture of membranes (ARM). Prolapse does not always cause cord compression. If the cervix is fully dilated, a vaginal birth may still be possible (see Chapter 17).

Entrapment of aftercoming head

Incidence: 0–8.5% at term (Cheng and Hannah, 1993).

It is thought that if the diameters of a baby's bottom are smaller than those of its head it is more likely to pass through a cervix that is not fully dilated. This is much more likely if the baby is premature, as the head-to-body ratio is different from that of a full term baby. This may result in the entrapment of the aftercoming head behind a partially open cervix.

However, the specific presentation of the breech baby appears significant. It has been suggested that the diameters of the term breech baby's bottom will be the same size as the head (Stevenson, 1993), with the bitrochanteric diameter measuring around 9 cm, similar to the average biparietal diameter of 9.5 cm (Frye, 2010).

- 'If the frank or complete breech passes easily through the pelvis, the head can be expected to follow without difficulty' (Hofmeyr, 2000).

- In a term baby, if the head is not going to pass through the cervix and pelvis, the buttocks would also be obstructed and labour will not progress (Hofmeyr, 2001 citing Gebbie, 1982).
- Entrapment is more common in a preterm baby (Stevenson, 1993) and may be related to maternal pushing being encouraged prior to, or following, misdiagnosis of full dilatation.

Deflexion and hyperextension (star gazing) of the baby's head

Incidence of hyperextension: 5% (Confino *et al.*, 1985).

Deflexion of the head may resolve spontaneously in the course of labour, or may require help at point of birth (by using the Mauriceau-Smellie-Veit manoeuvre – see later in chapter). If **hyperextension** (more extreme deflexion) of the head is detected by ultrasound scan (USS) at term, a CS is normally advised. However, whilst hyperextension is less likely to resolve, the diameters would be the same as a face presentation if the baby had been a cephalic presentation (Evans, personal communication).

Deflexion and hyperextension may occur due to:

- Cord around baby's neck
- Placental location
- Muscle spasm in baby
- Fetal or uterine abnormalities
- Unnecessary intervention during labour: spontaneous pushing, not traction, should be encouraged; traction may cause extension of the baby's arms and head (Hofmeyr, 2000).

Head and neck trauma

Forceful traction by the carer may cause iatrogenic brain and spinal injuries (Banks, 1998).

Premature placental separation

This may be linked to maternal position in the second stage of labour, especially where the woman adopts a standing position. This may be due to the centre of gravity being higher in a breech than in a cephalic birth, resulting in more traction being placed on the cord and placenta by gravity (Cronk, 1998).

Labour and birth

Preparation/birth planning

Frank and open discussion between the midwife, the woman and her partner, exploring all options available, will help the woman reach a decision about whether or not to have a vaginal breech birth. It may also clarify issues for the woman and enable her to develop an appropriate and individual birth plan.

Points to consider include the following:

- The baby is in a good position and not considered too large.
- A skilled and competent midwife should support the woman in a breech birth.
- The woman, her partner and the midwife are informed regarding the anticipated process and progress of a breech labour and birth.
- The woman has confidence in her body and her midwife.
- Good communication between the woman and the midwife at all times.

The midwife's role

- To support the woman and have confidence in her innate ability to birth her baby
- To act as advocate for the woman at all times
- To keep the atmosphere relaxed during labour and birth with an awareness of the hormonal physiology and how it affects labour
- Not to 'manage' the woman's care or labour process; to encourage and enable the woman to respond intuitively and express her own needs and wishes
- To ensure and maintain a sound knowledge of skills and techniques to assist a breech birth, should it become necessary
- To recognise, assess and respond to problems, should they occur

It is important that midwives ensure they have appropriate support for themselves. Having a colleague present who is experienced in non-medicalised breech birth will provide support for the midwife.

Mechanisms of a breech birth

Midwives should refer to a suitable textbook to familiarise themselves with the various mechanisms. Very detailed and comprehensive descriptions, supported by diagrams, can be found in the book by Anne Frye (2010), and in two articles by Jane Evans (2012a, b).

Onset of labour

Midwifery care and support is the same as for any labour: consent should be obtained at all stages.

- Palpate the abdomen to check presentation and position of the baby.
- A vaginal examination (VE) in early breech labour is often recommended to determine the presenting part and any cord, foot, knee or compound presentation. Cervical dilatation may be minimal at this stage. Evans (2012a), however, cautions against an early VE unless the information cannot be gained any other way, as it could disturb the woman and interrupt her labour. She suggests that if labour appears to be progressing well then the presenting part may not be important, and careful FH monitoring will usually pick up a problematic cord prolapse.
- The presenting part is often higher in the pelvis than the midwife would expect with a cephalic presentation, and the station is likely to go up and down more during labour (Cooper, 1992).

Box 14.1   Upright maternal positions for labour and birth.

In the absence of conclusive research in breech birth positions, the following are suggested:

Squatting
- Expands the pelvic outlet.
- Advocated by Odent (1984) as being mechanically efficient, gravity reduces the delay between delivery of the baby's umbilicus and its head. Less likely to need intervention to assist birth.
- Squatting (even supported) is tiring and may need to be practised during pregnancy.
- Squatting may increase blood loss (but this may be due to ease of measuring it).

Standing
- Believed by some to be more natural physiological position for labour as gravity aids descent.
- Cronk (1998) speculates, however, that standing for the birth itself:
  - Causes a quicker birth which may cause rapid head decompression.
  - May encourage the baby's arms to be swept over its head, complicating their delivery and risking Erb's palsy.
  - May increase traction on cord and placenta risking early separation and/or hypoxia.
- As the baby's body hangs straight down, this may encourage a deflexed head.
- May increase perineal tearing and blood loss.

Kneeling / hands and knees
- Complements the attitude and angle of the uterus.
- Gravity helps the baby descend.
- Allows the baby's body and arms to manoeuvre naturally (Evans, 2012a).
- Prevents undue traction or pressure on the placenta or cord.
- Facilitates the birth of the baby's head (Evans, 2012b).

- If the woman is examined in a semi-recumbent position, assist her into her chosen position immediately afterwards. An upright position (Box 14.1) avoids problems such as postural hypotension, fetal heart rate (FHR) irregularities and slowing of labour progress (Sleep *et al.*, 2000; Gupta *et al.*, 2007). However, Evans says that a woman might not wish to labour in an upright position, and '... where I have observed women lying down it has been for a reason that was not apparent until the actual birth' (personal communication).

Pain management

Encourage the woman to apply skills she may have learnt antenatally such as relaxation, visualisation, vocalisation and mobility. Use massage, TENS, and other means of labour support.

The use of a birthing pool is controversial and needs to be explored on an individual basis according to the wishes of the woman, the experience of the individual midwife and the place of the birth. The benefits of water are well documented (see Chapter 3), and those benefits, it could be argued, would be of use to a woman having a spontaneous vaginal breech birth, especially in the first stage of labour. This may prove challenging for both the woman and her carer where local guidelines on the use of a birthing pool exclude any presentation other than cephalic.

Midwives interested in exploring the use of water in breech presentation (and other unusual situations) may find work by Dr Herman Ponette in Belgium and Cornelia Enning in Germany helpful (see 'Useful contacts'). UK midwife breech experts Mary Cronk and Jane Evans do not recommend actually birthing in the pool. Evans (2012a) says:

> *'Although ... some practitioners ... support the practice of breech water births, I personally advise against actually giving birth in water when the baby is a breech presentation. This is because the buoyancy of the water works against gravity and impedes the mechanisms. If the breech presentation is undiagnosed and the woman is in the pool already, she will often instinctively adopt a semi-reclining position which allows the buoyancy of the water to lift the baby in a way similar to the Burns Marshall manoeuvre. When such a birth is progressing rapidly it is important to keep the birthing room very calm and just observe progress before disturbing the woman, by asking her to exit the pool. It may be better to proceed with an underwater birth than to interrupt it unless help is needed.'*

There is no evidence that the routine use of an epidural is appropriate in a vaginal breech birth; women should have a choice of analgesia (RCOG, 2006a). Obstetricians may recommend it believing that it may prevent the premature urge to push and also enable them to carry out obstetric manoeuvres. This may be acceptable to the woman and be part of her decision-making process. Evans (2012a), however, warns that an epidural may block the sensations that the woman's body and baby are sending her, and thus reduce the spontaneous movements she makes in response. Women need to be fully informed of the risks and benefits of an epidural including the restrictions it may place on them in terms of mobility and the inability to adopt upright positions to facilitate a spontaneous breech birth.

First stage

- Care and observations are the same as for a cephalic birth (see Chapter 1):
  - Avoid unnecessary VEs
  - Use midwifery skills to monitor external signs of progress
  - The woman should eat and drink as she wishes
  - Encourage regular emptying of the bladder
- There may be a long latent phase due to a lack of application of the presenting part to the cervix, but progress may escalate rapidly once an active first stage is reached.
- The woman may feel breathless during or after contractions due to the pressure of the baby's head against her diaphragm. She may experience the pain more in her back than the front.
- Multigravidae may experience little or no discomfort in early labour; it is not unusual for the cervix to be 4 cm dilated before they become aware they are in labour (El Halta, 2010).
- No ARM. If membranes rupture spontaneously, check the fetal heart for any effects of cord compression, and consider VE to exclude cord prolapse.

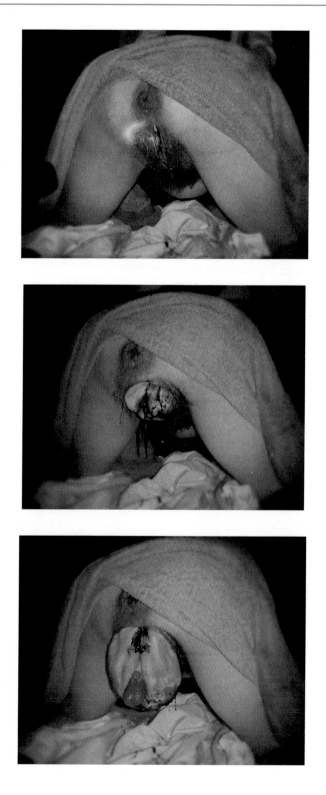

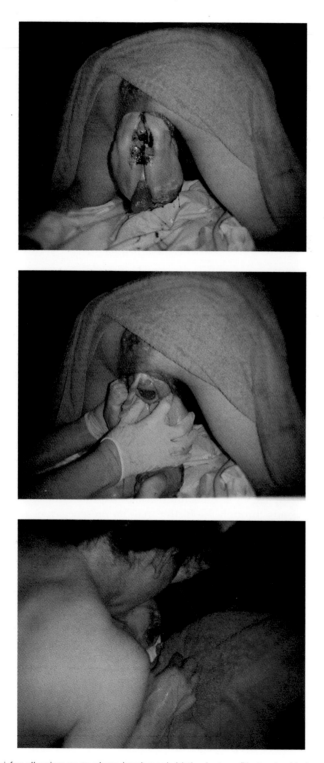

We thank Jacqui for allowing us to share her breech birth photos. *Photos by kind permission of Joy Horner (www.birthjoy.co.uk).*

- No augmentation of labour.
- The RCOG (2006a) states that continuous electronic fetal monitoring (EFM) should be offered to women with a breech presentation in labour, and local guidelines/policy may reflect this. Advancements in fetal monitoring equipment and the provision of systems that can provide continuous waterproof EFM have already been developed and are available (Price, 2001).
- A woman may choose or decline to comply with unit policy EFM. If used, do so in a way to encourage mobility rather than restrict it.
- Fetal blood sampling from the buttocks is not advised (RCOG, 2006a).
- A premature urge to push is unlikely in the term breech baby. The hip size in an extended or flexed term breech baby is likely to equal the head size (Stevenson, 1993). It is more likely to occur if the baby is in (or rotating from) a posterior positon. Suggest the woman adopts the knee–chest position and help her to breathe through the contractions until the urge to push has passed or her cervix is fully dilated.

Second stage

A latent phase may occur, as with cephalic birth, between full dilatation and the spontaneous urge to push. The woman will often doze during this period. Second-stage contractions are often less frequent, shorter and less powerful. Maternal anal dilatation and pressure may 'diagnose' the second stage, or a gentle VE may be used to confirm full dilatation. In principle, remember: 'hands off the breech'. Just watch, wait and support. If a baby requires assistance, refer to Table 14.2 for assisted breech delivery techniques.

- Multigravidae may experience the descent of the baby as feeling different from a previous cephalic baby.
- Frank 'toothpaste tube' meconium is to be expected due to the pressure on the baby as it descends through the birth canal. Its presence does not necessarily indicate that the baby is, or has been, distressed (Hulme, 1992). However, meconium-stained *liquor* should be assessed and responded to the same as for a cephalic baby. Frye (2010) suggests that if is evident prior to 6 cm dilatation, it should be considered as a possible sign of fetal compromise.
- When the buttocks reach the perineum, it may be necessary to do an episiotomy if it is tight or not stretching despite good contractions and maternal effort, or to expedite the birth for fetal compromise. The RCOG (2006a) supports the use of selective rather than routine episiotomy in breech birth. Ulander *et al.* (2004) found less perineal damage with a breech than with a cephalic presentation.
- Banks (1998) suggests that if the membranes are intact, they should be broken when the buttocks reach the perineum to allow any meconium to drain from the vagina. However, the close fit of the baby's bottom in the vagina usually prevents meconium from getting to the liquor around the baby's head, and the membranes usually release spontaneously as the legs are born.
- A rocking or up-and-down motion during the descent of the baby's bottom ('rumping') is the same process as that of 'crowning'.

The birth

- No touching unless absolutely necessary or there is a complication (see Table 14.2 for techniques to assist a breech birth).
- General observations of the baby throughout the birth should include the colour of the baby, the tone of the baby and the vitality of the cord, once it is visible. These should be recorded and the birth expedited and support called for if there appears to be a problem.
- The buttocks are born by lateral flexion. Simultaneously the body rotates so that the shoulders drop into the transverse diameter of the pelvic brim (the widest diameter).
- Descent continues as the pelvis, thighs, then knees emerge.
- The legs are released by the baby extending its pelvis round the maternal symphysis pubis (Evans, 2012a, 2012b). Extended legs look never-ending (see Figure 14.4) but usually flop out on their own, shortly followed by the arms (Cronk, 1998).
- Further rotation occurs so the head enters the pelvis, in the same diameter as if it were cephalic. Internal head restitution occurs, also in a similar way to a cephalic birth.
- As the arms are being born, the cord may be compressed between the baby's head and maternal pelvis (both bony). Wharton's jelly affords some protection but expect the FHR to be slower. The lower heart rate is also due to the reduction in the placental site and thought to be an automatic reflex to conserve oxygen in the baby (Stevenson, 1993).
- There is no evidence to support the practice of encouraging the mother to push the baby out in one sustained contraction following the birth of the baby to the umbilicus in an attempt to minimise the reduction of oxygen to the baby. This may actually cause damage or trauma to the mother and/or baby (Hofmeyr and Kulier, 1996).
- There is no evidence of any benefit in bringing down a loop of cord to relieve tension: this may in fact tighten a nuchal cord and/or cause the cord to go into spasm (Evans, 2012a).
- The arms will be born with spontaneous rotation of the baby. If this does not occur or there is delay Løvset's manoeuvre (Table 14.2) may be necessary to release the arms – remembering that the woman is upright, not semi-recumbent, so it is important to be very clear about the mechanism of arm delivery.
- Some midwives may want to poise a hand under the buttocks to prevent the baby delivering suddenly and falling to the floor/bed. Evans (2012a, 2012b) reports that many women spontaneously drop their bottom down so the baby is 'sitting' on the floor/bed, and suggests no additional support is necessary and may inhibit head flexion.
- Avoid the temptation to ausculate the fetal heart at this point: *hands off* unless there is an obvious clinical indication of a problem (Evans, 2012a, 2012b).
- A fit healthy baby makes a 'tummy scrunch' movement (flexing its legs up towards its abdomen and bringing its arms up to its shoulders as if trying to do a sit-up) to facilitate head flexion; the sensation of this movement often automatically causes the woman to drop from an upright kneeling position to a more horizontal position, thus moving her pelvis round the baby's flexing head. Assisted flexion is **only** required if this does not occur (Evans, 2012a, 2012b).

- If head flexion does not occur perform assisted flexion (chin-to-chest) by gently placing a finger on the back of the baby's head (occiput) and with the other hand gently placing two fingers on the baby's cheekbones. Inserting a finger in the baby's mouth is no longer recommended as traction on the jaw may cause dislocation (AAFP, 2012).

There is divided opinion over optimal positions for vaginal breech birth, as the subject has been under-researched. Midwives should encourage and enable the woman to adopt whatever position is best for her. Box 14.1 summarises upright positions.

Table 14.2   Techniques for an assisted vaginal breech delivery.

Burns Marshall manoeuvre
- ○ Baby 'hangs' by its own weight to encourage descent and flexion of the head. Avoid the head delivering too quickly.
- ○ When the nape of the neck and hairline are visible, grasp the baby's ankles in one hand and lift the body in an arc over the mother's abdomen.
- ○ Use the other hand to support the perineum and avoid sudden delivery of the head.
- ○ Once the mouth is clear, the baby will be able to breathe. Allow the rest of the head to deliver slowly.

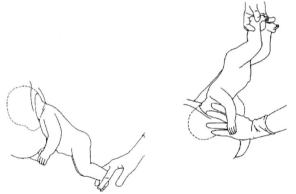

Mauriceau–Smellie–Veit manoeuvre
- ○ This is useful if the hairline does not become visible after the baby has been allowed to support its weight, i.e. the head may have become extended.
- ○ Straddle the baby on one arm – usually the left in a right-handed individual.
- ○ Gently place a finger on the back of the baby's head (occiput) and with the other hand gently place two fingers on the baby's cheekbones to assist flexion if necessary. Putting a finger in the baby's mouth is no longer recommended as it can cause jaw fracture (AAFP, 2012).
- ○ A second person can apply suprapubic pressure if necessary.
- ○ Now place two outer fingers of the other hand over the baby's shoulders with the middle finger on the occiput to assist and maintain flexion.

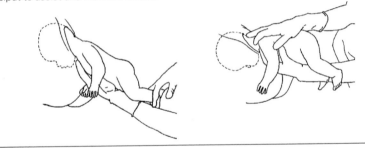

(continued)

Table 14.2   *(Continued)*

Extended legs
○ If the legs appear to be splinting the body, preventing lateral flexion of the trunk, place a finger in each of the baby's groins and apply gentle traction until the backs of the knees are visible. This should only be done if the delivery of the baby needs to be expedited for clinical reasons, since it interferes with the reflexes used by the baby during the birth and may cause the arms to extend over the baby's head (Evans, personal communication).
○ Apply popliteal pressure to abduct and flex the knees one at a time.

Extended arms: Løvset's manoeuvre
The arm(s) may be extended alongside, above or behind the head, sometimes due to rapid head delivery or when traction has been applied to deliver the trunk.

○ Grasp the baby's thighs with your thumbs over the sacrum, taking care to avoid the renal area.
○ Rotate the baby to bring the posterior shoulder anteriorly, beneath the symphysis pubis. Gentle traction may be applied but *rotation is more important than traction.*
○ Friction of the arm against the pelvic wall will bring the arm down to be released: use the 'cat lick' manoeuvre, gently sweeping the arm across the face and down the body.
○ Release the other arm by repeating the manoeuvre in the opposite direction.

N.B. Most of these manoeuvres have been designed for the woman in a semi-recumbent/lithotomy position, although they can be modified for upright birth. A clear understanding of anatomy and the mechanisms of a breech birth are essential.

Assisted breech delivery

Many midwives used to be taught that assisted breech manoeuvres were the only way to deliver a breech, and they are still favoured by many obstetricians, although even the RCOG (2006a) does not now recommend them routinely over spontaneous birth. However, these techniques may be used to assist the birth of the baby's head if legs, arms or head have become extended or if descent is very slow (Table 14.2). The midwife should be aware that once s/he has intervened s/he may well need to perform other manoeuvres to facilitate the birth.

The baby at birth

It is important to remember, and discuss with parents, that the mechanism of a breech birth is different from that of a cephalic baby and their appearance and response are likely to be different. This may be reflected in a lower 1-min Apgar score in breech babies born vaginally (Thorpe-Beeston *et al.*, 1992).

Cephalic babies often 'rest' between the birth of the head and the body allowing adjustment from compression to decompression of the head. Some suggest this does not occur with a breech birth, and this may be a factor in the occasional need for resuscitation. Evans, however, reports that there is often a pause in contractions between the birth of the body and the birth of the head. Whatever the cause, breech babies may be slower than cephalic babies to breathe spontaneously and may initially have lax muscle tone and poor reflexes whilst having a good heart rate. A bag and mask or a resuscitaire should be on hand and ready to use if necessary. If the cord is pulsating, the baby is receiving oxygen from the mother, so delayed cord clamping may have benefits, just as for any birth (see page 28, Chapter 1).

The best place to give supportive measures, if required, is in the mother's arms to enable her to stimulate the baby by voice and touch. If more extensive measures are required, they should be carried out close to the mother (see Chapter 18).

Third stage

This should be conducted according to the woman's wishes, subject to events and discussion (see Chapter 1). Oxytocics should be withheld until the birth of the baby's head is completed.

Summary

- *Hands off the breech* – manoeuvres are rarely required.
- No unnecessary VEs.
- No 'routine' ARM; if spontaneous rupture of membranes, check no cord/foot is presenting.
- Avoid epidurals.
- Enable women to adopt positions spontaneously.
- No augmentation: if there is poor progress, consider CS.
- Enable women to push spontaneously; give guidance if necessary.
- Frank meconium is to be expected.
- Check FHR regularly and act appropriately.
- Episiotomy only if felt necessary.
- Breech babies may be slower to breathe spontaneously than cephalic – be prepared.
- Ensure that you are well supported by like-minded people.
- Enjoy and celebrate the birth!

Useful contacts

Association for Improvements in the Maternity Services (AIMS) www.aims.org.uk
Birthspirit Ltd www.birthspirit.co.nz
Cornelia Enning (German midwife championing water birth) www.hebinfo.de/ (in German but online translation available)
Dr Herman Ponette (Belgian obstetrician with a medicalised approach to water birth, but still very interesting) www.helsinki.fi/~lauhakan/whale/waterbaby/p0.html
Independent Midwives Association www.independentmidwives.org.uk
National Childbirth Trust (NCT) www.nct.org.uk

Recommended reading

Evans, J. (2012a) Understanding physiological breech birth. *Essentially MIDIRS* 3(2), 17–21.
Evans, J. (2012b) The final piece of the breech birth jigsaw? *Essentially MIDIRS* 3(3) 46–9.

References

AAFP (American Academy of Family Physicians) (2012) *Advanced Life Support in Obstetrics (ALSO)*. Course Syllabus Manual. Leawood, Kansas, AAFP.

Alarab, M., Regan, C., O'Connell, M. P., Keane, D. P., O'Herlihy, M. D., Foley, M. (2004) Singleton vaginal breech delivery at term: still a safe option. *Obstetrics and Gynecology* 103, 407–12.

Banks, M. (1998) *Breech Birth Woman Wise*. Hamilton, New Zealand, Birthspirit Books.

Banks, M. (2001) *Breech Birth Beyond the Term Breech Trial*. Birthspirit. www.birthspirit.co.nz

Bragg, F., Cromwell, D., Edozien, L., Gurol-Urganci, I., Mahmood, T., Templeton, A., van der Meulen, J. (2010) Variation in rates of caesarean section among English NHS trusts after accounting for maternal and clinical risk: cross sectional study *British Medical Journal* 341, 5065. www.bmj.com/content/341/bmj.c5065.full

Carayol, M., Blondel, B., Zeitlin, J., Breart, G., Goffinet, F. (2007) Changes in the rates of caesarean delivery before labour for breech presentational term in France: 1972–2003. *European Journal of Obstetrics and Gynaecology and Reproductive Biology* 132(1), 20–6.

CESDI (2000) *Confidential Enquiry into Stillbirths and Deaths in Infancy*, 7th Annual Report. London, Maternal and Child Health Research Consortium.

Cheng, M., Hannah, M. (1993) Breech delivery at term: a critical review of the literature. *Obstetrics and Gynaecology* 82(4), 605–18.

CMACE (Centre for Maternal and Child Enquiries) (2011) *Perinatal Mortality 2009: United Kingdom*. London, CMACE. www.rcog.org.uk/files/rcog-corp/Perinatal%20Mortality%20Report%202008.pdf

Confino, E., Gleicher, N., Elrad, H., Isajovich, B., David, M. P. (1985) The breech dilemma – a review. *Obstetrical and Gynaecological Survey* 40(6), 330–7.

Cooper, M. (1992) *Twins, Breech and VBAC (Audiotape)*. Midwifery Today, Eugene, Oregon.

Coyle, M. E., Smith, C. A., Peat, B. (2005) Cephalic version by moxibustion for breech presentation. *Cochrane Database of Systematic Reviews*, Issue 2.

Cronk, M. (1998) Birthing a baby by the breech. *AIMS Journal* 10(3), 6–8.

Do, C., Smith, C., Dahlen, H., Bisits, A., Schmied, V. (2011) Moxibustion for cephalic version: a feasibility randomized controlled trial. *Complementary and Alternataive Medicine* 11, 18.

El Halta, V. (2010) Advanced midwifery seminar: moving midwifery forward: essays and outlines, workshop manual. Garden of Life, Dearborn MI. Care during labor and birth. In Frye, A. (ed.) *Holistic Midwifery. A Comprehensive Textbook for Midwives in Home Birth Practice*, Vol. 1. Portland, Oregon, Labrys Press.

Evans, J. (2012a) Understanding physiological breech birth. *Essentially MIDIRS* 3(2), 17–22.

Evans, J. (2012b) The final piece of the breech birth jigsaw? *Essentially MIDIRS* 3(3), 46–9.

Fitzpatrick, C., Robson, M., Hehir, M., OConnor, H., Coulter-Smith, S., Malone, F. (2011) The effect of the term breech trial on vaginal breech delivery 8 years on. *American Journal of Obstetrics and Gynecology* 204(1), S 334, Supplement to January 2011.

Frye, A. (2010) Care during labor and birth. In Frye, A. (ed.) *Holistic Midwifery. A Comprehensive Textbook for Midwives in Home Birth Practice vol 1*. Portland, Oregon, Labrys Press.

Glezerman, M. (2006) Five years to the term breech trial: the rise and fall of a randomized controlled trial. *American Journal of Obstetrics and Gynaecology* 194, 20–5.

Glezerman, M. (2012) www.expert-reviews.com 10.1586/EOG.12.2 Expert Reviews Ltd ISSN 1747-4108 P.159-167

Goffinet, F., Caroyal, M., Foidart, J. M., Alexander, S., Uzan, S., Subtil, D., Breart, G. (2006) PREMODA Study Group. Is planned vaginal delivery for breech presentation at term still an option? Results of an observational prospective study in France and Belgium. *American Journal of Obstetrics and Gynecology* 194, 1002–11.

Gupta, J., Hofmeyr, G., Smyth, R. (2007) Position in the second stage of labour for women without epidural anaesthesia. *Cochrane database of systematic reviews*, Issue 4.

Gyte, G. (2001) Planned caesarean section versus planned vaginal birth for breech presentation at term: a randomised multicentre trial. *MIDIRS Midwifery Digest* 11(1), 80–3.

Hannah, M. E., Hannah, W. J., Hewson, S. A., Hodnett, E. D., Saigal, S., Willan, A. R. (2000) Planned caesarean section versus vaginal birth for breech presentation at term: a randomised multicentre trial. *The Lancet* 356, 1375–83.

Hofmeyr, G. J. (2000) Suspected fetalpelvic disproportion and abnormal lie. In Enkin, M., Keirse, M. J. N. C., Neilson, J., Crowther, C., Duley, L., Hodnett, E., Hofmeyr, J. (eds) *A Guide to Effective Care in Pregnancy and Childbirth*, pp. 185–95. Oxford, Oxford University Press.

Hofmeyr, G. J. (2001) Abnormal fetal presentation and position. In Chamberlain, G. and Steer, P. (eds) *Turnbull's Obstetrics*, p. 557. Edinburgh, Churchill Livingstone.

Hofmeyr, G., Kulier, R. (1996) Expedited versus conservative approaches for vaginal delivery in breech presentation. *Cochrane Database of Systematic Reviews*. Issue 1.

Hofmeyr, G., Hannah, M., Lawrie, T. (2003) Planned caesarean section for term breech delivery. *Cochrane Database of Systematic Reviews* Issue 2, published online 2010. http://onlinelibrary.wiley.com/doi/10.1002/14651858.CD000166/pdf/standard

Hulme, H. (1992) Meconium aspiration syndrome: reflections on a midwifery subject. *MIDIRS Midwifery Digest* 2(2), 177.

Hutton, E., Hofmeyr, G. (2006) External cephalic version for breech presentation before term. *Cochrane Database of Systematic Reviews* 2006, Issue 1.

Hutton, E., Hannah, M., Ross, S., Delisle, M.-F., Carson, G., Windrim, R., *et al.* (2011) The Early External Cephalic Version (ECV) 2 Trial: an international multicentre randomised controlled trial of timing of ECV for breech pregnancies. *British Journal of Obstetrics and Gynaecology* 118, 564–77.

Impey, L., Lissoni, D. (1999) Outcome of external cephalic version after 36 weeks gestation without tocolysis. *Journal of Maternal and Fetal Medicine* 8, 203–7.

Lancet Correspondence (2001) Term breech trial. *The Lancet* 357(9251), 225–8.

Maier, B., Georgoulopoulos, G., Zajc, M., Jaeger, T., Zuchna, C., Hasenoehrl, G. (2011) Fetal outcome for infants in breech by method of delivery: experiences with stand-by service system of senior obstetricians and women's choices of mode of delivery. *Journal of Prenatal Medicine* 39, 385–90.

Michel, S., Drain, A., Closset, E., Deruelle, P., Ego, A., Subtil, D. (2011) Evaluation of a decision protocol for type of delivery of infants in breech presentation at term. *European Journal of Obstetrics and Gynecology and Reproductive Biology* 158, 194–98.

NICE (National Institute for Health and Clinical Excellence) (2002) *Technology Appraisal Guidance No 41: Guidance on the Use of Routine Anti-D Prophylaxis for RhD-negative Women.* London, NICE.

NICE (2003) *Clinical Guideline 6. Antenatal Care: Routine Care for the Healthy Pregnant Woman* London, NICE.

Neri, I., Airola, G., Contu, G., Allais, F., Fachinetti, F., Benedettoo, C. (2004) Acupuncture plus moxibustion to resolve breech presentation: a randomised controlled study. *Journal of Maternal, Fetal and Neonatal Medicine* 15(4), 247–52.

Odent, M. (1984) *Birth Reborn*. London, Souvenir Press.

Price, S. (2001) Electronic fetal monitoring equipment. *British Journal of Midwifery* 9(9), 579–82.

Robinson, J. (2000) Midwives need training in the lost art of breech birth. *British Journal of Midwifery* 8(7), 447.

Robinson, J. (2000/2001) Breech babies – caesarean or vaginal birth? *AIMS Journal* 12(4), 12–13.

RCOG (2001) Clinical Effectiveness Support Unit. *National Sentinel Caesarean Section Audit Report*. London, RCOG.

RCOG (2006a) *The Management of Breech Presentation. Guideline No. 20b*. London, RCOG.

RCOG (2006b) *External Cephalic Version and Reducing the Incidence of Breech Presentation. Guideline 20a*. London, RCOG.

RCOG (2007) TOG release: planned vaginal breech delivery births – choice or safety? *The Obstetrician and Gynaecologist*.

Schutte, J. M., Steegers, A. P., Santema, J., Schuitemaker, N., Van Roosemalen, J. (2007) Maternal deaths after elective caesarean section for breech presentation in the Netherlands. *Acta Ocstetrica et Gynecologica Scandinavica* 86(2), 240–3.

Sleep, J., Roberts, J., Chalmers, I. (2000) The second stage of labor. In Enkin, M., Keirse, M. J. N. C., Neilson, J., Crowther, C., Duley, L., Hodnett, E., Hofmeyr, J. (eds) *A Guide to Effective Care in Pregnancy and Childbirth*, 3rd edn, pp. 289–99. Oxford, Oxford University Press.

Stevenson, J. (1993) More thoughts on breech. *Midwifery Today*, 26, 24–5.

Thorpe-Beeston, J. G., Blanfield, P. J., Saunders, N. J. S. (1992) Outcome of breech delivery at term. *British Medical Journal* 305, 746–7.

Ulander, V. M., Gissler, M., Nuutila, M., Ylikorkala, O. (2004) Are health expectations of term breech infants unrealistically high? *ACTA Obstet Gynecol Scand* 83, 180–6.

Whyte, H., Hannah, M., Saigal, S., *et al.* (2004) Term Breech Trial Collaborative Group. Outcomes of children at 2 years after planned cesarean birth versus planned vaginal birth for breech presentation at term: The International Randomized Term Breech Trial. *American Journal of Obstetrics and Gynecology* 191(3), 864–71.

15 Twins and higher-order births

Jo Coggins

Introduction

The news of a multiple pregnancy is often met with delight by both mothers and midwives. The rarity of twins and higher-order births ensures that they remain a somewhat special phenomenon. However, it can be a daunting time for women as they may feel their choices are swept away by a plethora of obstetric concerns and interventions. Midwives have a key role in limiting this by advocating women's choices and ensuring that medical intervention is reserved only for those who need it.

Incidence and facts

- The ratio of UK multiple births to singletons was 1:64 in 2010.
- There were 169 UK triplet births in 2009 and just 6 quadruplet births (ONS, 2011).
- The proportion of multiple births is decreasing: 15.7 per 1000 women giving birth in 2010, compared with 16.4 per 1000 in 2009 (ONS, 2011). The number of in vitro fertilisation (IVF) multiple births has been dropping for some time (HFEA, 2001; RCM, 2011).
- UK triplets and higher-order births have decreased mainly due to the Human Fertilisation and Embryology Act 2008 which states that women undergoing IVF can only have two embryos transferred in each cycle, barring exceptional circumstances. Also the Human Fertilisation and Embryology Authority now promote just one

The Midwife's Labour and Birth Handbook, Third Edition. Edited by Vicky Chapman and Cathy Charles.
© 2013 John Wiley & Sons, Ltd. Published 2013 by John Wiley & Sons, Ltd.

embryo transfer, as it is more successful than multiple transfer (HFEA, 2011; RCM, 2011).

- Women aged 45 and over had the highest multiple pregnancy rate in 2010: 93.6 per 1000 pregnancies (ONS, 2011). This is partly because natural multiple birth conception increases with maternal age, and partly because older women more commonly request assisted conception.
- In the UK one third of twins are monozygotic (identical) and two-thirds are dizygotic (non-identical):
  - Monoygotic twins occur when one fertilised ovum splits during the early stages of pregnancy. There are no known causal factors.
  - Dizygotic twins occur when the mother produces two ova during her menstrual cycle, which are fertilised separately. Rates are influenced by age, parity, race and family history (Blickstein, 2005).
- Multiple pregnancies increase the risks for mothers and babies:
  - Maternal risks include pre-eclampsia, antepartum haemorrhage, preterm delivery and caesarean section (CS).
  - Neonatal risks: prematurity, low birth weight, neonatal intensive care unit (NICU) admission, chromosomal abnormalities, congenital malformation and perinatal pathology are more common in twin pregnancies; particularly in monozygotic twins (Chauhan *et al.*, 2010; Corsello and Piro, 2010). Twin-to-twin transfusion is a life-threatening condition affecting monozygotic dichorionic twins.
- There has, however, been a significant downward trend in the perinatal mortality rate for twin births in the UK since 2000 (CMACE, 2011):
  - Stillbirths down from 16.7 per 1000 total births in 2000 to 11.2 per 1000 in 2008.
  - Neonatal deaths down from 21.5 per 1000 live births in 2000 to 17 per 1000 in 2008.

Place of delivery

The risks associated with multiple pregnancies are generally greater than those of singletons. A recent survey by the National Perinatal Epidemiology Unit (NPEU) found that mothers of multiples have a higher risk of complications requiring hospital admission and are more likely to be induced. They are also twice as likely to have an epidural in labour although this may be due to hospital policies and guidelines rather than maternal choice (NPEU, 2011). Obstetricians counselling women emphasise these risks, hence most women choose consultant-led units for delivery (NPEU, 2011). For some, though, the idea of a hospital birth and the interventions likely to accompany it contradicts the ethos of 'normal birth', and they choose home birth. These women may benefit particularly from the care of an independent midwife, who may be more experienced in caring for women with multiple births at home.

Mode of delivery

Many women carrying twins can enjoy safe vaginal births (Wen *et al.*, 2004), although Cochrane review concludes that since the second-born twin has a higher risk of a poor perinatal outcome than the first-born, the optimal mode of delivery is unclear and likely to depend on individual circumstances (Hofmeyr *et al.*, 2011).

There is insufficient research into mode of delivery for higher-order births, and practice varies worldwide. In the UK where obstetricians are the lead caregiver, 60–80% of twins and higher order multiples are delivered by CS (Steer, 2007). This begs the question: are women offered true choice or are their decisions swayed by obstetricians who lean towards a more medical view of birth?

A woman's choice regarding twin birth is usually influenced by the presentation of the babies. Most commonly, they present vertex/vertex (40%), followed by vertex/non-vertex (30%), non-vertex/vertex (20%) and non-vertex/non-vertex (10%) (Blickstein, 2005). Historically, obstetricians have recommended CS for any woman whose leading twin is non-vertex. However, evidence suggests that other factors are of greater or equal importance in determining a safe vaginal delivery, such as predicted birth weights (Blickstein, 2005).

A Canadian multicentre study is underway comparing planned CS with planned vaginal birth, where the leading twin is cephalic and both twins are 1500–4000 g (Twin Birth Study, 2011). Unfortunately the research excludes a breech leading presentation. Researchers state that the Term Breech Trial (TBC) (Hannah *et al.*, 2000) has proven poorer outcomes for breech presentation, even though this trial has been critically challenged (see Chapter 14). One criticism of the TBC was the medicalised management of the vaginal breech group: women were often immobile, with epidurals, continuous monitoring, and with highly managed recumbent births. A similar danger may exist for this proposed Canadian study: while the researchers state that epidural is 'at the discretion' of the mother/caregivers, mandatory CTG monitoring is required. A midwife is unlikely to be managing these labours, as researchers request an experienced twin labour obstetrician. So will researchers once again be measuring only medically managed labours against planned CS? Also, if this trial results in promotion of CS for twins, just as CS is currently recommended by NICE for breech, then there is a danger that practitioners may lose their skills in multiple birth, and reduce choice for women.

In the UK, almost all triplets and quadruplets are delivered operatively (Steer, 2007). It is unclear whether this is based on a valid assessment of risk, or due to lack of an evidence base and fear of litigation. Interestingly, evidence from studies in other countries, including the USA, concludes outcomes for mothers and babies are improved by vaginal delivery, providing it is in a hospital and attended by appropriately skilled clinicians (Grobman *et al.*, 1998). This is mainly due to a reduction in post-operative complications for mothers and a lower incidence of respiratory distress syndrome in babies. Sheppard *et al.* (1999) support this, highlighting the fact that mothers recover more quickly following vaginal birth, and are therefore better placed to begin caring for their babies. Therefore it seems women in the UK may be disadvantaged if obstetricians continue to routinely advocate elective CS for triplets and higher-order births. Midwives should ensure women are sufficiently informed to make the choices that are right for them.

The woman's choice is likely to be influenced by the fact that multiple pregnancy does carry increased risks, even before labour has begun. Babies may have to 'compete' in the womb for space and position and sometimes for nutrients and oxygen. Babies who are multiples are more likely to have speech and language delay, visual perceptual problems, minor neuromotor dysfunction, learning disabilities and behaviour problems (TAMBA website), which can be daunting to prospective parents planning their birth. Not all risks are simply labour-related: many are specific to being a twin, or related to premature birth and/or low birth weight, which are irrelevant of mode of delivery. While the extra stress of labour may increase the risk to an already compromised baby, it is important that women are not simply counselled to believe that caesarean section produces safe outcomes while vaginal birth is inherently risky. As with all labours, multiple pregnancy labour should be approached with both vigilance and empathy.

Care in labour

Midwives' knowledge and understanding of normal birth is invaluable when caring for a mother carrying two or more babies in labour. This is sometimes a difficult role, as the midwife must act as an advocate for the mother whilst working alongside obstetric colleagues.

Most midwives get the opportunity to care for twin labours, whilst fewer will see triplets or higher-order vaginal birth. Care in labour is broadly the same whatever the number of babies, although anxieties will be significantly higher with triplet and higher-order birth than with twins.

If the birth is in hospital, women may wish to look around it at some stage during their pregnancy. A tour of NICU/SCBU may be appreciated as around 50% of twins and almost all triplets will require admission (TAMBA, 2006b). This is usually due to low birth weight resulting from prematurity. Prematurity is one of the most significant risks associated with multiple pregnancies, and midwives must be aware of the principles of care for preterm labour (see Chapter 13).

In hospital, when the woman is in labour the midwife should inform the relevant professionals. The birthing room should be prepared adequately with equipment checked and accessible. Additional equipment for instrumental or operative delivery should be discreetly available. Thompson (2010) highlights the importance of a positive, welcoming birth environment and the beneficial impact this has on women during labour. Likewise, for twin births in the absence of complications and/or prematurity concerns, there is little need for anyone other than the attending midwife to be in the room, usually joined by another midwife or two during the second stage. For non-cephalic presentations, also for triplets and higher order births there is likely to be much more obstetric and paediatric involvement, with theatre staff on high alert.

Care during the first stage of labour should be similar to that offered to any woman. A calm, kind midwife who offers appropriate explanations and plenty of praise and reassurance will help ensure the woman feels safe and confident. There are some special considerations for mothers with a multiple pregnancy:

- **Positioning.** The woman should be comfortable and able to mobilise freely, maintaining an upright position to aid labour progress. The increased uterine size in a multiple pregnancy can cause considerable discomfort, and frequent changes of position may be needed.
- **Intravenous (IV) cannulation.** An IV cannula is advised as oxytocin (Syntocinon) may be recommended promptly after the second twin if contractions are slow to resume, and also there is a higher postpartum haemorrhage (PPH) risk.

- **Fasting.** Some obstetricians advocate fasting to prevent gastric aspiration if a general anaesthetic is required. Cochrane review found no evidence for or against food/drink restriction in women at increased risk of anaesthesia (Singata *et al.*, 2010). Gastric aspiration may occur with poor anaesthetic technique and can happen even when women have fasted (O'Sullivan *et al.*, 2007). Offering a hydrogen ion inhibitor (e.g. ranitidine, cimetidine) to encourage rapid emptying of stomach contents may confer benefits, should an emergency CS be required (Johnson *et al.*, 2000).
- **Epidural analgesia.** Women may be advised to have an epidural because invasive procedures may be required to assist the second twin, and emergency CS is also a greater possibility. However, epidurals carry significant side effects reducing mobility, progress and pushing urge which can lead to malrotation and instrumental delivery (Lieberman *et al.*, 2005).

Monitoring the fetal heart rates

NICE (2007) guidelines advocate continuous electronic fetal monitoring (EFM) although some would challenge this (Beech Lawrence, 2001). See Chapter 3 for more information. EFM is often restrictive and uncomfortable for women and is associated with increased intervention and no improvement in outcomes (Grant, 2000; NICE, 2007). Intermittent auscultation is possible but it can be difficult to locate two or more heartbeats. In practice, midwives are usually under pressure to perform continuous EFM although this can also be technically difficult, and is particularly hard if there are three or more babies. Indeed difficulty of monitoring may be one reason why CS is so quickly resorted to in cases of higher order births. Ultimately, women have the right to choose and may decline EFM or prefer to have only periodic CTG traces. The following points offer some guidance for both methods:

- **Intermittent auscultation**
  - Both/all heartbeats must be heard simultaneously to ensure they are separate.
  - Another midwife or midwives can help using extra doppler device(s).
  - Midwives should 'listen in' for up to 1 min following a contraction approximately every 15 min in the first stage and every 5 min in the second stage (NICE, 2007).
- **Electronic monitoring**
  - CTG should only be used in active labour as it restricts mobility and may cause unnecessary anxiety.
  - To avoid accidentally monitoring the same FH with two transducers, CTG machines often have a twin facility which separates and prints out the individual fetal heart rate patterns of each baby. This is useful if both babies have similar baselines and are hard to audibly/visually differentiate.
  - Poor contact via abdominal transducers can be a problem during twin/multiple labours and may distract care away from the mother. A fetal scalp electrode may be indicated (see Chapter 3).
  - Electronic fetal monitoring does not require the woman to recline on the bed. Consider using a birthing ball or chair.

Second stage of labour

As the woman approaches the second stage, a second midwife should be informed. In an acute unit also inform the labour ward coordinator and obstetrician, although they do not need to necessarily be in the room. In many twin pregnancies and certainly higher multiple birth there is likely to be pressure for extra staff, e.g. paediatricians/neonatal practitioners, to be present, particularly for prematurity. But the majority of twins will be a good gestation, with fair predicted birthweights; if so they should stay outside the door unless required. The birthing environment should remain calm and quiet. Low lighting, relaxing music and use of a gentle, reassuring voice will convey an atmosphere of confidence and calm to anyone entering the room. On sensing this, they are likely to adopt similar behaviour, causing minimal disturbance to the woman at this pivotal moment.

Birth of the first baby

The birth of the first baby should take place as any other, and providing the mother and baby are well they can enjoy skin-to-skin contact immediately, leaving the umbilical cord unclamped and able to pulsate. *Do not give syntometrine.* It is now important to auscultate the other baby/babies' heartbeat(s) intermittently or by CTG as appropriate.

Birth of the second/subsequent baby

Contractions usually resume in due course and the presenting part of the next baby begins its descent into the pelvis. Evans (2000) postulates this interval between births is nature's way of giving the mother time to greet her first baby before the next is born. In the absence of complications, midwives should protect this special time between the woman and baby by ensuring that unnecessary interventions are avoided.

The interval between the birth of the first and second/subsequent babies is when emergency procedures are most often required (Levin and Levy, 2005). Complications at this stage usually derive from malpresentation or cord damage/prolapse. One study reported an emergency CS rate of 9.25% for a second twin, due mainly to malpresentation followed by fetal distress (Wen *et al.*, 2004). Another study found that with a cephalic presentation the main complications were cord prolapse and fetal distress, increasing the risk of CS and instrumental delivery rates to 6.3% and 8.3%, respectively (Yang *et al.*, 2005). It is arguable that this is often due to unnecessary intervention, e.g. clamping/cutting the first baby's cord or artificially rupturing the membranes (ARM) of the second/subsequent baby.

The risks as identified above are increased for higher order births, as the remaining babies may become entangled/obstructed, and cord proplapse risk is higher.

Midwives should consider proactive measures to aid normality:

- **Upright postures.** Help the woman to maintain an upright posture: this may aid the natural descent of the second baby/babies and reduce malpresentations and positional fetal heart rate (FHR) anomalies.
- **Listening to the fetal heart.** As the next baby descends, second-stage FHR changes may occur, e.g. variable decelerations. However, prolonged or persistent atypical

decelerations or bradycardia may indicate malpresentation or cord prolapse. A vaginal examination (VE) may help determine this.

- **Determining the lie/presentation of the next baby.** Palpation and VE are commonly performed at this stage and occasionally a quick scan: this is often the key moment for a multiple birth. If the baby is cephalic the pressure is off! For higher order births, the same interest over lie and presentation occurs with each following baby.
- **Time interval between the births.** Research is mainly confined to twins. If the FHR of the second twin is normal, evidence suggests 30 min is a safe cut-off due to the gradual deterioration in the arterial cord pH, although one study showed babies still had good outcomes up to an hour (McGrail and Bryant, 2005). Another study found that birth interval was only a significant predictor of low Apgar score for larger breech second twins >1900 g, and that gestational age was the single most important predictive factor overall (Evrim *et al.*, 2003). A large 15-year German study (Stein *et al.*, 2008) found similar findings of poorer Apgars, acidaemia and adverse short-term outcomes in larger and/or non-cephalic second twins.They also measured delivery intervals for over 8000 twin births:
  - 75.8% delivered within 15 minutes
  - 16.4% delivered in 16–30 minutes
  - 4.3% delivered in 31–45 minutes
  - 1.7% delivered in 46–60 minutes
  - 1.8% delivered after more than 60 minutes: (72 instances)

  There is very little research into birth intervals for higher-order births other than twins.
- **Avoid ARM for the second baby.** This is often undertaken by obstetricians. ARM has no clear benefits (Smyth *et al.*, 2007) and can cause cord compression and/or prolapse (Prabulos and Philipson, 1998); FHR anomalies (Smyth *et al.*, 2007); accidental rupture of the first baby's cord; malpresentation/malposition of the second baby since the presenting part may not have had opportunity to fully engage. As the risks outweigh the benefits, this practice should be avoided.

After birth each baby and their cord should be labelled 'twin/baby 1, twin/baby 2, baby 3, etc.' in case anomalies are detected when examining the placentae and membranes or if cord pHs are needed. Cord clamps can be used (i.e. one for baby 1, and two for baby 2, etc.); however, an alternative initial method is necessary for a physiological third stage, where cord clamping is contraindicated. Following this the midwife should assist the mother into a comfortable position in which she can greet her babies and initiate their first feed.

Third stage of labour

Mothers experiencing multiple birth are often encouraged to have an actively managed third stage due to the increased risk of postpartum haemorrhage resulting from a larger placental site (Levin and Levy, 2005). The placental site is likely to be larger still for triplet and higher order births, where there may be an increased cause for concern.

Active management

- IV syntocinon infusion is often prepared in advance of delivery as a precaution: it should only really be commenced if a PPH, although sometimes it is put up prophylactically.
- Administer oxytocic of choice, e.g. Syntometrine, after birth of the final baby.
- Delivering twin placentas by controlled cord traction is straightforward: following the administation of an oxytocic, guard the uterus with one hand and apply controlled cord traction to both/all cords simultaneously.

Physiological third stage

A minority of women wish to avoid the side effects of oxytocics and following a straightforward labour (without epidural or oxytocics) opt instead for a physiological third stage. (See Chapter 1.) In the absence of heavy bleeding, there is no indication to augment this stage, although helping the woman into a comfortable position to breastfeed her babies is helpful.

Following the delivery of the placenta(s) the uterus will feel larger and higher than those following a singleton birth – but should still feel well contracted. Examination of the placenta(e) and membranes is crucial to ensure nothing is retained (Figure 15.1). Many women are intrigued by their placenta(s).

It is a common misconception that two placentae means that twins are dizygotic and one means they are monozygotic. Visual inspection alone can not always be relied upon to determine zygosity!

- Monozygotic (identical) twins develop from one zygote that splits, forming two embryos, usually with a single shared placenta. HOWEVER, if monzygotic

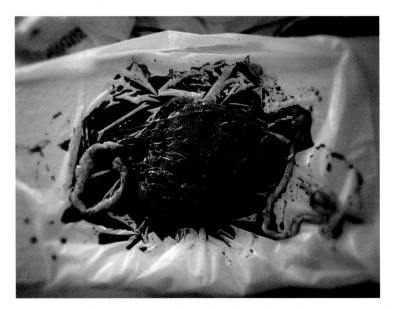

Fig. 15.1 Twin placenta, delivered uneventfully and physiologically. This is a monozygotic (identical twin) placenta – but zygosity is not always possible to tell by visual inspection alone.

twins separate early they have separate sacs and placentas: this occurs in 18–30% of cases.

- Dizygotic (fraternal/non-identical) twins develop from two separate eggs fertilised by different sperm resulting (theoretically) in two individual placentas. HOWEVER, dizygotic twin placentas may appear to fuse as they grow, appearing as one.

Care after the birth

Care immediately following the birth should allow for the mother's private time with her new family. Inspection for perineal trauma and any necessary repair can wait if she is not bleeding. If breastfeeding, she may require help and extra pillows to achieve a comfortable position in which the babies can enjoy skin to skin and root and find the breast.

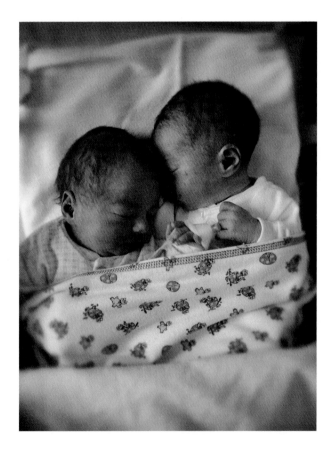

Documentation

The midwife is responsible for contemporaneous record keeping throughout the woman's labour and delivery. In the event of an emergency or circumstances preventing documentation in real time, it is important to record events in retrospect.

Summary

- Women with multiple pregnancies often need extra emotional/psychological support and should not have their choices swept away by obstetric concerns.
- In the UK, CS is advocated for triplets and higher-order births, yet studies in other countries conclude better maternal/neonatal outcomes with vaginal delivery.
- Multiple births carry increased risks for mothers and babies. The second/subsequent baby/babies particularly risk potential second-stage complications, i.e. hypoxia, cord prolapse and malpresentation.
- Give special consideration to positioning, analgesia and fetal monitoring in labour.
- After first baby is born: stay calm, don't rush; auscultate FH of next baby and check presentation.
- Avoid ARM of the second or subsequent babies.
- NICE recommends CTG in active labour although the evidence base is poor. Monitoring multiples can present practical difficulties and an FSE may be required.
- Protect the woman's choice and ask extra staff to wait outside the room.
- Mothers of twins/multiples may require extra support following the births to find a comfortable position for skin-to-skin and breastfeeding.

Useful contacts

Association of Independent Midwives www.aims.org.uk
Multiple Births Association www.multiplebirths.org.uk
Twins and Multiple Births Association www.tamba.org.uk
Twins UK www.twinsuk.co.uk

References

Beech Lawrence, B. (2001) Electronic fetal monitoring: do NICE's new guidelines owe too much to the medical model of childbirth? *The Practising Midwife* 4(7), 31–3.

Blickstein, I. (2005) Definition of multiple pregnancy. In Blickstein, I., Keith, L. (eds) *Multiple Pregnancy: Epidemiology, Gestation and Perinatal Outcome*, 2nd edn. London, Taylor and Francis.

Chauhan, S. P., Scardo, J. A., Hayes, E., *et al.* (2010) Twins: prevalence, problems and pre-term births. *American Journal of Obstetrics and Gynaecology* 203(4), 305–15.

CMACE (Centre for Maternal and Child Enquiries) (2011) *Perinatal Mortality 2009: UK.* London, CMACE. www.rcog.org.uk/files/rcog-corp/Perinatal%20Mortality%20Report%202008.pdf

Corsello, G., Piro, E. (2010) The world of twins: an update. *Journal of Maternal Fetal and Neonatal Medicine.* Oct 23, Suppl 3, 59–62.

Dickersin, K. (2000) Control of pain in labour. In Enkin, M., Keirse, M. J. N. C., Neilson, J., Crowther, C., Duley, L., Hodnett, E., Hofmeyr, J. (eds) *A Guide to Effective Care in Pregnancy and Childbirth*, 3rd edn. Oxford, Oxford University Press.

Evans, J. (2000) *Can a Twin Birth be a Positive Experience?* [updated online version]. http://www.radmid.demon.co.uk

Evrim, E., Tamer, M., Tapisiz, O. L., Ustunyurt, E., Caglar, E. (2003) Effect of inter-twin delivery time on Apgar score of the second twin. *Australian and New Zealand Journal of Obstetrics and Gynaecology* 43(3), 203–6.

Grant, A. (2000) Care of the fetus during labour. In Enkin, M., Keirse, M. J. N. C., Neilson, J., Crowther, C., Duley, L., Hodnett, E., Hofmeyr, J. (eds) *A Guide to Effective Care in Pregnancy and Childbirth*, 3rd edn., pp. 267–80. Oxford, Oxford University Press.

Grobman, W. A., Peaceman, A. M., Haney, E., Silver, R., MacGregor, S. (1998) Neonatal outcomes in triplet gestations after a trial of labour. *American Journal of Obstetrics and Gynecology* 179(4), 942–5.

Hannah, M. E., Hannah, W. J., Hewson, S. A., Hodnett, E. D., Saigal, S., Willan, A. R. (2000) Planned caesarean section versus vaginal birth for breech presentation at term: a randomised multicentre trial. *The Lancet* 356, 1375–83.

HFEA (Human Fertilisation and Embryology Authority) (2011) http://www.hfea .gov.uk/6458.html

Johnson, C., Keirse, M., Enkin, M., Chalmers, I. (2000) Hospital practices – nutrition and hydration in labour. In Enkin, M., Keirse, M. J. N. C., Neilson, J., Crowther, C., Duley, L., Hodnett, E., Hofmeyr, J. (eds) *A Guide to Effective Care in Pregnancy and Childbirth*, 3rd edn, pp. 255–66. Oxford, Oxford University Press.

Jolly, M., Sebire, N., Harris, J., Robinson, S., Regal, L. (2000) The risks associated with pregnancy in women over 35. *Human Reproduction* 15(11), 2433–7.

Lieberman, E., Davidson, K., Lee-Parritz, A., Shearer, E. (2005) Changes in fetal position during labor and their association with epidural analgesia. *Obstetrics and Gynecology* 105(5), 974–98.

Levin, D., Levy, R. (2005) Epidemiology of bleeding and haemorrhage in multiple gestations. In Blickstein, I. and Keith, L. (eds) *Multiple Pregnancy: Epidemiology, Gestation and Perinatal Outcome*, 2nd edn. London, Taylor and Francis.

McGrail, C. D., Bryant, D. R. (2005) Intertwin time interval: how it affects the immediate neonatal outcome of the second twin. *American Journal of Obstetrics and Gynecology* 192(5), 1420–22.

National Institute for Health and Clinical Excellence (NICE) (2007) *Clinical Guideline 55: Intrapartum Care*. London, NICE. www.nice.org

National Perinatal Epidemiology Unit (2011) *Maternity Care for Women having A Multiple Birth* [online] https://www.npeu.ox.ac.uk

ONS (Office for National Statistics) (2011) *Live Births in England and Wales by Characteristics of Birth, 2010*. ONS. Statistical bulletin: Nov www.ons.gov.uk.ons/dcp171778_241936.pdf

O'Sullivan, G., Liu, B., Shennan, A. (2007) Oral intake in labor. *International Anaesthesiology Clinics* 45(1), 133–47.

Prabulos, A. M., Philipson, E. H. (1998) Umbilical cord prolapse – is time from diagnosis to delivery critical? *Journal of Reproductive Medicine* 43(2), 129–32.

RCM (Royal College of Midwives) (2011) IVF multiple birthrates falling, HFEA reports. *Midwives* 4, 9.

Singata, M., Tranmer, J., Gyte, G. M. L. (2010) Restricting oral fluid and food intake during labour. *Cochrane Database of Systematic Reviews*, Issue 1.

Sheppard, C., Malinow, A., Alger, L. (1999) Vaginal delivery versus cesarean section for triplets and quadruplets: no difference in immediate measures of neonatal outcome. *American Journal of Obstetrics and Gynecology* 180 (1S–II) Supplement.

Smyth, R. M. D., Allderd, S. K., Markham, C. (2007) Amniotomy for shortening spontaneous labour. *Cochrane Database of Systematic Reviews*, Issue 4.

Steer, P. (2007) Perinatal death in twins *British Medical Journal* 334 (7593), 545–6.

Stein, W., Misselwitz, B., Schmidt, S. (2008) Twin-to-twin delivery time interval: influencing factors and effect on short-term outcome of the second twin. *Acta Obstet Gynecol Scand* 87(3), 346–53.

TAMBA (Twins and Multiple Births Association) (2006a) *Multiple Births Fact Sheet.* http://www.tamba.org.uk

TAMBA (2006b) *A Midwife's Guide to Twins, Triplets and More* [online]. http://www .tamba.org.uk

TAMBA (2007) *Multiple Births Factsheet* [online]. www.tamba.org.uk

Thompson, G. (2010) Psychology and labour experience: Birth as a peak experience. In Walsh, D., Downe, S. (eds) *Essential Midwifery Practice: Intrapartum Care.* Oxford, Wiley-Blackwell.

Twin Birth Study (2011) *http://sunnybrook.ca/research/content/?page=sri_proj_cmicr_trial_tbs_ home*

Wen, S., Fung, K., Oppenheimer, L., Demissie, K., Yang, Q., Walker, M. (2004a) Occurrence and predictors of cesarean delivery for the second twin following vaginal delivery of the first. *American Journal of Obstetrics and Gynecology* 103(3), 413–9.

Wen, S., Fung Kee, K., Oppenheimer, L., Demissie, K., Yang, Q., Walker, M. (2004b) Neonatal mortality in second twin according to cause of death, gestational age and mode of delivery. *American Journal of Obstetrics and Gynecology* 191(3), 778–83.

Yang, Q., Wen, S. W., Chen, Y., Krewski, D., Fung Kee Fung, K., Walker, M. (2005) Occurrence and clinical predictors of operative delivery for the vertex second twin after normal vaginal delivery of the first twin. *American Journal of Obstetrics and Gynecology* 192(1), 178–84.

16 Haemorrhage

Sheila Miskelly

Introduction

Haemorrhage may be defined as blood loss sufficient to cause haemodynamic instability (American Academy of Family Physicians (AAFP), 2012).

Heavy bleeding in the antenatal, intrapartum or immediate post-delivery period can become a serious emergency requiring rapid action. It is a comparatively common occurrence, and every midwife will face at least one serious haemorrhage at some time in his/her career. It can be terrifying for a woman and her partner (Mapp and Hudson, 2005). Timely and methodical management usually resolves the situation, but occasionally the haemorrhage can be catastrophic, even leading to death (CMACE, 2011).

Incidence and facts

- The UK maternal death rate from haemorrhage is approximately 0.39 per 100 000 (CMACE, 2011). The Centre for Maternal and Child Enquiries (CMACE, 2011) reported nine deaths in 2006–2008 directly due to haemorrhage (five postpartum haemorrhages (PPH), two placental abruptions, two placenta praevia).
- Haemorrhage can occur prior to, during or following birth; it can be dramatic and sudden or slow and incipient. Slow, continuous bleeding often goes unnoticed, but may still lead to maternal death (AAFP, 2012; RCOG, 2011a).
- Women may appear relatively unaffected by significant *initial* blood loss depending on weight, haemoglobin level and haemodilution, but once they have lost 20–40%

The Midwife's Labour and Birth Handbook, Third Edition. Edited by Vicky Chapman and Cathy Charles.
© 2013 John Wiley & Sons, Ltd. Published 2013 by John Wiley & Sons, Ltd.

blood volume they are likely to become symptomatic (RCOG, 2011a, b; Mukherjee and Arulkumaran, 2009).

- Early recognition and prompt action are the principles of haemorrhage management, whatever the setting (RCOG, 2009).
- Accurate visual estimation of blood loss is known to facilitate timely resuscitation (Bose *et al.*, 2006). Blood loss >300 ml is often underestimated, with greater inaccuracy as volume increases (WHO, 2006).
- A woman's haemorrhage risk should be assessed antenatally by the midwife; those with increased risk should be advised to give birth in an obstetric unit with an on-site blood bank (NICE, 2007; RCOG, 2009; CMACE, 2011).
- Each unit should have a multidisciplinary massive haemorrhage protocol and regularly rehearsed drills (CMACE, 2011; CNST, 2012). Practical sessions with real blood spillages may improve blood loss estimation (Bose *et al.*, 2006).
- All women who are Rhesus negative should receive anti-D immunoglobulin if they experience bleeding (Neilson, 2010).
- Suggested categorisation of **antepartum haemorrhage** by the RCOG (RCOG, 2011c), as follows, may be considered useful in conjunction with the wider clinical picture.
  - **Spotting:** staining, streaking or blood spotting noted on underwear or sanitary protection
  - **Minor haemorrhage:** blood loss <50 ml that has settled
  - **Major haemorrhage:** blood loss 50–1000 ml, with no signs of clinical shock
  - **Massive haemorrhage:** blood loss >1000 ml and/or signs of clinical shock.

Placenta praevia

Placenta praevia is the abnormal implantation of the placenta, either partially or fully in the lower uterine segment (Neilson, 2010; RCOG, 2011b), with partial or complete coverage of the cervical os. Haemorrhage is a significant risk, especially likely in the third trimester with the development of the lower segment and uterine contractions (Neilson, 2010).

Incidence and facts

- Placenta praevia presents in 0.4% of term pregnancies (AAFP, 2012): the risk increases to 2.3% for women who have three caesarean sections (CS).
- Placenta praevia accounted for two maternal deaths in the 2011 CMACE report.
- Women with placenta praevia who have had a previous CS have up to a 10% risk of placenta accreta/percreta (AAFP, 2012).
- Placenta praevia (and also accreta/percreta) is more common in women with a uterine scar, previous uterine surgery and multiparity (AAFP, 2012); all women whose placenta lies under their CS scar should have ultrasound imaging or MRI (NICE, 2008).
- A low-lying placenta identified at 20/40 anomaly scan usually resolves as the lower segment grows; however, if it partially/fully covers the internal os, a rescan at 32 weeks is recommended: transvaginal scan gives greatest accuracy (NICE, 2008).
- If the placental edge is <2 cm from the internal os in the third trimester, CS is likely (RCOG, 2011b). If the os is covered then CS is the only safe option. Elective CS

delivery in asymptomatic women is not recommended before 38/40 for placenta praevia, or before 36–37/40 for suspected placenta accreta (RCOG, 2011b).

- Antenatal discussion should take place between the woman, partner and an obstetrician, including mode and timing of delivery, risk of haemorrhage, possible blood transfusion and hysterectomy (CMACE, 2011; RCOG, 2011b). Advice will depend on location of the placenta, position/station of the baby and the woman's wishes (RCOG, 2011b).
- Senior obstetric and anaesthetic staff should be available in case of severe haemorrhage (NPSA, 2010).
- Women declining blood products should have alternatives discussed. Insufficient evidence supports autologous blood donation (RCOG, 2011b) but intra-operative blood cell salvage may be an option. These women should be advised to deliver where cell salvage, critical care and interventional radiology facilities are available (CMACE, 2011: RCOG, 2008). For diagnosis of placenta praevia see Table 16.1 and for care of a woman with placenta praevia see page 256.

Table 16.1   Diagnosis of placenta praevia and placental abruption.

	Placenta praevia	Placental abruption
Pain	Usually painless	Varies from mild to severe
		Uterine pain or back pain if placenta posterior or concealed abruption (AAFP, 2012)
Uterus	Soft / usually relaxed	Tense/tender
	25% experience variable strength contractions (Lockwood, 1996)	Hypertonus generally seen in severe cases when the baby has died and with concealed abruption (AAFP, 2012)
Bleeding	Usually visible (AAFP, 2012)	Usually visible but 20% present with concealed bleeding (Frazer & Watson, 2000; AAFP, 2012)
Symptoms of shock (see page 287)	May be present	May be present
Baby	Commonly non-engaged, ballotable presenting part	Usually normal lie and presentation
	35% present as unstable lie (Lockwood, 1996)	
Vaginal examination	Contraindicated: may exacerbate bleeding (Frazer & Watson, 2000)	Not contraindicated
Ultrasound scan (US)	All women who have had previous CS must have placental site identified and magnetic resonance imaging may indicate whether the placenta is accreta or percreta (CMACE, 2011) Review US reports for placental location and fetal gestation Transvaginal US may confirm placental edge (AAFP, 2012) & enhance placental image quality (RCOGa, 2011)	US to exclude placenta praevia. Differentiation between fresh bleeding and placental tissue can be difficult as haematomas become hypoechoic after a week (Nyberg, 1997)

Vasa praevia

Vasa praevia is a condition where fetal vessels from the placenta encroach on or cross the cervical os. The estimated incidence varies from 1:2000 to 1:6000 pregnancies and is probably under-reported (RCOG, 2011b).

Two types are identified:

- Velamentous cord insertion (Figure 16.1) in either single or bipartite (bilobed) placenta;
- Fetal vessels connecting succenturiate (accessory) placental lobes.

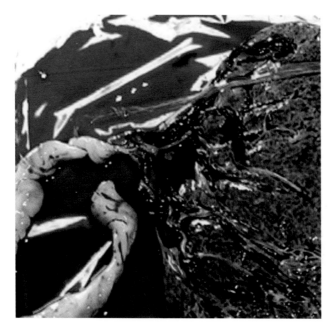

Fig. 16.1   Velamentous insertion of the cord.

Risk factors include multiple gestation, fetal anomalies, bilobed placenta, succenturiate lobes, second trimester low-lying placenta and in vitro fertilisation (AAFP, 2012).

Vasa praevia may be identified by transvaginal colour Doppler ultrasound, but may not be evident until sufficient cervical dilatation in labour to detect pulsations of vessels; if identified, CS delivery is indicated (RCOG, 2011b).

Vasa praevia presents no real risk to the mother, but significant haemorrhage risk to the fetus, and should be considered at membrane rupture if fresh bleeding is evident (RCOG, 2011b). A fetus only has 250 ml of blood (AAFP, 2012); therefore even minor fetal blood loss incurs risk.

Placental abruption

Placental abruption is the partial or total separation of the placenta from the uterus during pregnancy or labour (Neilson, 2009). It is a major cause of perinatal mortality (McGeown, 2001).

Incidence and facts

- Estimated incidence is 6.5:1000 births (Neilson, 2009).
- Recurrence is 4–5% in subsequent pregnancies (Nielson, 2009) and up to 25% in women who have abrupted in two previous pregnancies (RCOG, 2011b).
- Two maternal deaths were attributed to placental abruption in the latest CMACE (2011) report.
- The fetal mortality rate is 119:1000 abruptions, mainly attributable to sudden fetal hypoxia and/or premature delivery (Neilson, 2012).
- The stillbirth risk is proportionate to the degree of placental separation (AAFP, 2012).
- Many cases are mild and the pregnancy uneventful. Severe cases require the coordinated care of obstetricians, midwives, anaesthetists and haematologists (McGeown, 2001).
- Abruption should be considered in any woman with abdominal or back pain, with or without bleeding. Ultrasound scan may assist diagnosis (AAFP, 2012).
- Accumulating blood can exacerbate the situation by causing further placental separation (Neilson, 2012).
- For smaller bleeds, facilitating vaginal delivery (inducing/augmenting labour if required, and using continuous electronic fetal monitoring (EFM)) may reduce the CS rate by 50% without effecting perinatal mortality (Fraser and Watson, 2000).
- One third of women with abruption and fetal demise will develop coagulopathy as thromboplastins from the placental site are released, potentially activating the clotting cascade (AAFP, 2012). Disseminated intravascular coagulation (DIC) may follow (AAFP, 2012).

Risk factors for placental abruption

- Hypertension
- Abdominal trauma, e.g. domestic violence, road traffic incident
- High parity (AAFP, 2012)
- Oligohydramnios (AAFP, 2012), prolonged/premature rupture of membranes (RCOG, 2011c)
- Uterine overdistension, e.g. polyhydramnios, multiple gestation (AAFP, 2012; RCOG, 2011c)
- Tobacco, cocaine or methamphetamine use (AAFP, 2012)
- Some thrombophilias (McGeown, 2001)
- Intrauterine infection (RCOG, 2011c)
- Pregnancy following assisted reproductive techniques (RCOG, 2011c)

Care of a woman with placenta praevia or placental abruption

For diagnosis see Table 16.1.

Abruption/low-grade placenta praevia may be managed expectantly if bleeding is mild/moderate, settling (AAFP, 2012) and/or the baby is very preterm and the mother is stable (Fraser and Watson, 2000). With severe placenta praevia CS delivery is likely.

- **Assess and record blood loss.**
- **Note location of tenderness:** may relate to placental site, e.g. back pain associated with posterior placenta (AAFP, 2012).
- **Monitor vital signs:** tachycardia >90 bpm with systolic BP <100 mmHg and/or diastolic <50 mmHg may indicate impending hypovolaemic shock (WHO, 2003). Record vital signs on a labour chart or Modified Early Obstetric Warning Scoring (MEOWS) chart if not in labour (RCOG, 2009). See Table 16.2.
- **Perform EFM** (AAFP, 2012). If cardiotocograph (CTG) is suspicious/pathological delivery may need to be expedited (AAFP, 2012) (see Chapter 3).
- **Palpate/monitor contractions.** Abruption may cause a high resting tone and super-imposed small frequent contractions (AAFP, 2012).
- **Site large gauge IV cannula.** Check full blood count and blood group. If bleeding persists give IV fluids, and site a second large gauge cannula (RCOG, 2011b) Maintain a fluid balance chart.
- Ensure **cross-matched blood** (4 units) ordered.
- **Consider clotting studies** as DIC may develop (AAFP, 2012): fibrinogen levels, prothrombin time/international normalised ratio/activated partial thromboplastin time.
- **Perform Kleihauer test** if woman is rhesus negative (Crowther and Keirse, 2002) to detect fetal cells in the maternal circulation.
- **Inform team:** obstetrician, anaesthetist, paediatrician, neonatal intensive care unit and theatres and if maternal condition serious inform intensive therapy unit (ITU) (NPSA, 2010). Consider Situation, Background, Assessment, Recommendation (SBAR) system of communication (Box 16.1).

In labour

- **Analgesia and support.** Placental abruption can be very painful. Support, reassurance and analgesia are essential. Assist the woman to get comfortable, use bean bags/pillows, massage, touch and pharmacological analgesia.
- **Monitor labour progress.** Continue EFM throughout (AAFP, 2012), monitor contractions and document fluid balance, blood loss and maternal vital signs. Rapid intervention may be required.
- **Give regular antacids**/hydrogen ion inhibitors in anticipation of possible anaesthetic (NICE, 2007).
- **Expedite delivery** if bleeding is heavy, ongoing or greater than infusion ability (AAFP, 2012), if there is evidence of compromise to mother or baby (Hayashi, 2000) or labour is not progressing (AAFP, 2012).
- **If haemorrhage continues**
  - **Site a second large gauge cannula.**
  - A **central venous pressure** line may be sited to accurately monitor fluid volume.

Table 16.2   Modified Early Obstetric Warning Score Chart (MEOWS). *Modified from RCOG (2009) by permission of Vicky Tinsley, Great Western Hospital NHS Foundation Trust.*

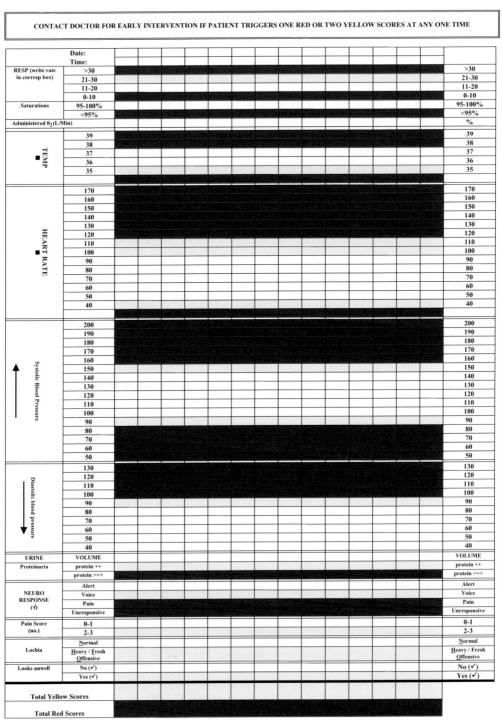

Name: DOB: /   /   Ward

Box 16.1 Situation, Background, Assessment, Recommendation (SBAR).

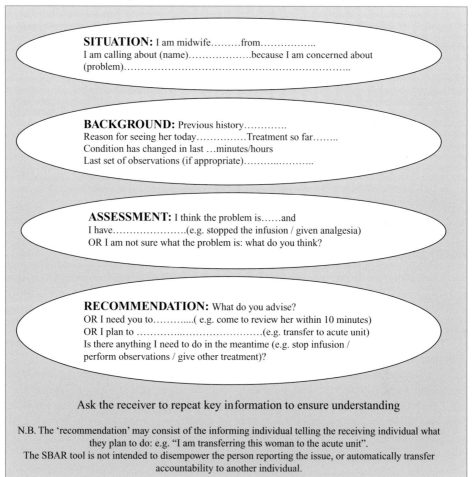

SITUATION: I am midwife..........from.................
I am calling about (name)...................because I am concerned about
(problem)..

BACKGROUND: Previous history.............
Reason for seeing her today...............Treatment so far........
Condition has changed in last ...minutes/hours
Last set of observations (if appropriate).....................

ASSESSMENT: I think the problem is......and
I have.....................(e.g. stopped the infusion / given analgesia)
OR I am not sure what the problem is: what do you think?

RECOMMENDATION: What do you advise?
OR I need you to.............(e.g. come to review her within 10 minutes)
OR I plan to ....(e.g. transfer to acute unit)
Is there anything I need to do in the meantime (e.g. stop infusion /
perform observations / give other treatment)?

Ask the receiver to repeat key information to ensure understanding

N.B. The 'recommendation' may consist of the informing individual telling the receiving individual what
they plan to do: e.g. "I am transferring this woman to the acute unit".
The SBAR tool is not intended to disempower the person reporting the issue, or automatically transfer
accountability to another individual.

The SBAR Tool originated in the US Navy and was adapted for use in health care by Dr M. Leonard and colleagues
from Kaiser Permanante, Colorado, USA. Modified from NHS Institute for Innovation and Improvement (2011).

○ **Record hourly urine volume** via catheter. Output should be ≥30 ml/hour (AAFP, 2012).
○ **Order blood** urgently: platelet and fresh frozen plasma infusion may be required prior to operative delivery if coagulopathy present (AAFP, 2012).

See also basic care for shock, Chapter 17, page 286.

Third-stage management

- **Active management is recommended** to reduce PPH risk.
- **Leave the baby's cord long** to enable umbilical cord catheterisation if required.
- **Take paired cord blood samples** for pH testing. If the mother is rhesus negative, a **direct Coombs test** from umbilical cord blood may indicate antibody presence; consequent haemolysis may cause neonatal hyperbilirubinaemia.
- Have **syntocinon infusion** ready in case of PPH.
- **Remember** blood loss is frequently underestimated (WHO, 2006).

Postpartum haemorrhage

The World Health Organization defines PPH as 500 ml blood loss in first 24 hours post-delivery (WHO, 2003; Mousa and Alfirevic, 2007). However, any blood loss that causes the woman's condition to deteriorate is considered a PPH (WHO, 2006). It is suggested that PPH >1000 ml constitutes major PPH (RCOG, 2009). Early summoning of quality and senior help by the midwife can save valuable time and prevent a situation getting out of control.

Women who suffer a PPH usually find the experience frightening and traumatic. The memories of fear and pain may increase their anxiety in any future birth. The woman's birth partner may experience feelings of helplessness and concern, sometimes manifested as quiet anxiety, asking many questions or occasionally showing panic or aggression.

Incidence and facts

- PPH occurs in up to 18% of births (AAFP, 2012) and 4–8% of CS (RCOG, 2004).
- Five cases of maternal death from PPH are reported in CMACE report (2011). Lack of routine observation in the postpartum period was cited as a major failure in three cases.
- Genital tract tears were implicated in two maternal PPH deaths (CMACE, 2011).
- The National Patient Safety Agency reports 23 maternity incidents of patient harm between 2006 and 2010 due to delayed provision of blood in haemorrhage incidents (NPSA, 2010).
- Clinicians should ensure a management plan is discussed with the woman, documented and that she is advised to deliver in an acute unit (CMACE, 2011; NICE, 2007). However, PPH is unpredictable and can occur in women with no identifiable risk factors (Mousa and Alfirevic, 2009).
- Management and treatment of primary PPH requires a multidisciplinary approach (Mousa and Alfirevic, 2009).
- Insidious blood loss can be fatal if not recognised early (CMACE, 2011).

The 4Ts: Tone, Tissue, Trauma, Thrombophilias

PPH has four causes, the 4Ts: Tone (uterine atony), Tissue, Trauma and, rarely, Thrombophilias (clotting problems).

Incidence: 70% tone, 20% trauma, 10% tissue and 1% thrombin (AAFP, 2012).

Tone (uterine atony)

Most PPHs are caused by uterine atony (Mousa and Alfirevic, 2009). Predisposing factors include any situation that weakens or over-distends the uterus. The aim of care is to deliver the placenta, if in situ, and ensure the uterus is well contracted.

Use of uterotonics is recommended; however, no particular uterotonic drug can be recommended over another (NICE 2007), use of misoprostol as a first line treatment of primary PPH is not currently recommended (Mousa and Alfirevic, 2009).

For management see Box 16.2.

Box 16.2   Management of PPH.

Women considered at high risk of PPH should be advised to have a large 14 gauge IV cannula sited (CMACE, 2011). Recent haemoglobin result should be available and blood cross-matched (CMACE, 2011).

Call for help
- At a home birth, call for a paramedic ambulance and follow transfer guidelines in Chapter 6, p. 113.
- In hospital summon more midwives and an obstetrician.

Deliver the placenta if in situ
- If the placenta is completely adhered there is usually no bleeding.
- If separation is partial the bleeding can be copious and delivery of an incomplete placenta may occur.
- Always check the placenta for completeness.

Rub up a contraction
- Rub the fundus in a firm circular motion: keep rubbing if required for up to a minute. The uterus should feel hard, not 'boggy'/soft.
- Regularly re-assess and re-rub if the uterus starts to relax under the fingers.

Give oxytocics/site IV
- Administer a second oxytocic agent: either:
  - IM syntometrine
  - IV oxytocin (syntocinon) bolus
  - IM (or cautiously IV) ergometrine
- Be wary of oxytocic overload and antidiuretic effects (AAFP, 2012).
- Warn the woman she may feel sick / vomit.

Further treatment
- Site large gauge cannula; take emergency bloods: full blood count, urea and electrolytes, group, cross match (4 units), coagulation screen (RCOG, 2009).
- Commence IV syntocinon 30–40 IU in 500 ml fluid (Hartmanns/normal saline) as per local protocol.
- Monitor vital signs and record on MEOWS Chart.

- Protect airway and breathing; give oxygen 10–15 litres per minute, regardless of maternal oxygen saturation levels; contact anaesthetist if consciousness compromised (RCOG, 2009).

Catheterisation
- Ensures no impediment to uterine contractility and enables renal function assessment.
- Satisfactory urine output is at least 100 ml in 4 hrs (WHO, 2006).

Reassess
- **By this point, most bleeding is controlled and responding to oxytocics.** If so, continue to observe.
- If not, call a more senior obstetrician and anaesthetist immediately. **DO NOT DELAY.**
- Consider a detailed genital tract examination (Campbell & Lees, 2000).

Ongoing haemorrhage/replace blood loss
- Site a *second* large 14 gauge cannula if not already sited (RCOG, 2009).
- Commence IV fluids: infuse 3 ml for every ml of blood loss (WHO, 2003). Options are: (a) crystalloid infusion, e.g. Ringer's Lactate; (b) colloid infusion, e.g. gelofusine: this will remain within the circulatory vessels for longer; BUT beware of potential fluid overload.
- Infuse maximum 3.5 litres clear fluid while awaiting compatible blood (RCOG, 2009).
- Infuse blood products as necessary.
- Consider further drugs: misoprostol (orally, vaginally or rectally) or carboprost/hemabate IM (kept in fridge): these may make the woman feel unwell.

Continued severe haemorrhage
- In hospital conduct bimanual compression (Box 16.3); prepare the woman for theatre to undergo exploration of the uterine cavity and surgical management of the haemorrhage.
- At home conduct bimanual compression until surgical intervention. In extreme maternal collapse with a retained placenta, the midwife may perform urgent manual removal of the placenta (NMC, 2004) (see Box 16.3).
- Large fluid volumes should be warmed.
- Consider blood products to replace clotting factors: recombinant activated factor VII (rFVIIa) may be used in consultation with a haematologist (RCOG, 2009).
- IV fluids of balanced electrolyte solution should be continued at 1 litre 6 hourly for the following 48 hours, although individual cases will vary (WHO, 2003).

Tissue

Retained tissue in the uterus can consist of either placental fragments or an adherent placenta (RCOG, 2009). The uterus cannot contract efficiently due to retained tissue, resulting in haemorrhage. The placenta must be delivered to allow uterine contraction.

Always check the placenta and membranes after delivery for completeness.

See page 265 for management of retained placenta.

Trauma

Trauma may consist of lacerations of the cervix, vagina, perineum or anus, episiotomy, pelvic haematomas and uterine inversion/rupture (AAFP, 2012). Occasionally large blood vessels are involved. Predisposing risk factors include any situation where the birth outlet is severely stretched, e.g. macrosomia, malpositions or use of any instrument, e.g. forceps or scissors. An episiotomy if large, or performed too early before the perineum has thinned, can cut through blood vessels resulting in uncontrolled bleeding. Episiotomy also increases the risk of third- and fourth-degree tears (Sleep *et al.*, 2000).

Despite heavy blood loss, the uterus usually feels well contracted and does not gush blood when pressed. Many midwives choose to give a precautionary dose of an oxytocic if they remain unsure of the source of the bleeding.

Treatment of trauma

External bleeding

- Locating the source of the bleeding can be very painful – Entonox can be offered. Talk through what you are doing and suggest the woman says if she needs you to stop at any time.
- A bleeding vessel can be hidden behind clots or oozing blood loss. Methodically check the area: the clitoris, labia, perineum and vagina – dabbing firmly with gauze.
- A bleeding vessel is obvious as when dabbed clear it instantly oozes or pumps blood, obscuring the view. Apply pressure to the bleeding point using sterile gauze or similar material; hold firmly for at least five minutes. This may be sufficient but keep checking the area in the following hours.
- If still oozing, the bleeding vessel should be clamped and will require tying off promptly (see Figure 16.2).
- If the bleeding is internal, or excessive, contact a senior obstetrician (CMACE, 2011).

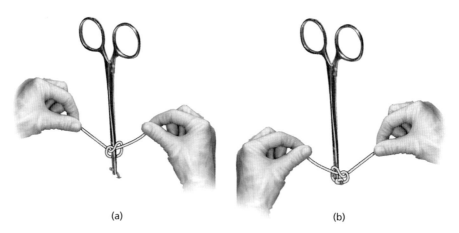

(a)   (b)

Fig. 16.2 Tying off a bleeding vessel. Bleeding vessels can be awkward to reach and tying them off may be painful for the woman. Grasp the vessel with a pair of forceps, then loop some thread around the forceps (this may require the aid of an assistant). Tie one throw of a knot – left thread over right (a) and slip the knot down past the end of the forceps to encircle the vessel. Pull the knot right and then tie a second throw – right thread over left (b). The knot should be square and not slip. Trim the thread and then release the forceps carefully.

Internal bleeding

- Contact an experienced obstetrician to carry out further examination.
- If at a home birth or birthing centre, the midwife must undertake this examination, as prompt arrest of bleeding is essential.
- Bleeding from the cervix or deep in the vagina requires a speculum examination using a good light source and plenty of gauze. Use a clamp or sponge holder forceps wrapped in gauze for dabbing the blood away, allowing a view of the bleeding point.
- If the bleeding is high up, apply direct pressure or pack with gauze; the woman will require suturing under anaesthesia. Sutures should not be placed blindly deep in the vaginal fornix as they can cause uterine injury. Occasionally, very high tears need repairing via the abdomen (Kean, 2000).
- Compression of the abdominal aorta, just above and to the left of the umbilicus, may be necessary in extreme cases (AAFP, 2012).
- Keep a count of gauze swabs used before and after, as one could easily become 'lost' (NPSA, 2010).

Haematoma

This is a solid swelling formed by blood trapped/concealed in the tissues. An acute haematoma is rare, approximately 1:1000 births. The volume of blood is often underestimated (Kean, 2000). Episiotomy is a related factor in 85–90% of haematomas (Kean, 2000).

Signs and symptoms of haematoma

- Visible bleeding may be minimal, there may be no external signs or apparent distortion of the vagina and rectum (AAFP, 2012).
- Internal examination may be intolerable due to severe vaginal/vulval/rectal pain or unrelenting pressure.
- Signs of hypovolaemic shock.

Treatment

- For small haematomas <3 cm, offer analgesia and observe (Kean, 2000; AAFP, 2012).
- Most large haematomas require not only analgesia but prompt surgical intervention (AAFP, 2012), i.e. incision, drainage and stemming of any bleeding vessel, followed by packing or suturing depending on tissue friability (Kean, 2000).
- Treat any hypovolaemia promptly (see basic treatment for shock, page 286).

Thrombophilias/clotting problems

Thrombophilias and clotting problems directly account for only 1% of PPHs as most are identified and treated antenatally (AAFP, 2012). The clotting cascade once triggered can lead to DIC (AAFP, 2012).

Some pregnancy-related conditions result in clotting problems: e.g. large placental abruption (classically accompanied by fetal demise), severe pre-eclampsia/eclampsia, intrauterine death, amniotic fluid embolism and sepsis (AAFP, 2012). Some uncommon conditions, e.g. thrombocytopenia and von Willebrand's disease, can also affect clotting.

Signs and symptoms

- Continued bleeding and lost blood does not clot.
- Oozing from puncture sites.

Treatment

- Care should involve senior anaesthetic, obstetric, midwifery and haematology staff.
- Treat the underlying disorder (AAFP, 2012). ITU admission may be required. Take blood urgently for cross match, full blood count and clotting studies.
- Give urgent fluid and blood product replacement, depending on diagnosed coagulopathy (AAFP, 2012) (see basic treatment for shock, page 286).
- On haematologist advice consider additional options for treating thrombin PPH, e.g. intravenous (IV) tranexamic acid (an antifibrinolytic agent) or recombinant activated factor VII (rFVIIa) (RCOG 2007; Mousa and Alfirevic, 2009).

Retained placenta

A retained placenta and manual removal can have a negative effect on the quality of contact the woman has with her newborn, reducing time spent feeding and getting to know the new baby, and can leave the woman anaemic, tender and sore. Rarely, the placenta may be truly adherent and imbedded due to scanty or absent decidua, resulting in placenta accreta/increta or percreta. More severe cases can result in primary or secondary PPH, infection, hysterectomy and even maternal death (RCOG, 2009).

Incidence and facts

- A retained placenta occurs in up to 3% vaginal births (AAFP, 2012).
- There is a moderate level of evidence that an actively managed third stage of ≥30 minutes is associated with an increased incidence of PPH (NICE, 2007).
- A physiological third stage lasts <60 minutes in 95% women (NICE, 2007).
- NICE (2007) therefore defines a *prolonged third stage* (not necessarily a retained placenta) if the placenta is undelivered after 30 minutes of active management or 60 minutes of expectant management.
- Active management is recommended if physiological management has been unsuccessful after 60 minutes (NICE, 2007). Only if active management has been unsuccessful would more interventionist procedures be used, and the term 'retained placenta' be appropriate.

- For suspected placenta accreta/percreta urgent manual removal is indicated in theatre since both lead to adverse outcomes including maternal death (CMACE, 2011). This high-risk situation should be managed by the consultant obstetrician, consultant anaesthetist and involve the haematologist to ensure the best outcome (RCOG, 2009).
- Occasionally non-bleeding placenta accreta/percreta is managed conservatively, leaving it in situ to undergo re-absorption. This may reduce the risks of manual removal, such as hysterectomy (http://www.ncbi.nlm.nih.gov/pubmed/19772011).
- Bleeding may be minimal with a totally adherent placenta, but increases with partial adherence (RCOG, 2009).
- In the absence of medical aid and in an extreme emergency, manual removal of the placenta can be undertaken by a midwife (NMC, 2004): see Box 16.3.

Box 16.3   Manual removal of the placenta and bimanual compression.

Manual removal: only conducted by a midwife in an extreme emergency (NMC, 2004)
Manual removal is likely to be very painful for the woman and risks infection and uterine rupture if performed too roughly. The woman should be offered Entonox. The procedure should be explained to her and her birth partner, who may wish to stay and give support, or leave the room (Crafter, 2002).

- Wear sterile gloves.
- Place the external hand on the fundus, to prevent it moving away.
- Insert the fingers, then the hand into the vagina, through the os and trace the cord to locate the placenta.
- Locate the edge of the placenta (cleavage plane) and using a side-to-side movement gently coax the placenta away from the uterus (Crafter, 2002), cupping the separated cotyledons in the palm of the hand (AAFP, 2012).
- Aim to deliver the placenta intact (AAFP, 2012).
- Once separated deliver the placenta by cord traction.
- Keep the hand inside the uterus to 'brush' gently over the placental site and dislodge any possible fragments left behind (Crafter, 2002).

Bimanual compression

This is extremely painful and should only be performed if bleeding continues and medical assistance is not available. Rub up a contraction with the external hand on the fundus. Insert the other hand and make a clenched fist shape, pushing up against the anterior fornix of the vagina, while pressing down with the external hand, thereby pressing the walls of the uterus together (Crafter, 2002).

Role of the midwife in delivering a retained placenta

Provided blood loss is normal, the midwife can try the following:

- **Observation of vital signs:** pulse, blood pressure, respirations, vaginal loss, colour and general physical condition.
- **Breastfeeding and nipple stimulation.** This stimulates natural oxytocin, which helps the uterus contract.
- **Proceed to active management** of third stage if the placenta does not deliver with physiological management. NICE (2007) recommends active management after

60 minutes; however, some midwives may question the strength of the evidence and wait for longer if the woman is not bleeding and is happy to continue.

- **Controlled cord traction.** If an oxytocic has been administered, attempt to deliver the placenta by applying cord traction and guarding the uterus. If any heavy bleeding occurs, stop cord traction.
- **Maternal position.** Assist the mother to remain upright, e.g. squatting/kneeling or sitting on the toilet/bedpan.
- **Encourage active pushing.** The woman may experience contractions as period-type pains and they may be infrequent. Encourage her to push with these pains. Anecdotally, midwives who recommend this report that pushing may take a while and require many attempts but that it is often successful.
- **Palpable bladder.** A full bladder may displace the uterus. Offer a bedpan/toilet. However, urination is often unachievable, and if the bladder is palpable discuss passing a catheter. Offer entonox during any catheterisation.
- **Establish IV access.** Oxytocin infusion should not be used to facilitate delivery of the placenta (NICE, 2007); however, it should be commenced promptly if any active bleeding or if the woman is transferring from home/birthing centre.

If the placenta remains undelivered, inform the obstetrician who may:

- Perform a vaginal examination to determine degree of separation, if any, as sometimes the placenta has separated and is lying in the vagina/cervix.
- Attempt removal by fundal pressure and/or cord traction.
- Inject 20IU oxytocin in 20 ml saline directly into the umbilical vein of the clamped and cut cord (NICE, 2007). *Caution*: ensure that the baby is separated from the mother's cord before attempting this.
- If unsuccessful, proceed to digital manual removal of the placenta (MROP) in theatre under adequate regional (occasionally general) anaesthesia (NICE, 2007). IV oxytocin infusion, prophylactic antibiotics and close observation for signs of PPH or infection are recommended post-procedure (NICE, 2007).

Summary

Placenta praevia and placental abruption

- Monitor vital signs, pain, uterine tone and FH
- Take blood and treat hypovolaemia
- If severe, prepare for emergency delivery, possibly CS
- Remember the risk of PPH

Postpartum haemorrhage

Tone (uterine atony) (see Box 16.2).
Tissue (partial or complete retention of placenta):

- Try to deliver placenta
- Check placental completeness
- Control haemorrhage

Trauma:

- Apply pressure over bleeding point
- Clamp and tie off bleeding vessel
- Serious trauma/haematomas will go to theatre

Thrombophilias/clotting disorders:

- A rare cause of haemorrhage
- Bleeding from puncture sites; blood does not clot
- Treat underlying causes

Retained placenta:

- Bleeding worse if partial rather than full adherence
- Give IV fluids and oxytocics as per local protocol
- Injecting cord with oxytocic may help but MROP usually required
- A midwife may perform MROP in an extreme emergency

References

Alexander, J., Thomas, P., Sanghera, J. (2008) Treatments for secondary postpartum haemorrhage. *Cochrane Database of Sytematic Reviews*, Issue 2.

American Academy of Family Physicians (AAFP) (2012) *Advanced Life Support in Obstetrics (ALSO) Course Syllabus Manual, Revised*. Leawood, Kansas, AAFP.

Bose, P., Regan, F., Paterson-Brown, N. (2006) Improving the accuracy of estimated blood loss at obstetric haemorrhage, using clinical reconstruction. *British Journal of Obstetrics and Gynaecology* 113(8), 919–24.

Campbell, S., Lees, C. (2000) Obstetric emergencies. In Campbell, S., Lees, C. (eds) *Obstetrics by Ten Teachers*, 17th edn, pp. 303–17. London, Edward Arnold.

Centre for Maternal and Child Enquiries (CMACE) (2011) *Saving Mothers' Lives. The Eighth Report of Confidential Enquiries into Maternal Deaths in the United Kingdom*. London, RCOG Press. http://onlinelibrary.wiley.com/doi/10.1111/j.1471-0528.2010.02847.x/pdf

CNST (2012) *Maternity Clinical Risk Management Standards*. NHS Litigation Authority. www.nhsla.com

Crafter, H. (2002) Intrapartum and primary postpartum haemorrhage. In Boyle, M. (ed.) *Emergencies around Childbirth: A Handbook for Midwives*, pp. 11–26. Oxford, Radcliffe Medical Press.

Crowther, C., Keirse, M. J. N. C. (2002) Anti D Administration in pregnancy. *Cochrane Database of Systematic Reviews*, Issue 4.

Fraser, R., Watson, R. (2000) Bleeding in the latter half of pregnancy. In Enkin, M., Keirse, M. J. N. C., Neilson, J., Crowther, C., Duley, L., Hodnett, E. and Hofmeyr, J. (eds) *A Guide to Effective Care in Pregnancy and Childbirth*, 3rd edn, pp. 178–84. Oxford, Oxford University Press.

Hayashi, R. (2000) Obstetric collapse. In Kean, L. H., Baker, P. N., Edelstone, D. I. (eds) *Best Practice in Labor Ward Management*, pp. 415–33. Edinburgh, WB Saunders.

Kean, L. (2000) Other problems of the third stage. In Kean, L. H., Baker, P. N., Edelstone, D. I. (eds) *Best Practice in Labour Ward Management*, pp. 435–50. London, WB Saunders.

Lockwood, C. (1996) Third trimester bleeding. In Queenan, J. T., Hobbins, J. C. (eds) *Protocols for High Risk Pregnancies*, 3rd edn, pp. 568–72. Oxford, Blackwell Science.

Mapp, T., Hudson, K. (2005) Feelings and fears during obstetric emergencies. *British Journal of Midwifery* 13(1), 30–5.

McGeown, P. (2001) Practice recommendations for obstetric emergencies. *British Journal of Midwifery* 9(2), 71–3.

Mousa, H., Alfirevic, Z. (2009) Treatment for primary postpartum haemorrhage. *Cochrane Database of Systematic Reviews*, Issue 1.

Mukherjee, S., Arulkumaran, S. (2009) Postpartum haemorrhage. *Obstetrics and Gynaecology Reproductive Medicine* 19(5), 121–6.

NICE (2005) *Intra-operative Blood Cell Salvage in Obstetrics: Interventional Procedure Guidance 144*. London, NICE. www.nice.org.uk

NICE (2007) *Clinical Guideline 55: Intrapartum Care*. London, NICE. www.nice.org.uk

NICE (2008) *Clinical Guideline 62: Antenatal Care: Routine Care for the Healthy Pregnant Woman*. London, RCOG Press. www.nice.org.uk

National Patient Safety Agency (NPSA) (2010a) *Transfusion of Blood and Blood Components in an Emergency*. www.npsa.nhs.uk

National Patient Safety Agency (NPSA) (2010b) *Reducing Risk of Retained Swabs after Vaginal Birth and Perineal Suturing*. www.npsa.nhs.uk

National Patient Safety Agency (2010c) *National Reporting and Learning Service. 'How to use the placenta praevia after caesarean section care bundle'* www.npsa.nhs.uk

NHS Institute for Innovation and Improvement. www.institute.nhs.uk

Neilson, J. P. (2010) Interventions for suspected placenta praevia. *Cochrane Database of Systematic Reviews*, Issue 1.

Neilson, J. P. (2012) Interventions for treating placental abruption. *Cochrane Database of Systematic Reviews*, Issue 2.

Nursing and Midwifery Council (NMC) (2004) *Midwives Rules*. www.nmc-uk.org

Nyberg, D. A. (1987) Ultrasound scanning and placental abruption. *American Journal of Roentgenology* 148(1), 161–4.

Prendiville, W., Elbourne, D. (2000) The third stage of labor. In Enkin, M., Keirse, M. J. N. C., Neilson, J., Crowther, C., Duley, L., Hodnett, E., Hofmeyr, J. (eds) *A Guide to Effective Care in Pregnancy and Childbirth*, 3rd edn, pp. 300–9. Oxford, Oxford University Press.

RCOG (2004) *Caesarean Section Guideline No. 13*. London, RCOG.

RCOG (2007) *Blood Transfusion in Obstetrics. Green Top Clinical Guideline No 47*. London, RCOG.

RCOG (2009) Prevention and management of postpartum haemorrhage. *Green Top Clinical Guideline No 52*. London, RCOG.

RCOG (2011a) Maternal collapse in pregnancy and the puerperium. *Green Top Clinical Guideline No 56*. London, RCOG.

RCOG (2011b) Placenta praevia, placenta accreta and vasa praevia: diagnosis and management. *Green Top Clinical Guideline No 27*. London, RCOG.

RCOG (2011c) Antepartum haemorrhage. *Green Top Clinical Guideline No 63*. London, RCOG.

Sleep, J., Roberts, J., Chalmers, L. (2000) The second stage of labor. In Enkin, M., Keirse, M. J. N. C., Neilson, J., Crowther, C., Duley, L., Hodnett, E., Hofmeyr, J. (eds) *A Guide to Effective Care in Pregnancy and Childbirth*, 3rd edn, pp. 289–99. Oxford, Oxford University Press.

WHO (World Health Organization) (2003) *Integrated Management of Pregnancy and Childbirth: Managing Complications in Pregnancy and Childbirth: A Guide for Midwives and Doctors.* Geneva, WHO.

WHO (World Health Organization) (2006) Managing postpartum haemorrhage. In *Midwifery Education Modules*, 2nd edn. Geneva, WHO.

17 Emergencies in labour and birth

Sheila Miskelly

Introduction

A small but significant proportion of women develop complications which may threaten their lives or those of their babies. Emergency situations can be very disturbing and provoke a range of emotional responses and consequences for all involved (WHO, 2003). Acute units must have comprehensive multidisciplinary facilities for rapid response to obstetric emergencies. In birth centres and at home births the midwife is responsible for emergency measures and prompt transfer (DoH, 2004). Regular skills drills, included in training packages such as PROMPT and ALSO have been shown to improve outcomes (Paxton *et al.*, 2005; AAFP 2012).

Clear, calm explanation will help to reduce anxiety for the woman and her partner. Be respectful of the woman's dignity, be aware that her choices may be reduced, acknowledge her fears and give sensitive responses to her needs (WHO, 2003).

> *'Even when serious emergencies occur, midwives can do much to create an environment which respects the woman as a person with feelings and emotions rather than an object to be rushed to theatre'* (Weston, 2001).

The National Patient Safety Agency (NPSA, 2006) and Clinical Negligence Scheme for Trusts (CNST, 2012) recommend that emergencies are reviewed and analysed to identify improvements in practice (see Chapter 22).

The Midwife's Labour and Birth Handbook, Third Edition. Edited by Vicky Chapman and Cathy Charles.
© 2013 John Wiley & Sons, Ltd. Published 2013 by John Wiley & Sons, Ltd.

Snapped cord

A short or friable cord can snap at, or following, birth. It occurs in 3% of vaginal births (Prendiville and Elbourne, 2000). Grasp and clamp the baby's end *immediately* – see page 126–7. If the cord snaps, or starts to 'give' under traction then, providing there is no haemorrhage, encourage placenta delivery by maternal effort. Pushing in an upright position often succeeds unless the placenta is truly adhered. Ensure an empty bladder. If no success after an hour, see retained placenta page 265–7.

Cord prolapse and cord presentation

Cord presentation is the presence of umbilical cord between the fetal presenting part and the cervix, with or without membrane rupture (RCOG, 2008). Cord prolapse occurs when the umbilical cord prolapses through the cervix, either occult (alongside the presenting part) or, more dangerously, overt/frank (past the presenting part) in the presence of membrane rupture (RCOG, 2008). The cord may even be visible outside the vagina. Asphyxia can result, primarily from poor blood flow to/from the fetus due to cord compression (RCOG, 2008).

Incidence and facts

- Cord prolapse occurs in 0.1 to 0.6% of births: with 0.4% in vertex presentation but 1% in breech presentation (RCOG, 2008): of all breech cord prolapses, 46% are complete breech, 15% footling breech, 0.5% frank breech (AAFP, 2012).
- 50% of cord prolapse cases occur following obstetric manipulation, including artificial rupture of membranes (ARM) (RCOG, 2008).
- Cord prolapse is associated with poor perinatal outcomes, even when emergency delivery facilities are available (Prabulos and Philipson, 1998).
- Prognosis is worse if it occurs outside a maternity hospital (Draycott *et al.*, 2008).
- Mortality is predominantly associated with prematurity and congenital abnormities rather than birth asphyxia per se (Squire, 2002).
- Electronic fetal monitoring (EFM) aided the diagnosis of cord prolapse in only 41% cases (Murphy and MacKenzie, 1995).

See Table 17.1 for causes and associated factors for cord prolapse.

Table 17.1   Risk factors for cord prolapse (RCOG, 2008).

General	Procedure related
Multiparity	Artificial rupture of membranes
Low birthweight <2.5 kg	Vaginal manipulation of fetus with ruptured membranes
Prematurity <37 weeks	During external cephalic version
Fetal congenital abnormalities	Internal podalic version
Breech presentation	Stabilising induction of labour
Transverse, oblique or unstable lie	Insertion of uterine pressure transducer
Second twin	
Polyhydramnios	
Unengaged presenting part	
Low-lying placenta, abnormal placentation	

Signs and symptoms of cord prolapse

- Visible cord protruding from vagina.
- Cord felt (often pulsating) on vaginal examination (VE).
- Fetal bradycardia/prolonged variable decelerations particularly following rupture of membranes.

Practice recommendations/manoeuvres

- Speculum and/or VE should be performed at preterm gestations when cord prolapse is suspected (RCOG, 2008).
- **Call for help.** If at home/birthing centre, call paramedic ambulance even if delivery appears imminent; if in second stage, also call midwife ventouse/forceps practitioner (if available). Communicate accurately: the Situation, Background, Assessment, Recommendation (SBAR) tool is helpful. See page 260.
- **Fetal heart monitoring.** Continuous EFM is recommended (RCOG, 2008).
- **Maintain pressure on presenting part.** Manually elevate the presenting part using fingers or hand inserted in the vagina. (AAFP, 2012). If achievable maintain pressure during ambulance journey and/or while the woman is transferred to a birth room/theatre (AAFP, 2012).
- **Remain calm.** Explain to the woman and her partner what is happening and what is required of them. The clinician conducting internal pressure is ideally situated to offer supportive reassurance and explanations to the woman and her partner.
- **Position the mother.** The *all fours/knee-chest* position reduces pressure caused by the presenting part (see Figure 17.1). It is possibly the most effective position, but can be uncomfortable and undignified for the woman. Cover her lower half for modesty.

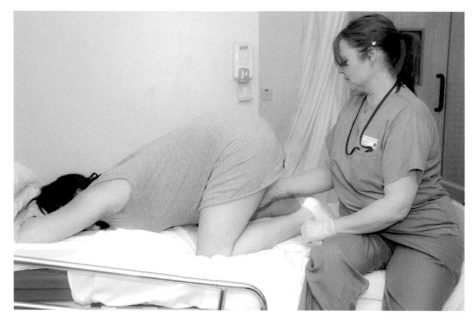

Fig. 17.1   Knee-chest position. *Photo by Debbie Gagliano-Withers.*

- **Alternative positions:**
  - **Trendelenburg.** The woman lies on her back with a 30° tilt using a wedge to prevent aortocaval compression with a head down tilt, if possible, to relieve pressure.
  - **Exaggerated Sims.** The woman lies on her left side with her upper leg flexed and the knee resting on the bed; a useful position for emergency transfer by ambulance.
- **Cord handling.** Opinion varies as to whether the cord should be replaced into the vagina (RCOG, 2008). Touching/cooling the cord may cause vasoconstriction. Wrapping the cord with warm saline-soaked swabs is of unproven benefit (Goswami, 2007).
- **Fill the bladder.** This may relieve cord compression and inhibit uterine activity if a theatre is not immediately available (RCOG, 2008). Consider instilling 500–750 ml saline into the bladder via a Foley catheter attached to an intravenous (IV) giving set (AAFP, 2012). Ensure bladder is emptied prior to delivery and avoid prolonged bladder distension.
  - **Tocolysis.** Terbutaline 0.25 mg subcutaneously may be used to reduce contractions and therefore alleviate bradycardia (RCOG, 2008).
- **Deliver urgently.** If birth is not imminent CS is recommended, as it is associated with reduced perinatal mortality/Apgar <3 at 5 minutes. However, if birth is imminent vaginal birth gives similar or better neonatal outcomes. Therefore, vaginal delivery (often forceps or ventouse, particularly for a primigravida) can be attempted if full dilatation is present and a rapid delivery is likely (RCOG, 2008).
- **Assistance with resuscitation.** Babies may need resuscitation after cord prolapse: 21% have low one-minute Apgar scores, and 7% low five-minute scores (Murphy and Mackenzie, 1995). Summon paediatric support, or an experienced second midwife at a birthing centre or at home. Analyse paired cord bloods for pH and base excess level if possible (RCOG, 2008).

Amniotic fluid embolism

Amniotic fluid embolism (AFE) is a rare but catastrophic, condition. It is unpredictable, unpreventable, rapidly progressive, and often fatal (AAFP, 2012; CMACE, 2011). A woman may collapse suddenly with no clear diagnosis at the time. AFE is an anaphylactic type reaction to amniotic fluid that has entered the woman's circulation (AAFP, 2012). This results in left ventricular failure and pulmonary vasospasm resulting in acute lung injury. Clotting factors are also activated with disseminated intravascular coagulation (DIC) commonly resulting (Davis, 1999; Fahy, 2001; AAFP, 2012). The rapidly deteriorating situation can be extremely stressful for staff and birth partners, particularly as death often results. However, high quality, rapid intensive multi-professional care can increase survival and improve outcomes (CMACE, 2011; Knight *et al.*, 2010).

Incidence and facts

- The UK AFE maternal mortality rate is 0.57 per 100 000 maternities: 13 women died between 2006 and 2009 (CMACE, 2011). There is a high perinatal mortality rate, and around 60% babies sustain some degree of neurological damage (AAFP, 2012; Knight *et al.*, 2010).

- Risk factors include advanced maternal age, placental abnormalities, operative delivery, eclampsia, polyhydramnios, cervical lacerations, uterine rupture (AAFP, 2012).
- Rapid full effective resuscitation should take place irrespective of the diagnosis for the initial collapse (CMACE, 2011).
- The more knowledgeable clinicians become about AFE, the more frequently it is diagnosed (Fahy, 2001).
- A detailed post-mortem including immunochemistry/histochemistry should be undertaken in the event of death (CMACE, 2011). Diagnosis is confirmed by the presence of fetal squames and lanugo hair in the pulmonary vasculature (CEMACH, 2004).
- AFE diagnosis will rely on clinical observations if the woman survives or if autopsy is unavailable (CMACE, 2011).
- All cases of AFE, whether the woman survives or not, should be reported to the UK AFE Register at UK Obstetric Surveillance System (UKOSS) which was commenced in 2000.

Signs and symptoms of AFE

See Table 17.2.

Table 17.2   Signs and symptoms of amniotic fluid embolism (Fahy, 2001).

Sign/symptom	% of women
Hypotension (shock)	100
Fetal distress (if undelivered)	100
Pulmonary oedema or adult respiratory distress syndrome	93
Cardiopulmonary arrest	86
Cyanosis	83
Coagulopathy	83
Dyspnoea (difficult or laboured breathing)	49
Seizure	48

Symptoms may be non-specific and overlap with/indicate other conditions, e.g. pulmonary embolism, eclampsia, DIC, haemorrhage, septic or anaphylactic shock (RCOG, 2011; CMACE, 2011). The woman may gasp for breath and develop rapid hypotension and shock symptoms. Her behaviour may change as hypoxic/toxic confusional state develops. She is then likely to collapse and experience cardiac arrest (AAFP, 2012; RCOG, 2011).

Practice recommendations

- **Call for help/transfer to hospital.**
- **Think ABC.** Airway, Breathing and Circulation (see Box 17.4 and Chapter 18).

- **Early input** of coordinated care from the resuscitation team and consultant anaesthetist, obstetrician and haematologist (RCOG, 2011). Rapid intensive therapy unit transfer is recommended and may increase survival (CMACE, 2011; RCOG, 2011).
- **Deliver baby** by CS as rapidly as possible in the event of maternal cardiac arrest (MOET, 2003). Obstetricians do not need to prepare a sterile field (RCOG, 2011).
- **Aftercare.** The woman will require intensive care with supportive treatment (CMACE, 2011).

Uterine rupture

Uterine dehiscence is defined as disruption of the uterine muscle with intact serosa (RCOG, 2007). The more serious condition of *uterine rupture* is defined as disruption of the uterine muscle extending to and involving the uterine serosa, or disruption of the uterine muscle with extension to the bladder or broad ligament (RGOG, 2007). Occasionally these events occur antenatally, but more often during labour, birth or prior to delivery of the placenta (RCOG, 2007).

Incidence and facts

- Uterine rupture is rare: 111 cases were reported to UKOSS from April 2009 to January 2010; roughly 17:100 000 UK maternities (Knight *et al.*, 2010).
- Incidence in UK women with an unscarred uterus is reported as <2:10 000 and with a scarred uterus 22–74:10 000 deliveries (RCOG, 2007).
- One maternal death was attributed to uterine rupture in the 2011 CMACE report. However, other morbidity is significantly higher, e.g. catastrophic haemorrhage, fetal hyoxia, or both.
- 86% cases occurred in women with a previous CS (CMACE, 2011).
- There is no single clinical feature indicative of uterine rupture: diagnosis is ultimately confirmed at CS or postpartum laparotomy (RCOG, 2007).
- Early recognition and diagnosis may improve outcomes (AAFP, 2012).

Associated risk factors

- Caesarean section, inappropriate use of prostaglandins/oxytocin to induce/augment labour (NICE, 2004), trauma caused by high-cavity forceps, manual manipulation for unstable lie, manual removal of placenta, road traffic incident or other blunt trauma including physical assault (Kroll and Lyne, 2002).

Signs and symptoms of uterine rupture are given in Box 17.1.

Practice recommendations

- Midwifery care: call for help/transfer to hospital.
- Discontinue IV oxytocin if in progress (AAFP, 2012).
- Administer 100% oxygen and IV fluids rapidly.

Box 17.1 Signs and symptoms of uterine rupture.

Pain
- Sudden uterine or scar pain (AAFP, 2012).
- Chest or shoulder tip pain (RCOG, 2007).
- A feeling of 'giving way' (Silverton, 1993).
- Lower abdominal pain may come with a contraction, or be constant and unrelenting (AAFP, 2012).
- The woman may find it too painful to have her uterus touched or palpated.
- Pain may decrease after the rupture (WHO, 2003).

Uterus/contractions
- Solid, tonic uterus or abnormal uterine shape (WHO, 2003).
- Contractions may stop or dwindle (AAFP, 2012).

Fetus
- Abnormal CTG may occur (RCOG, 2007) culminating in prolonged fetal bradycardia (AAFP, 2012).
- Recession of presenting part (RCOG, 2007) or suprapubic bulging (AAFP, 2012).
- Easily palpable fetal parts (WHO, 2003).

Shock
- Tachycardia (AAFP, 2012).
- Hypotension (RCOG, 2007).
- Sudden onset shortness of breath (RCOG, 2007).

Bleeding
- Fresh vaginal bleeding or blood-stained amniotic fluid may be seen.
- Haematuria may develop (RCOG, 2007).
- Following delivery a ruptured uterus may rise as it fills with blood.

The woman may
- Look cold and clammy.
- Appear restless, agitated or withdrawn.
- Say she is frightened and that something is wrong.
- Vomit.

Obstetricians are likely to:

- Deliver the baby by instrumental means or proceed to urgent CS (AAFP, 2012).
- Repair the uterus immediately in theatre. Haemorrhage is likely. If bleeding is uncontrollable, hysterectomy may be necessary (Bakshi and Meyer, 2000).

Aftercare

- Closely monitor the woman following surgery as she is at risk of postpartum haemorrhage (RCOG, 2007). An IV oxytocin infusion is advisable post-delivery. In severe cases the mother and baby may require intensive care. Perinatal mortality/morbidity is more common in cases of complete displacement of the baby into the abdominal cavity due to uterine rupture (AAFP, 2012).

Shoulder dystocia

Shoulder dystocia is one of the most serious birth emergencies. It is caused by the impaction of the anterior shoulder of the fetus against the maternal symphysis pubis, or less commonly the posterior fetal shoulder on the sacral promontory, after delivery of the head (RCOG, 2008), requiring additional obstetric manoeuvres to release the shoulders (RCOG, 2008). Shoulder dystocia cannot be predicted (WHO, 2003); all midwives must be able to recognise and manage this emergency promptly (Brown, 2002).

Incidence and facts

- Shoulder dystocia occurs in 0.3–1% of babies weighing 2.5–4 kg. AAFP (2012) and 5–9% of babies weighing 4–4.5 kg (Baxley and Gobbo, 2004; AAFP, 2012).
- Over 50% of shoulder dystocias occur in normal sized babies with no identifiable risk factors (AAFP, 2012).
- Preconception and prenatal risk factors have extremely poor predictive value and therefore in clinical practice do not facilitate accurate, reliable prediction of shoulder dystocia (Gherman, 2002).
- Obesity increases occurrence by three times (Cedergren, 2004).
- Morbidity for the baby includes obstetric brachial plexus palsy (OBPP) injuries in 7–20% following dystocia, with 1–2% of those sustaining permanent injury (AAFP, 2012). Hypoxia, fractures of the clavicle/humerus, bruising and soft tissue damage may occur, and in severe cases, fetal death may result.
- Morbidity for the woman includes trauma, blood loss, bruising to the perineum/ genital tract and surrounding tissues, episiotomy/serious tears. Psychologically, post-traumatic stress syndrome, postnatal depression (Baxley and Gobbo, 2004) including, in severe cases, grief at the death of her baby.
- Litigation may result from brachial plexus injury.
- Simulated training sessions improve performance in shoulder dystocia management (Deering *et al.*, 2004).

Associated risk factors

All shoulder dystocia associated risk factors have poor predictive value in clinical practice (WHO, 2003).

Antenatal associated risks

- Macrosomia (AAFP, 2012).
- Maternal diabetes, short stature and abnormal pelvic anatomy (AAFP, 2012).
- Post-dates pregnancy (AAFP, 2012).
- Previous shoulder dystocia (Baskett and Allen, 1995).

Intrapartum-associated risks

- Prolonged first or second stage of labour (RCOG, 2008).
- Birthing semi-recumbent on a bed can restrict the movement of the coccyx and sacrum contributing to 'bed-birth dystocia' (Mortimore and McNabb, 1998; McGeown, 2001).

- Oxytocin augmentation (RCOG, 2008).
- Instrumental delivery (AAFP, 2012).

Recognising shoulder dystocia

Shoulder dystocia is usually preceded by a slow 'bobbing' delivery of the baby's head; the baby's chin then retracts against the perineum and 'turtlenecks' (AAFP, 2012). With the next contraction the baby will not deliver as its anterior shoulder is impacted against the symphysis pubis bone, due to the shoulder (bisacromial) diameter exceeding the diameter of the pelvic inlet (AAFP, 2012).

Beware of overdiagnosing shoulder dystocia. Sometimes anxious clinicians start to worry after only 1 or 2 minutes. Think: 'has there been a contraction yet?' Two minutes can seem like a long time, but no baby will be compromised at this point: this is quite normal. Spontaneous restitution of the shoulders may take one or two contractions. Premature traction without a contraction may give the false impression that dystocia is occurring.

Practice recommendations

Upright birthing positions improve the alignment of the mobile pelvic bones and improve the shape and capacity of the pelvis, optimising the chances of a 'good fit' between baby and pelvis (Simpkin and Ancheta, 2005). Common sense suggests that any woman at risk of shoulder dystocia should be discouraged from birthing in the semi-recumbent position.

Changing the woman's position in itself can be beneficial in preventing/shifting impacted shoulders.

Do not clamp and cut a nuchal cord. This will cut off the only oxygen supply the baby has, and hypoxia will rapidly follow.

Avoid excessive traction. Once shoulder dystocia is diagnosed do not put overzealous traction on the head. An OBPP injury following a head-to-body delivery of, say, only 2–3 minutes could be judged in court to have been due to overzealous intervention, and possibly excessive traction (Johnson, 2005). Performing the manoeuvres correctly will certainly take more than 2–3 minutes. A previously healthy fetus may withstand up to 10 minutes of complete anoxia before there is a significant risk of brain damage (Pasternak, 1993); however, an already compromised fetus's tolerance may be reduced significantly.

Avoid fundal pressure which could increase shoulder impaction and cause serious injuries, including uterine rupture, haemorrhage and even maternal death.

Use of systematic manoeuvres. Most shoulder dystocias will resolve with these manoeuvres. Prophylactic use of McRoberts or other manoeuvres prior to clinical diagnosis of shoulder dystocia requires further evaluation (Poggi, 2004). Many midwives might respond, however, that prevention happens all the time: optimal positioning in the second stage, e.g. squatting/all fours (which might be described as physiological McRoberts positions), widens the pelvic diameters (see Chapter 1), and therefore logically must reduce the chances of shoulder dystocia. Indeed the all fours position appears so successful in managing shoulder dystocia (Kovavisarach, 2006) that Walsh (2007) has even suggested that it should be the first mnemonic option for shoulder dystocia.

The HELPERR drill

The AAFP (2012) states that HELPERR manoeuvres serve to:

- Increase the functional size of the bony pelvis.
- Decrease the bisacromial (fetal shoulder) diameter.
- Change the relationship of the bisacromial diameter within the bony pelvis.

(See also Figures 17.2, 17.3, 17.4.)

HELPERR is a clinical tool providing a structured framework and an accepted approach to shoulder dystocia management (AAFP, 2012). Unfortunately when reciting the mnemonic, the assumption appears to be that all women give birth lying semi-recumbent or in lithotomy, and therefore it is important to stress the importance of individual clinical judgement as to which manoeuvre is employed first.

H   Help!
E   Evaluate for episiotomy
L   Legs hyperflexed (McRoberts manoeuvre)
P   Pressure suprapubic
E   Enter the vagina for internal manoeuvres
R   Remove the posterior arm
R   Roll on to all fours

Whilst AAFP (2012) suggests that there is no indication that one manoeuvre is superior to another, suggestions are that McRoberts is the most successful (RCOG, 2008), whilst Kovavisarach (2006) suggests that the all fours position is extremely effective. However, the order of each manoeuvre is left to the attending clinicians' discretion with importance attributed to the effective application of each manoeuvre (AAFP, 2012) rather than to the order in which the manoeuvres are conducted. Thirty to sixty seconds is the recommended time span allocated to each manoeuvre (AAFP, 2012). All manoeuvres can be repeated if delivery is not achieved.

Help summoned immediately. Activate emergency bell, call emergency team via switchboard or dial 999 if at homebirth/birthing centre.

Evaluate for episiotomy. Episiotomy can improve access to conduct manoeuvres, but it will not in itself release the bony impaction of the shoulder (Nocon, 2000; AAFP, 2012). Episiotomy causes perineal trauma, and is almost impossible to perform once the head has delivered; some midwives therefore question its necessity (Gaskin, 1990). The

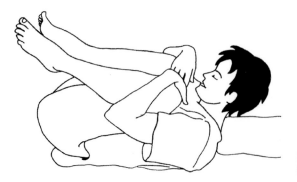

Fig. 17.2 McRoberts manoeuvre (side view).

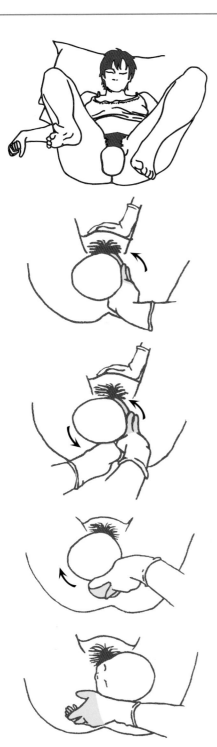

(a) **McRoberts manoeuvre** (end view)
The woman is encouraged to abduct her thighs towards her chest.

(b) **McRoberts and Rubins I** (suprapubic pressure)
- An assistant stands on the same side as the fetal back to apply downward, lateral pressure or rocking above the lateral shoulder.

Internal manoeuvres/Rubins II
- Approach the anterior shoulder from behind.
- Push it towards the fetal chest to reduce the shoulder girdle or move into the oblique diameter.

(c) **McRoberts, Rubins II and the Woods screw manoeuvre**
- Use both hands, place two fingers behind the anterior shoulder and two in front of the posterior shoulder.
- Attempt to rotate the shoulders as indicated, into the oblique diameter.

(d) **Reverse Woods screw manoeuvre**
- Place the fingers behind the posterior shoulder.
- Attempt rotation as shown.

(e) **Removal of posterior shoulder**
- Insert a well-lubricated hand.
- Locate the fetal arm and flex at the elbow; sweep arm out across the fetal chest.

Fig. 17.3 Manoeuvres for shoulder dystocia with the woman in a semi-recumbent position and the fetal position left occipitoanterior (LOA).

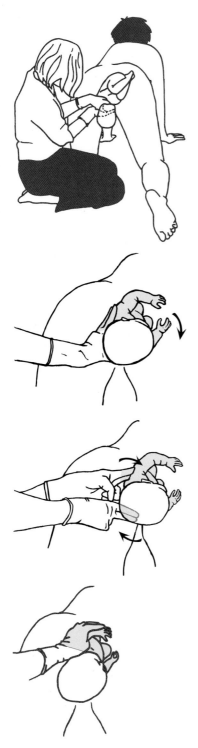

(a) The midwife checks restitution has occurred and attempts delivery of the posterior shoulder. In this position the posterior shoulder is uppermost.

(b) **Rubins II**
- Approach the posterior shoulder from behind.
- Push it towards the fetal chest to reduce the shoulder girdle.

(c) **Rubins II and Woods screw manoeuvre**
- Use both hands; place two fingers behind the anterior shoulder and two fingers in front of the posterior shoulder.
- Attempt to rotate the shoulders as indicated, into the oblique diameter.

(d) **Removal of posterior shoulder**
- Insert a well lubricated hand.
- Locate the arm and flex at the albow, sweep arm out across the fetal chest.

Fig. 17.4   Manoeuvres for shoulder dystocia with the woman in an all fours position and the fetal position left occipitoanterior (LOA).

Management of Obstetric Emergencies and Trauma group (MOET, 2003) recommends using an individual clinical judgement approach.

Legs hyperflexed (McRoberts manoeuvre). The woman lies in a flat supine position and abducts her thighs, pulling her knees to her chest, thus raising her coccyx off the bed and flattening her sacral promontory (see Figures 17.2 and 17.3a). The McRoberts manoeuvre facilitates delivery in over 40% of cases, and over 50% when used in conjunction with external pressure (AAFP, 2012).

Pressure applied externally suprapubically (also known as Rubins I manoeuvre). The clinician stands on the same side as the baby's back and directs pressure towards the maternal midline (Coates, 1995; AAFP, 2012) in a downward, lateral pressure, or rocking with the palm of the hands over the baby's anterior shoulder in order to reduce the bisacromial diameter and shift the impacted shoulder. If the direction of pressure is incorrectly applied towards the symphysis bone it will only impact the baby's shoulder further on the pelvic bone. Suprapubic pressure and McRoberts manoeuvre employed together can improve success rates (Gherman *et al.*, 1997).

Enter. Internal manoeuvres can be attempted whatever the mother's position and include Woods screw and Rubins II (Figures 17.3 and 17.4). These manoeuvres are painful for the woman and difficult and uncomfortable for the midwife.

- **Rubins II** (see Figures 17.3b,c and 17.4b,c). Insert the lubricated fingers of one hand (always posteriorly as there is more space) and apply pressure on the impacted anterior shoulder from behind, thus pushing the anterior shoulder towards the fetal chest and reducing the bisacromial diameter. Apply Rubins I external pressure simultaneously unless the woman is on all fours.
- **Woods screw** manoeuvre can be combined with Rubins II (AAFP, 2012). Insert the fingers of the second hand so that they are in front of the posterior shoulder (see Figures 17.3c and 17.4c). You can internally push/rotate the baby towards the symphysis pubis, thus rotating the baby into the oblique which frees the anterior shoulder from the pubic bone.
- **Reverse Woods screw.** Place fingers from behind on to the posterior aspect of the posterior shoulder and attempt to rotate the baby towards the symphysis pubis (see Figure 17.3d).

Remove the posterior arm. To deliver the posterior shoulder, insert the whole lubricated hand posteriorly into the vagina to locate the baby's posterior arm and elbow. Flex the arm at the elbow and sweep across the fetal chest and out (see Figures 17.3e and 17.4d). Avoid excessive traction on the arm if possible, as the shoulder should have now disimpacted and delivery should normally follow (AAFP, 2012).

Roll onto all fours. Depending on the woman's mobility, midwives may consider this position change before the more interventionist manoeuvres, as it is so successful (Walsh, 2007; RCOG, 2008). Turning onto all fours, sometimes referred to as the Gaskin manoeuvre, may dislodge the impacted shoulder (AAFP, 2012) by allowing unrestricted movement of the pelvis including the coccyx. The baby's weight on the symphysis helps widen the anterior-posterior pelvic diameter. The posterior shoulder (now nearest the ceiling) usually delivers first in this scenario. Anecdotally, in all fours delivery position, midwives report that there is sometimes enough room to insert the hand, along the curve of the sacrum and to splint, then free, the posterior shoulder. The all fours position may be impossible/impractical for women with a dense epidural block.

Last resort procedures

Whilst being unpleasant to undertake, these procedures are preferable to fatality.

- **Clavicle fracture (cleidotomy).** Press upwards on the centre of the clavicle (AAFP, 2012); try using two fingers placed on the clavicle and pushing with the thumb between them. The bone should snap easily (Davis, 1997; RCOG, 2008), allowing release of the shoulder.
- **Cephalic replacement/Zavanelli manoeuvre** (RCOG, 2008). Turn the baby's head back to occipitoanterior or occipitoposterior (depending on the baby's original position for delivery). Flex the baby's head, push it back into the vagina and proceed to immediate CS. This manoeuvre has delivered varying success.

Aftercare

Post-birth counselling. The couple may benefit from debriefing at a time that is appropriate (Mapp, 2005). They may prefer to discuss this with the person(s) present at the delivery, and may wish to see a consultant obstetrician to discuss any long-term effects and the prospects for future pregnancies.

Documentation. Solicitors can frequently find fault in the documented management of shoulder dystocia, questioning whether the care followed recognised manoeuvres. Good practice and documentation help prevent litigation.

One individual acting as scribe throughout the procedure will aid good record-keeping. AAFP (2012) recommends that documentation should include:

- Team members present
- Manoeuvres performed and duration of event
- Venous and arterial cord PH recordings
- On which of the baby's arms manoeuvres were performed.

RCOG (2008) also recommends recording

- Time of delivery of the head
- The direction the head is facing after restitution
- Time of delivery of the body
- Condition of the baby (Apgar score)
- What time attending staff arrived.

Inverted uterus

This is the inversion of the uterus into the vagina during the third stage of labour. It is a rare but life-threatening complication due to the risk of significant haemorrhage and shock (AAFP, 2012).

Incidence and facts

- 1:2000 to 1:50 000 UK births (Kroll and Lyne, 2002).
- Kroll and Lyne (2002) suggest that the variation in statistics is dependent on third-stage management and the level of reporting.

Associated risk factors

- Mismanagement of the third stage of labour (Peña-Martin, 2007), e.g. fundal pressure and overzealous cord traction.
- Uterine atony, fundal implantation of the placenta or congenital weakness of the uterus has been identified as risk factors (AAFP, 2012), also placenta accreta or a short umbilical cord (Kroll and Lyne, 2002).

Signs and symptoms

See Box 17.2.

Box 17.2   Signs and symptoms of uterine inversion.

Uterus
Inability to palpate uterus abdominally (WHO, 2003).
The uterus may be visible as a shiny, bluish-grey mass protruding at the vagina (AAFP, 2012).

Haemorrhage
The most common sign is haemorrhage, but the woman's rapid collapse appears to be out of proportion to the amount of blood lost (AAFP, 2012).

Profound shock
Rapid shock may be partially attributed to a vasovagal, neurogenic response due to traction of the ovaries and fallopian tubes (AAFP, 2012) (see Box 17.4).

Pain
Intense lower abdominal pain caused by traction on the ovaries and peritoneum and may be accompanied by a bearing-down sensation (Kroll & Lyne, 2002), although occasionally women report very little pain.

Practice recommendations

Treatment for uterine inversion consists of two main components: replacement of the uterus and treatment of shock (Beringer and Patteril, 2004).

- **Call for help** and/or transfer to hospital.
- **Replace the uterus promptly** (see Box 17.3). If not, or if attempts fail, a cervical restriction ring and/or an oedematous womb may result, preventing replacement (Kroll and Lyne, 2002). Betamimetics (uterine muscle relaxants) or general anaesthesia may then be required (AAFP, 2012).
- **Do not attempt to remove the placenta if it is adherent** to the uterus, as this may cause haemorrhage (WHO, 2003).
- **Treat for shock** (see Box 17.4).
- If immediate replacement of uterus is unsuccessful:
  - **Prepare for theatre.**
  - **Place the uterus in the vagina** if possible or hold by hand close to the vagina to minimise pulling on internal structures.
  - **Withhold oxytocics** until the uterus is replaced (WHO, 2003).
  - **Administer strong analgesia**, e.g. morphine.

Box 17.3   Replacing an inverted uterus.

Prompt manual replacement
- Apply gentle pressure with three or four fingers at the centre of the fundus and push up until the uterus reverts (AAFP, 2012).
- Ensure the entire uterus is completely fed up through the cervix and hold in place for at least 5 minutes or until a firm contraction occurs (Kroll & Lyne, 2002).
- Women normally find inversion painful and replacement can be agonising (Kroll & Lyne, 2002).

Placenta
Only after the uterus is replaced can an oxytocic be administered and the placenta carefully delivered (Campbell & Lees, 2000; Magill-Cuerden, 2001).

Aftercare

- An indwelling catheter for 24 hours avoids distension of the bladder (Silverton, 1993).
- Refer for physiotherapy to discuss pelvic floor muscle care and lifting/straining strategies.
- The mother may remember little of events, but her partner will have seen her sudden collapse. Offer the couple the option of seeing an obstetrician to discuss what happened, and why and to discuss any long-term effects of her collapse and future pregnancies.

Maternal collapse/shock

Shock is characterised by circulatory failure to maintain adequate perfusion of the vital organs (WHO, 2003). Blood is directed to vital organs; the peripheral circulation shuts down and if not corrected rapid progressive deterioration occurs. Due to increased circulatory volume during pregnancy initial compensation occurs, but by the time the BP drops and tachycardia and tachypnoea are evident the situation is serious.

The types of shock in pregnancy and after birth can be broadly divided into two categories:

Haemorrhagic

- Ante/postpartum haemorrhage (commonest cause)
- Uterine inversion or rupture.

Non-haemorrhagic

- Pulmonary or amniotic embolism
- Endotoxic shock (septicaemia)
- Hypotension (regional anaesthesia or anaphylaxis).

Box 17.4   Basic care for shock.

(1) Summon help.
(2) Ascertain the possible cause of shock:
   * Commence appropriate treatment. If PPH see management page 261.
   * Deliver the baby.
   * If at home/birthing centre, arrange urgent paramedic ambulance to hospital.
(3) Physical care:
   * Site two large gauge cannulae (a priority).
   * Take emergency bloods for:
     ○ group and cross-matching
     ○ full blood count
     ○ clotting studies; fibrinogen levels, prothrombin time (international normalised ratio) (PT(INR))/activated partial thromboplastin time (APTT)
   * Commence IV fluids.
   * Administer facial oxygen.
   * Observations:
     ○ pulse and respiration rate
     ○ blood pressure (BP)
     ○ pulse oximetry
(4) Serious collapse (see maternal resuscitation, Chapter 18).
   Stay calm, think ABC:
   A = Airway
   B = Breathing
   C = Circulation
(5) Documentation. In hospital it is usually possible to assign a person to perform documentation of:
   * Vital signs.
   * Fluids charted, in and out including estimated blood loss.
   * Drugs given, dosages and times.
(6) Transfer to high-dependency area/intensive care unit:
   * Urinary catheter with urometer.
   * Central venous pressure line.
(7) In complete cardiac arrest of a pregnant woman, deliver the baby within 5 minutes. Obstetricians do not need to prepare a sterile field and should go for the quickest incision possible (Bobrowski, 1994).
(8) Communicate with the family.

Possible signs and symptoms of shock

* Pallor, blueness, central cyanosis, feeling cold to touch
* Tachycardia ± hypotension
* Anxiety and agitation, possibly vomiting
* Gasping for air (if severe)
* Drowsiness or unconsciousness
* Cardiac arrest can rapidly follow.

See Box 17.4 for management of shock.

Summary

Cord prolapse

* Call for help.
* VE to apply pressure to presenting part until delivery.

- Woman to adopt the all fours/knee-chest position, exaggerated Sims or Trendelenburg.
- If at home/birthing centre, transfer to a consultant unit.
- Explain to the woman calmly what is happening and why.
- Consider as a last resort filling the woman's bladder with 400–700 ml saline.
- Emergency delivery: probable CS in first stage, or instrumental birth in second stage.

Amniotic fluid embolism

- Main symptoms: breathlessness, shock, followed by cardiac arrest (Fahy, 2001).
- Treat for sudden shock/collapse.
- High maternal mortality: proceed to urgent delivery of the baby.

Uterine rupture

- Prepare for theatre.
- Emergency delivery of baby.
- Haemorrhage control.
- Uterine repair in theatre.

Shoulder dystocia

Consider HELPERR mnemonic as a guide:

- H = Call for help
- E = Evaluate for episiotomy
- L = Legs hyperflexed (McRoberts manoeuvre)
- P = Pressure applied externally suprapubically
- E = Enter for internal manoeuvres
- R = Roll onto all fours
- R = Remove posterior arm

Uterine inversion

- Call for help.
- Replace the uterus promptly (see Box 17.3).
- Treat for shock (see Box 17.4).
- Offer analgesia.
- Withhold oxytocics until delivery of placenta.
- If unable to replace uterus prepare for theatre.

References

American Academy of Family Physicians (AAFP) (2012) *Advanced Life Support in Obstetrics (ALSO). Course Syllabus Manual* Leawood, Kansas, AAFP.

Athukorala, C., Middleton, P., Crowther, C. A. (2006) Intrapartum interventions for preventing shoulder dystocia. *Cochrane Database of Systematic Reviews*, Issue 4.

Bakshi, S., Meyer, B. A. (2000) Indications for and outcomes of emergency peripartum hysterectomy: a five-year review. *Journal of Reproductive Medicine* 45(9), 733–7.

Baskett, T. F., Allen, A. C. (1995) Perinatal implications of shoulder dystocia. *Obstetrics and Gynaecology* 86, 14–17.

Baxley, E. G., Gobbo, R. W. (2004) Shoulder dystocia. *American Family Physician* 69(7), 1707–4. Pub med.

Beringer, R. M., Patteril, M. (2004) Puerperal uterine inversion and shock. *British Journal of Anaesthesia* 92(3), 439–41.

Bobrowski, R. (1994) In James, D. K., Steer, P. J., Weiner, C.P., Goink, B. (eds) *High Risk Pregnancy: Management Options*, 2nd edn, pp. 959–82. London, W.B. Saunders.

Brown. L. (2002) Shoulder dystocia: auditing the development of guidelines for shoulder dystocia. *British Journal of Midwifery* 10(11), 671–5.

Campbell, S., Lees, C. (2000) Obstetric emergencies. In Campbell, S., Lees, C. (eds) *Obstetrics by Ten Teachers*, 17th edn, pp. 303–17. London, Edward Arnold.

Cedergren, M. I. (2004) Maternal morbid obesity and the risk of adverse pregnancy outcome. *Obstetrics and Gynaecology* 103(2), 219–24.

CNST (2012) *Clinical Negligence Scheme for Trusts, Maternity Risk Management Standards*. NHS Litigation Authority. www.nhsla.com

Coates, T. (1995) Shoulder dystocia. In Alexander, J., Levy, V., Roch, S. (eds) *Aspects of Midwifery Practice*. Basingstoke, Macmillan.

Confidential Enquiry into Maternal and Child Health (CEMACH) (2004) *Why Mothers Die 2000–2002 The Sixth Report of Confidential Enquiries into Maternal Deaths in the United Kingdom*. London, RCOG Press.

Centre for Maternal and Child Enquiries (CMACE) (2011) *Saving Mothers' Lives. The Eighth Report of Confidential Enquiries into Maternal Deaths in the United Kingdom*. London, RCOG Press. http://onlinelibrary.wiley.com/doi/10.1111/j.1471-0528.2010.02847.x/pdf

Davis, E. (1997) *Hearts and Hands: A Midwife's Guide to Pregnancy and Birth*, 3rd edn. Berkeley, California, Celestial Arts.

Davis, S. (1999) Amniotic fluid embolism and isolated disseminated intravascular coagulation. *Canadian Journal of Anaesthesia* 46(5), 456–9.

Deering, S., Poggi, S., Cedonia, C., Gherman, R., Satin, A. (2004). Improving resident competency in the management of shoulder dystocia with simulation training. *Obstetrics and Gynaecology* 103(6), 1224–8.

DoH (Department of Health) (2004) *The National Service Framework for Children, Young People and Maternity Services* (Standard 11). London, DoH.

Draycott, T., Winter, C., Crofts, J., Barnsfield, S. (2008) *PROMPT: Practical Obstetric Multiprofessional Training Course Manual*. London: RCOG Press. www.prompt-course.org

Enkin, M. (2000) Labour and birth after a previous caesarean section. In Enkin, M., Keirse, M. J. N. C., Neilson, J., Crowther, C., Duley, L., Hodnett, E., Hofmeyr, J. (eds) *A Guide to Effective Care in Pregnancy and Childbirth*, 3rd edn, pp. 359–71. Oxford, Oxford University Press.

Fahy, K. M. (2001) Amniotic fluid embolism: a review of the research literature. *Australian Journal of Midwifery* 14(1), 9–13.

Gaskin, I. (1990) *Spiritual Midwifery*. Summertown, Tennessee, The Book Publishing Co.

Gherman, R. B. (2002) Shoulder dystocia: an evidence based evaluation of the obstetrical nightmare. *Clinical Obstetrics and Gynaecology* 45, 345–61.

Gherman, R. B., Goodwin, T. M., Souter, I., Neumann, K., Ouzounian, J. G., Paul, R. (1997) The McRoberts manoeuvre for the alleviation of shoulder dystocia: how successful is it? *American Journal of Obstetrics and Gynecology* 176(3), 656–61.

Goswami, K. (2007) Umbilical cord prolapse. In Grady, K., Howell, C., Cox, C. (eds) *Managing Obstetric Emergencies and Trauma: the MOET Course manual*, 2nd edn, pp. 233–7. London, RCOG Press.

Johnson, A. (2005) Obstetric brachial plexus palsy: the medico-legal view. *The Obstetrician and Gynaecologist 7*, 259–65.

Knight, M., Tuffnell, D., Brocklehurst, P., Spark, P.,Kurinczuk, J. J. (2010) Incidence and risk factors for amniotic-fluid embolism.*Obstetrics and Gynaecology* 115(5), 910–17.

Kovavisarach, E. (2006) The "all-fours" manoeuvre for the management of shoulder dystocia. *International Journal of Gynaecology and Obstetrics* 95(2), 153–4.

Kroll, D., Lyne, M. (2002) Uterine inversion and uterine rupture. In Boyle, M. (ed.) *Emergencies around Childbirth – A Handbook for Midwives*, pp. 89–95. Oxford, Radcliffe Medical Press.

Magill-Cuerden, J. (2001) Clinical file: case study. *The Practising Midwife* 4(1), 29.

Managing Obstetric Emergencies and Trauma (MOET) (2003) *Course Manual*, Cox, C., Johanson, R., Grady, K., Howell, C. (eds). London, RCOG Press.

Mapp, T. (2005) Feelings and fears post obstetric emergencies. *British Journal of Midwifery* 13(1), 36–40.

McGeown, P. (2001) Practice recommendations for obstetric emergencies. *British Journal of Midwifery* 9(2), 71–4.

Mortimore, V., McNabb, M. (1998) A six year retrospective analysis of shoulder dystocia and delivery of the shoulders. *Midwifery* 14, 162–73.

Murphy, D. J., MacKenzie, I. Z. (1995) The mortality and morbidity associated with umbilical cord prolapse. *British Journal of Obstetrics and Gynaecology* 102(10), 826–30.

NICE (National Institute for Health and Clinical Excellence) (2004) *Caesarean Section. Clinical Guideline 13*. London, London.

NICE (2007) *Clinical Guideline 55: Intrapartum Care*. National Institute for Health and Clinical Excellence. London, NICE. http://guidance.nice.org.uk/CG55/Guidance

NPSA (2006) *Seven Steps to Patient Safety for Primary Care*. London, NPSA. www.npsa.nhs.uk

Nocon, J. J. (2000) Shoulder dystocia and macrosomia. In Kean, L. (ed.) *Best Practice in Labour Ward Management*, pp. 167–86. Edinburgh, WB Saunders.

Pasternak, J. F. (1993) Hypoxic-ischaemic brain damage in the term infant. Lessons from the laboratory. *Pediatric Clinician North America* 40, 1061–72.

Paxton, A., Maine, D., Freedman, L., Fry, D., Lobis, S. (2005) The evidence for emergency obstetric care. *International Journal of Gynaecology and Obstetrics* 8(2), 181–93.

Peña-Martin, G., Comunián-Carrasco, G. (2007) Fundal pressure versus controlled cord traction as part of the active management of third stage of labour. *Cochrane Database of Systematic Reviews*, Issue 4.

Poggi, S. (2004) In Athukorala, C., Middleton, P., Crowther, C. A. Intrapartum interventions for preventing shoulder dystocia. *Cochrane Database of Systematic Reviews*, Issue 4.

Prabulos, A. M., Philipson, E. H. (1998) Umbilical cord prolapse. Is time from diagnosis to delivery critical? *Journal of Reproductive Medicine* 43(2), 129–32.

Prendiville, W., Elbourne, D. (2000) The third stage of labour. In Enkin, M., Keirse, M. J. N. C., Neilson, J., Crowther, C., Duley, L., Hodnett, E., Hofmeyr, J. (ed.) *A Guide to Effective Care in Pregnancy and Childbirth*, 3rd edn, pp. 300–9. Oxford, Oxford University Press.

RCOG (2007) *Birth After Previous Caesarean. Green Top Guideline No. 45*. London, RCOG.

RCOG (2008) *Umbilical Cord Prolapse. Green Top Guideline No. 50*. London, RCOG.

RCOG (2011) *Maternal Collapse in Pregnancy and the Puerperium. Green Top Guideline No. 56*. London, RCOG.

RCOG (2012) *Shoulder Dystocia. Green Top Guideline No. 42*. London, RCOG.

Silverton, L. (1993) *The Art and Science of Midwifery*. London, Prentice Hall International.

Simpkin, P., Ancheta, R. (2005) *The Labor Progress Handbook*, 2nd edn. Oxford, Blackwell.

Squire, C. (2002) Shoulder dystocia and umbilical cord prolapse. In Boyle, M. (ed.) *Emergencies Around Childbirth – A Handbook for Midwives*. Abingdon, Radcliffe Medical Press.

UKOSS (UK Obstetric Surveillance System) Source: National Perinatal Epidemiology Unit, University of Oxford. marian.knight@npeu.ox.ac.uk ukoss@npeu.ox.ac.uk

Walsh, D. (2007) Managing shoulder dystocia: 'on your back' or 'all-fours'? *British Journal of Midwifery* 15(5), 254.

Weston, R. (2001) When birth goes wrong. *The Practising Midwife* 4(8), 10–2.

WHO (World Health Organization) (2003) Integrated management of pregnancy and childbirth. *Managing Complications in Pregnancy and Childbirth: A Guide for Midwives and Doctors*. Geneva, WHO.

18 Neonatal and maternal resuscitation

Nick Castle

Introduction

Midwives must be able to resuscitate both the newborn baby and the mother, and therefore they require annual neonatal and maternal resuscitation training. This training should also cover standard adult resuscitation.

Incidence and facts

- In the developed world around 5–10% of newborn babies require some degree of intervention at birth; typically active stimulation. This number is higher in the developing world (Ergenekon *et al.*, 2000).
- 1% of babies >2.5 kg require assisted ventilation and 20% of these need intubation.
- Occasionally babies are born unexpectedly 'flat', but this can be managed effectively by basic resuscitation techniques (Palme-Kilander, 1992). Only 0.2% of 'low-risk birth' babies require assisted ventilation, and only 10% of these require intubation (Palme-Kilander, 1992).
- It has been estimated that up to 800 000 newborn babies who currently die could be saved by timely basic resuscitation techniques (Zideman *et al.*, 1998), primarily prompt aerating of the lungs (Richmond and Wyllie, 2010; Wyllie *et al.*, 2010).
- Anticipation is the most important aspect of resuscitation; equipment and personnel should be assembled as soon as possible for suspected problems.

The Midwife's Labour and Birth Handbook, Third Edition. Edited by Vicky Chapman and Cathy Charles.
© 2013 John Wiley & Sons, Ltd. Published 2013 by John Wiley & Sons, Ltd.

Risk management: anticipation

Many situations may result in a newborn baby requiring active resuscitation (Box 18.1) including unexpected births in the community or the emergency department, although usually these deliveries are uneventful.

Box 18.1   Resuscitation anticipation: risk factors.

Antenatal risk factors
- Maternal diabetes
- Pre-eclampsia/essential hypertension
- Chronic maternal illness (e.g. cardiovascular, thyroid, pulmonary, renal, neurological)
- Previous stillbirth or neonatal death
- Antepartum haemorrhage
- Oligo/polyhydramnios
- Size versus dates discrepancy
- Reduced fetal movements
- Alcohol or drugs misuse
- Other drugs (e.g. lithium carbonate, magnesium, adrenergic-blocking drugs)
- No antenatal care

Intrapartum risk factors
- Preterm birth
- Prolonged rupture of membranes or infection (e.g. chorioamnionitis)
- Abnormal fetal heart rate (e.g. bradycardia, tachycardia, prolonged decelerations)
- Meconium-stained liquor (especially thick, fresh particulate)
- Breech or malpresentation
- Recent maternal opioid analgesia (<4 hours) or general anaesthetic
- Cord prolapse
- Placenta praevia / abruption
- Fetal abnormality
- Instrumental or operative delivery

(RCPGH & RCOG, 1997; AHA *et al.*, 2000)

Once a 'high-risk' birth is identified, a clinician trained in newborn resuscitation (e.g. paediatrician or advanced neonatal practitioner) should be summoned before birth (RCPCH and RCOG, 1997). Midwives caring for women at home or in a birthing centre should be aware of factors that can influence the baby's condition at birth and that may necessitate transfer. For a list of community midwife's resuscitation equipment, see Box 18.2.

Basic neonatal resuscitation

The 2010 international resuscitation guidelines (Wyllie *et al.*, 2010) supersede previously published guidelines. Successful neonatal resuscitation is based on anticipation, environmental control, assessment, stimulation, effective ventilation and, rarely, cardiac compressions with intubation and drug administration. Resuscitation involves a number of processes that occur simultaneously. Each step will be considered separately, although the initial assessment and stimulation should occur as one swift action (see Figure 18.1).

Box 18.2   Resuscitation equipment for home birth.

Baby resuscitation equipment
- Suction device with suction catheters (soft and yankauer)
- Self-inflating 500 ml bag-mask-valve (BVM) with blow-off valve set at 40 cm H_2O. The traditional 240 ml BVM device is no longer recommended as it is difficult to provide a slow constant inflation pressure (Ziderman *et al.*, 1998)
- Oxygen cylinder with variable flow meter
- Stethoscope
- Towel

Maternal resuscitation equipment
- Suction device
- Oxygen mask (medium concentration)
- Pocket mask with one-way valve and various oral airways
- BVM device (optional – as the above pocket mask using oxygen is effective for basic life support)
- Oxygen cylinder with variable flow meter

Miscellaneous: towels, torch, watch/stop watch, stethoscope (see home birth chapter)
Access to phone to call for assistance
Full list at http://www.resus.org.uk/pages/HomBeqip.htm

Environment

It is essential that the newborn baby does not become cold, as acidosis is worsened by hypothermia (Tyson, 2000). Skin-to-skin contact immediately following birth is effective at maintaining/increasing the baby's body temperature (see pages 25 and 212). In a hospital or birthing centre, an overhead heater as part of the resuscitaire should be available. Such equipment is not available in the community, so the attending midwife should minimise draughts and warm the delivery area and have warmed towels available. The baby should be dried, and any damp towels removed from contact with the body. Although this is common sense, it is typically simple procedures that are forgotten during the initial phase of any resuscitation attempt.

Assessment

A rapid assessment of tone, colour, respiratory rate, heart rate, and gut instinct that things are not right will indicate the need to instigate resuscitation procedures. A stepwise approach is recommended in the assessment of the newborn that may require resuscitation to include active stimulation and opening the airway.

ABC of neonatal resuscitation

(A) Airway. Place the newborn on a firm surface with the head in a neutral position. The newborn has a large head and a small neck, which can lead to airway obstruction. A gentle chin lift/jaw thrust may help.

(B) Breathing. Assess rate, rhythm and depth of ventilation – if the baby is apnoeic administer 'inflation breaths' (see Figure 18.1). Routine supplementary oxygen therapy is no longer recommended and should ideally be administered in

Newborn Life Support

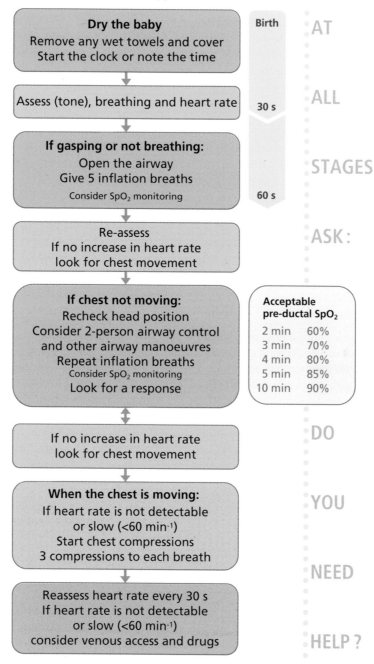

Fig. 18.1 Neonatal life support algorithm. *Reproduced with the permission of the Resuscitation Council (UK).*

accordance with pulse oximetry (Richmond and Wyllie, 2010). Refer to Figure 18.1 for optimal oxygen saturation (SpO_2).

(C) Circulation. Observe the baby's colour: if floppy and pale, circulation is inadequate. Record the baby's heart rate, ideally using a stethoscope as palpation is unreliable if the heart rate is <100 bpm (Owen and Wyllie, 2004). Commence compression if heart rate is <60 bpm.

Stimulation

Drying and warming the baby provides adequate stimulation whilst preventing heat loss, but if this fails to generate a response then instigate resuscitation procedures (Richmond and Wyllie, 2010) (Figure 18.1). Avoid more aggressive forms of stimulus: they are not a substitute for effective resuscitation.

Suction

There is no role for routine suctioning as it delays ventilation, causes airway trauma and may lead to vagal-induced bradycardia (Richmond and Wyllie, 2010). Consider suction only if ventilation is unsuccessful.

The initial five breaths

These 'inflation breaths' are designed to inflate and expand the lungs and remove amniotic fluid (Richmond and Wyllie, 2010). If delivered effectively, these initial breaths can restore spontaneous breathing. They are delivered slowly with constant pressure, with maximum pressure 30–40 cm of water (Richmond and Wyllie, 2010) (normally 20–25 cm for preterm babies) held for 2–3 seconds. This is difficult to do with a bag-valve-mask device; a T-piece device, e.g. Tom Thumb, may be more effective (Wyllie *et al.*, 2010). Do not deliver short, sharp, fast ventilations as this is ineffective and a common reason for failed initial resuscitation (see Tables 18.1 and 18.2).

Table 18.1   Means of ventilation.

Device	Advantages	Disadvantages	Comments
Mouth-to-mouth	Easy to learn Provides a good seal	Socially unpleasant Difficult to provide additional oxygen	This is a priority skill to learn, but in a hospital basic airway devices should be available
Pocket mask (adult ventilation only)	Easy to learn Provides a good seal Can be used by one person Some types have O_2 ports	Requires training to use effectively Maximum O_2: 50% at 10–15 l/min	Ideal first response device as it is easy and effective Ideal for community midwifery use
Bag-valve-mask (BVM) device	Can provide high flow O_2 Less tiring for rescuer	Difficult to use: often results in under-ventilation Usually less available at the bedside	This can be used by a single person or as a two-person technique, i.e. one securing mask to face, the other slowly squeezing the bag

Table 18.2   Reasons for no response to assisted ventilation.

Problem	Possible cause	Action
Poor technique	Ventilating too fast	Slow down: administer the first breaths over 2-3 seconds, then subsequent breaths at 30 breaths/minute
Chest not rising	Poor seal	Readjust mask position
	Wrong size bag-valve-mask (BVM) device or facemask	Use a 500 ml BVM: re-measure size of facemask
		Reposition head: consider chin lift/jaw thrust
	Airway obstructed	Consider suction if thick meconium – although no proof of its efficacy (Resuscitation Council UK, 2010)
		Consider an oral airway
Pressure release valve activated (this valve reduces the risk of pulmonary barotrauma)	Airway obstructed	As above: reposition head, consider suction and/or oral airway
	Ventilating too fast	Slow down (see 'poor technique' above)
		NB: Occasionally you may need to override the pressure relief valve by pressing on the valve (some BVMs have a clip for this purpose). However, this is rarely required, especially with a 500 ml BVM

Initial breaths should be administered using air, with the need for supplementary oxygen being directed by pulse oximetry (Richmond and Wyllie, 2010; Figure 18.1). At this point the baby will either (a) have improved and be spontaneously breathing/crying, (b) remain apnoeic but with a heart rate >60 bpm or (c) be apnoeic with a heart rate <60 bpm.

Ventilation should continue at a faster rate of 30 breaths/min (allow 1 second for inspiration and 1 second for expiration). Commence cardiac compressions if the baby has a heart rate <60 bpm; reassess the baby every 30 seconds and reconsider the need for supplementary oxygen.

Ongoing neonatal resuscitation/complications

Compressions

Cardiac compressions should be commenced once effective ventilation has been instigated but the heart rate remains <60 bpm. The ratio of breaths to compression is set at 3:1 although it is difficult for the single-handed resuscitator to maintain an effective respiratory rate whilst also performing compression (Whyte *et al.*, 1999). The presence of a second trained person improves resuscitation performance. Endotracheal intubation facilitates asynchronised compression/ventilations which improves coronary artery perfusion, but it is rarely required and should only be performed by a skilled intubator.

Cardiac compression technique

- **Two-finger method** (Figure 18.2): Place the tips of two overlaid fingers just below the nipple line in the centre of the baby's chest: this is the preferred technique for the single-handed midwife.

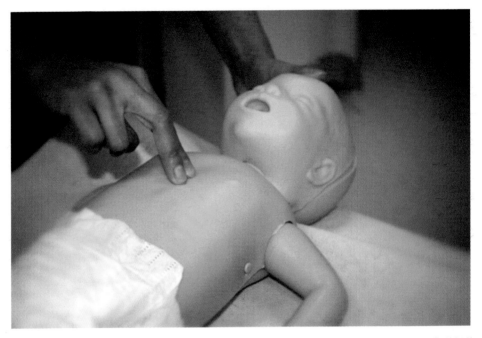

Fig. 18.2   Cardiac compressions: single person two-finger method. *Reproduced from Jevon, P. (2012) Paediatric Advanced Life Support, 2nd edn, with permission from Wiley.*

- **Two-thumb method** (Figure 18.3): Encircle the baby's chest with your hands, placing two overlaid thumbs just below the baby's nipples in the centre of the chest. The two-thumb technique is the preferred method for resuscitating all babies <1 year old (Biarent *et al.*, 2005).

  All midwives should be able to perform both resuscitation techniques.

The umbilical cord

Well babies benefit from delayed cord cutting (DCC) for >3–5 mins (RCM, 2012), and vigorous preterm babies for up to 3 mins (Richmond and Wyllie, 2010). DCC for non-vigorous babies is unclear; resuscitation is the priority, although extra cord oxygen may particularly benefit these babies. Richmond and Wyllie (2010) suggest possible DCC until the baby is breathing. Perhaps bring the bag-valve-mask device to the baby for the first inflation breaths at least, with the cord uncut. If needing to move baby to resuscitaire, consider 'milking' the cord towards the baby before cutting (see page 26). Leave the cord long (≥3 cm) as this facilitates umbilical venous and/or arterial access.

Meconium aspiration

Suctioning the baby prior to shoulder delivery is ineffective and no longer recommended (Vain *et al.*, 2004; Richmond and Wyllie, 2010). Only consider suction for the apnoeic baby where thick meconium obstructs the airway, although there is no evidence that even this prevents meconium aspiration (Richmond and Wyllie, 2010).

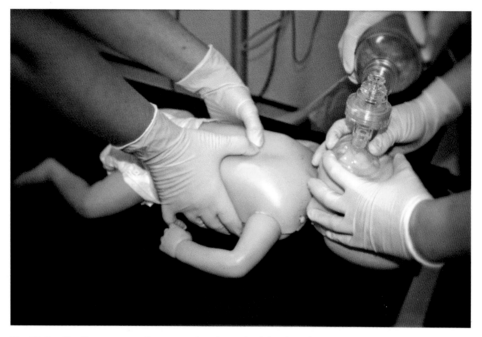

Fig. 18.3 Cardiac compressions: two-thumb method (preferred method but requires two people). *Reproduced from Jevon, P. (2012) Paediatric Advanced Life Support, 2nd edn, with permission from Wiley.*

Intubation

Intubation is rarely required (Palme-Kilander, 1992). It is a complex skill to learn and difficult to maintain. Therefore the emphasis is on effective ventilation and not intubation. Despite this there are still a number of situations where intubation remains useful:

- Prolonged ventilation/difficult ventilation
- Surfactant administration
- Special circumstances, e.g. diaphragmatic hernia.

The infrequency of neonatal intubation reduces the opportunity for staff to maintain clinical skills. In circumstances where BVM ventilation is proving ineffective/impossible, a laryngeal mask airway (Richmond and Wyllie, 2010; Wyllie *et al.*, 2010) or similiar intermediate airway device may be used.

Drugs

Drugs have a limited role in neonatal resuscitation (see Table 18.3).

- **Normal saline** is the preferred fluid for use in the resuscitation of the newborn (Richmond and Wyllie, 2010). A fluid challenge should be administered over at least 5 minutes if hypovolaemia is suspected or where initial attempts at resuscitation have failed.

Table 18.3   Neonatal resuscitation drugs (based on American Heart Association *et al.*, 2000).

Drug	Dose/concentration	Route	Typical dose (IV/IO)
Adrenaline	10–30 µg/kg 0.1–0.3 ml/kg of 1:10 000 (1 mg in 10 ml) Via ET-tube: increase to 50–100 µg/kg	Intravenous (IV) Intraosseous (IO) ETT	0.3–0.9 ml of 1:10 000
Sodium bicarbonate	1–2 ml/kg of 4.2% solution	IV only	3–6 ml of 4.2% solution
0.9% saline	10–20 ml/kg	IV only	10–50 ml
Naloxone	10 µg/kg (IV) 60 µg/kg (IM)	IV dose can be repeated A single one of dose of 200 µg IM can be given	30 µg IV bolus or A single 200 µg IM dose
10% dextrose	2.5 ml/kg	IV only	5–7.5 ml

- **10% Dextrose** should be administered to 'flat babies' who have a capillary blood sugar <2 mmol and are not responding to ventilation.
- **Naloxone** is rarely required and should only be considered once the baby has been effectively ventilated with a good cardiac output but remains apnoeic and where the mother has received opioids in labour. However, do not give it if there is a history of maternal opioid abuse (AHA *et al.*, 2000).
- **Adrenaline** is the main resuscitation drug for the neonate who, despite effective ventilation and cardiac compressions, has a heart rate <60 bpm (Richmond and Wyllie, 2010). Adrenaline should be administered intravenously (umbilical vein or cannula) or via the intraosseous route as administration via the endotracheal tube (ETT) is less effective and requires a higher dose (Richmond and Wyllie, 2010).
- **Sodium bicarbonate** is reserved for a baby who has not responded to effective ventilation, cardiac compressions and adrenaline (Richmond and Wyllie, 2010). There is little evidence to support its routine use.

Extremely preterm babies

Babies born under 28 weeks should be managed differently at birth. These babies should not be dried but covered in 'food-grade' plastic wrap/bag up to the baby's neck or over the head with the face exposed and then placed under a radiant heater (Richmond and Wyllie, 2010). The baby should remain fully wrapped until the baby's temperature has been recorded. See Chapter 13 for more information on preterm birth.

Terminating resuscitation

This is an emotive issue as neonatal intensive care has improved the outcome for even the smallest newborn (Van Reempts and Van Acker, 2001) (see Chapter 13). Refer to local policy on very low birth weight babies and babies born around the 24th week. If in doubt implement resuscitation as estimated gestational dates may be inaccurate.

Termination of neonatal resuscitation

The likelihood of successful neurological outcome following 10 minutes of advanced neonatal life support is extremely low (Haddad *et al.*, 2000), and therefore termination of resuscitation efforts in the lifeless baby is typically considered at this point (Wyllie *et al.*, 2010).

Maternal resuscitation

Incidence and facts

- Cardiac arrest in pregnancy has been estimated at 1:30 000 pregnancies.
- In the UK, the peri-mortem/post-mortem caesarean section (CS) rate is 1:170 000 deliveries: road traffic accident is the most common reason (Whitten and Montgomery, 2000).

Basic life support

The emphasis of basic life support (BLS) during pregnancy is on cardiac compressions and assisted ventilations (Soar *et al.*, 2010). The anatomical and physiological changes associated with pregnancy make resuscitation more difficult (see Box 18.3) with the main difficulties being an increased risk of aspiration/regurgitation, high oxygen demand with compressions/airway management complicated by the need for the woman to be in the left lateral tilted position and this therefore requires a change in resuscitation procedures (Soar *et al.*, 2010).

Box 18.3   Pregnancy factors affecting maternal resuscitation.

Difficult intubation
- Full dentition
- Large breasts
- Raised thoracic cage or flared rib cage
- Neck obesity/oedema
- Supraglottic oedema

Difficult chest compression
- Left lateral tilt positions (to avoid inferior vena caval occlusion)
- Flared rib cage
- Raised diaphragm

Respiratory
- Increased tidal volume requirements and O_2 demand
- Reduced chest compliance
- Reduced functional residual capacity

Cardiovascular
- Incompetent gastro-oesophageal sphincter
- Increased intragastric pressure
- Increased risk of regurgitation

UNRESPONSIVE?
▼
Shout for help
▼
Open airway
▼
Not breathing normally?
▼
Call 999 / summon resuscitation team
▼
30 chest compressions
▼
2 rescue breaths & 30 compressions (compression rate 100–120 per minute)

Fig. 18.4 Adult basic life support.

The ABC of maternal resuscitation

(Refer to Figure 18.4.)

(A) Airway. Check for foreign bodies and open the airway with a 'head tilt-jaw lift' manoeuvre. The jaw thrust manoeuvre can be used in conjunction with an airway adjunct (e.g. oropharyngeal airway) to facilitate effective ventilation.

(B) Breathing. Breaths should be delivered over one second to reduce the risk of gastric distension (Handley and Colquhoun, 2010) as well as minimising delays in compressions. When assessing cardiac arrest beware of gasping/agonal breathing.

(C) Circulation. The compression/ventilation ratio is 30:2 prior to intubation with a compression rate of 100–120 per minute. Following intubation, ventilation and cardiac compression are performed asynchronously at a rate of 100–120 (Soar *et al.*, 2010) and a respiratory rate of 10–12 per minute.

The left lateral tilt position or manual displacement of the uterus

After 20 weeks gestation (or earlier in multiple fetuses) the pregnant uterus can cause compression of the inferior vena cava (IVC) reducing the effectiveness of chest compressions. The previously recommended technique of physically placing the pregnant woman in a 'tilted' position can delay chest compression if the woman suffers cardiac arrest on the floor or a standard bed. The European Resuscitation Council and the American Heart Association now recommend (in the first instance) manual displacement of the uterus to the left, using one or two hands. This should be the first manoeuvre employed in association with chest compressions. However, if the woman is on a firm surface such as an operating table with tilting mechanism or on a spinal board then she should be tilted to a 15–45° (ideally 30°) left-sided tilt. Emphasis is therefore on prompt chest compression, early defibrillation and rapid caesarean section if circulation is not promptly restored. For more information see: www.resus.org.uk/pages/faqALS.htm#Q12

Advanced life support

The technique is the same regardless of the woman being pregnant (see Figure 18.4), with one significant change: emergency peri-/post-mortem CS. The choice of drugs

Table 18.4   Adult resuscitation drugs.

Drug	Dose/route	Rationale	Frequency
Adrenaline	1 mg 1:10 000 IV or double dose via endotracheal tube (ETT)	To improve cerebral and coronary artery perfusion	1 mg every 3 minutes
Atropine	No longer recommended during resuscitation. Uses now limited to the management of symptomatic bradycardia (with a pulse)	To increase heart rate by blocking the parasympathetic nervous system	To a maximum dose of 3 mg (in 0.5–1 mg boluses)
Amiodarone	300 mg IV bolus, then further 150 mg if required	To increase reversal of ventricular fibrillation (VF) or ventricular tachycardia (VT) following defibrillation	One or two doses if resistant VF/VT
Calcium chloride	10 ml/10% solution IV only	To protect the heart from hyperkalaemia or magnesium overdose	Until QRS complexes narrow
Sodium bicarbonate	1 mmol/kg (1 ml/kg of 8.4%) typically 50 ml bolus IV of 8.4%	Treatment of acidosis in intubated patients during prolonged cardiac arrest, treatment of hyperkalaemia and to treat tricyclic antidepressant overdose	Depending on clinical situation

remains the same regardless of pregnancy. Drugs for maternal resuscitation are given in Table 18.4.

Advanced airway management

Airway protection during maternal resuscitation is vital to reduce the risk of pulmonary aspiration. Pregnancy increases the difficulties of intubation (Box 18.3) so an experienced intubator and equipment for failed intubation must be available.

Defibrillation

Immediate defibrillation to reverse ventricular fibrillation (VF) or pulseless ventricular tachycardia (VT) remains vital, as no other intervention will be successful in restoring a normal cardiac rhythm. The risk to the unborn baby is extremely low and is greatly outweighed by the maternal benefits.

Emergency caesarean section

Emergency CS is directly linked to the successful resuscitation of the mother as well as the newborn and is an integral part of maternal resuscitation (Whitten and Montgomery, 2000). It is vital that there is no delay in performing this emergency procedure by moving the mother to an operating theatre, as this will waste time and adversely affect BLS. Equipment should be brought to the woman. Equally, full theatre-style sterility will not be possible and will also waste time. It has been suggested that delivery of the baby within four minutes of cardiac arrest may save the life of the baby (Boyle, 2002), although the mother's condition is of paramount importance.

Summary

For a midwife to be able to safely perform resuscitation of both the mother and the newborn baby, a combination of training, clinical assessment skills and the ability to identify and treat the at-risk mother/baby are vital.

Infant resuscitation

- Anticipation of problems allows for preparation.
- Warm, draught-free environment.
- Towels for drying the newborn.
- **Airway**
  - Place baby on firm surface and open the airway.
- **Breathing**
  - First five breaths (2–3 seconds): slow, constant pressure to inflate lungs.
  - Consider gentle suction only if ventilation unsuccessful.
- **Circulation**
  - Cardiac compressions if heart rate <60 bpm.
  - Compression rate 3 : 1; preferably use the two-thumb method.
  - Intubation rarely required and should only be performed by trained staff.

Maternal resuscitation

- Emergency CS aids resuscitation and may save the baby.
- Position in left lateral tilt.
- Airway: head tilt and jaw lift.
- Breathing: ventilation slowly and effectively delivered.
- Circulation: cardiac compressions at a ratio of 30 : 2.

References

American Heart Association (AHA), Resuscitation Council (UK), European Resuscitation Council *et al.* (2000) International guidelines 2000 for cardiopulmonary resuscitation and emergency cardiovascular care – an international consensus on science. *Resuscitation* 46 (special issue) xix–xx, 293–301, 401–16.

Biarent, D., Bingham, R., Richmond, S., Maconochie, I., Wyllie, J., Simpson, S., Nunez, A., Zideman, D. (2005) European guidelines council guidelines for resuscitation, Section 6. Paediatric Life Support. *Resuscitation* 67 (Suppl. 1), S97–S134.

Boyle, M. (2002) *Emergencies Around Childbirth: A Handbook for Midwives.* Abingdon, Radcliffe.

Ergenekon, E., Koc, E., Atalay, Y., Soysal, S. (2000) Neonatal resuscitation course experience in Turkey. *Resuscitation* 45(3), 225–7.

Esmail, N., Saleh, M., Ali, A. (2002) Laryngeal mask airway versus endotracheal intubation for Apgar score improvement in neonatal resuscitation. *Egypt Journal of Anesthesiology* 18, 115–21.

Haddad, B., Mercer, B., Livingstone, J., Sibai, B. (2000) Outcomes after successful resuscitation of babies born with Apgar scores of at 1 and 5 min. *American Journal of Obstetrics and Gynecology* 182, 1210–14.

Handley, H., Colquhoun, M. (2010) Adult Basic Life Support guidelines. *Resuscitation Council (UK)* http://www.resus.org.uk/pages/bls.pdf

National Institute for Health and Clinical Excellence (NICE) (2007) *Clinical Guideline 55: Intrapartum Care.* London, NICE.

Owen, C., Wyllie, J. (2004) Determination of heart rate in the baby at birth. *Resuscitation* 60, 213–7.

Palme-Kilander, C. (1992) Methods of resuscitation in low Apgar score newborn infants – a national survey. *Acta Paediatrica* 81, 739–44.

RCM (2012) Clamping update to be delivered *Midwives* 5, 15. www.rcm.org.uk

RCPCH and RCOG (Royal College of Paediatrics and Child Health and Royal College of Obstetricians and Gynaecologists) (1997) *Resuscitation of Babies at Birth.* London, BMJ Publishing.

Richmond, S., Wyllie, J. (2010) *Newborn Life Support. Resuscitation Council (UK).* http://www.resus.org.uk/pages/nls.pdf

Soar, J., Perkins, G. D., Abbas, G., Alfonzo, A., Barelli, A., Bierens, J. L., Brugger, H., Deakins, G. D., Dunning, J., Georgiou, M., Handley, A. J., Lockey, D. J., Paal, P., Sanroni, C., Karl-Christian, T., Zideman, D. A., Nolan, J. P. (2010) Cardiac arrest in special circumstances. *Resuscitation* 81, 1400–33.

Tyson, J. (2000) Immediate care of the newborn infant. In Enkin, M., Keirse, M. J. N. C., Neilson, J., Crowther, C., Duley, L., Hodnett, E., Hofmeyr, J. (eds) *A Guide to Effective Care in Pregnancy and Childbirth,* 3rd edn, pp. 417–28. Oxford, Oxford University Press.

Vain, N., Szyld, E., Prudent, L., Wiswell, T., Aguilar, A., Vivas, N. (2004) Oropharyngeal and nasopharyngeal suctioning of meconium-stained neonates before delivery of their shoulders: multicentre, randomised controlled trial. *Lancet* 364, 597–602.

Van Reempts, P., Van Acker, K. (2001) Ethical aspects of cardiopulmonary resuscitation in premature neonates: where do we stand? *Resuscitation* 51(3), 225–32.

Whitten, W., Montgomery, L. (2000) Postmortem and perimortem caesarean sections: what are the indications? *Journal of the Royal Society of Medicine* 93, 6–9.

Whyte, S., Sinha, A., Wyllie, J. (1999) Neonatal resuscitation – a practical assessment. *Resuscitation* 40(1), 21–5.

Wyllie, J., Perlman, J., Kattwinkel, J. *et al.* (2010) Part 11: Neonatal Resuscitation. *Resuscitation* 2010; 81s: 260–87.

Zideman, D., Bingham, R., Beattie, T., Bland, J., Bruinsstanssen, M., Frei, F. (1998) Recommendations on resuscitation of babies at birth. *Resuscitation* 37(2), 103–10.

19 Induction of labour

Mary-Lou Elliott

Introduction

Induction of labour (IOL), although a common procedure, can present challenges for both mothers and clinicians (NICE, 2008). The recommendation of IOL can begin a worrying time for many women who have planned for a normal labour and birth. Feelings of disappointment and loss of control can also occur if their intended place of birth changes from home/birthing centre to an unfamiliar consultant unit. The midwife has an important role to play in counselling women about IOL and providing the information needed to make informed choices about whether/when to consent to procedures, possible interventions and the support available during labour and birth.

Once women have passed their due date, frustration, anxiety and boredom can leave them vulnerable to the suggestion of induction. Midwives can be of great support during this time, encouraging positive thinking and suggesting natural methods for stimulating labour.

The Midwife's Labour and Birth Handbook, Third Edition. Edited by Vicky Chapman and Cathy Charles.
© 2013 John Wiley & Sons, Ltd. Published 2013 by John Wiley & Sons, Ltd.

Definition

IOL can be viewed as any procedure or intervention that initiates labour rather than allowing it to commence spontaneously. Although natural and alternative methods of induction can be used, the term IOL in this chapter refers to surgical and/or pharmacological methods.

Incidence and facts

- Approximately 20% of UK pregnancies are induced (NICE, 2008).
- 33% of women induced stated they would have valued more information about the reasons for and process of IOL (Nuutulia *et al.*, 1999).
- Despite an increased risk of operative delivery and sometimes a more painful labour, women undergoing IOL for premature rupture of membranes (PROM) tend to have fewer negative comments than those undergoing expectant management, and feel more satisfaction and less worry with the experience (Hodnett *et al.*, 1997). This could stem from a decrease in anxiety and the relief obtained from a proactive approach to finally getting their baby born.
- NICE (2008) recommends IOL should be offered to all women with uncomplicated pregnancies between 41 and 42 weeks.
- IOL for post-41/40 nulliparous pregnancies may reduce perinatal mortality without increasing caesarean section (CS) rates (NICE, 2008), but the evidence base is controversial.

IOL is usually recommended when it is agreed that the risk of continuing the pregnancy outweighs the risk of intervention to induce birth. An exception, however, is IOL for maternal request, where the mother's desire for delivery may be at odds with clinical opinion. IOL should only be considered when vaginal birth is felt to be the appropriate mode of delivery.

Risks and side effects

The concept of IOL as 'routine' is a dangerous one; it should always be approached with caution. In women with particular risk factors, induction should not take place on an antenatal ward but on a labour ward where the woman and baby can be more closely monitored. This is advisable for women with relevant risk factors including suspected fetal growth compromise, previous CS and high parity.

One less easily measurable risk of IOL may be the effect on a woman's sense of control. Once she has initially consented to IOL, she may be offered little subsequent choice in continuing on to the next 'inevitable' procedure, leading to a cascade of interventions (RCM, 2005). Anxiety and loss of control may lead to increased stress levels which can have physiological consequences for labour (see Chapter 1). However, prolonged pregnancy can also be stressful, so for some women induction actually gives them a sense of relief.

Other risks/issues

- Membrane sweeping can cause minor bleeding but does not increase membrane rupture or infection (NICE, 2008).

- Repeated vaginal examination (VE) can be painful, so only perform when essential. Hibitane obstetric cream is not recommended for VE: chlorhexidine can cause soreness.
- Prostin sometimes causes vaginal soreness; while there is no conclusive evidence that prostaglandin-induced labour is more painful than spontaneous onset (NICE, 2008), some anecdotal accounts suggest otherwise. Intravenous (IV) oxytocin infusion appears to cause more painful contractions, perhaps due to their more intense onset, and as a result many women in this situation will opt for epidural anaesthesia.
- Hypertonic uterine contractions caused by oxytocics and/or prostaglandins can lead to fetal oxygen deprivation, uterine rupture and maternal and/or perinatal death (Smith *et al.*, 2004). Close fetal and maternal surveillance is therefore essential. Induction and labour for women with high parity or previous CS carries a small but significant risk of uterine rupture even in the absence of hypertonic contractions (see Chapter 12).
- Response to prostaglandins and oxytocics is unpredictable, and midwives should observe women for tachycardia, nausea, vomiting, diarrhoea, water intoxication and headache (Hawkins, 2000).
- The CS risk evidence is controversial. Some studies suggest that IOL for uncomplicated post-term pregnancies increases the risk of CS delivery, length of hospital stay, use of epidural and other analgesia, neonatal resuscitation, neonatal intensive care unit admission and phototherapy (Seyb *et al.*, 1999; Maslow and Sweeny, 2000; Boulvain *et al.*, 2001). One large US study found the CS risk doubled, with low risk primigravidae with an unfavourable cervix having highest risk (Ehrenthal *et al.*, 2010). Cochrane meta-analysis (Gulmezoglu *et al.*, 2006) and NICE (2008), however, state that a policy of routine IOL for post-term pregnancies >41/40 is associated with no difference in CS delivery compared with conservative management.

Information giving and informed consent

Midwives are in a unique position to fully explain what IOL entails and answer any questions the woman and her partner may have. MIDIRS provides an informed choice leaflet 'Prolonged Pregnancy' (www.infochoice.org); most trusts provide information leaflets, containing contact numbers, should women have further questions following the initial discussion.

An obstetrician's recommendation of IOL can be difficult to refuse, but women should be made aware that they have the right to decline. NICE (2008) clearly state that if a woman chooses not to have induction, her decision should be respected.

If a woman declines post-dates IOL, conservative management should be offered, i.e. maternal vigilance of fetal movements, and twice weekly liquor volume scans and cardiotocographs (CTGs) (NICE, 2008).

Determining expected date of delivery (EDD)

Midwives will be familiar with the various methods of determining EDD. A first trimester ultrasound scan <16 weeks provides the greatest accuracy (NICE, 2008). This also reduces the proportion of births considered post-term (Gardosi *et al.*, 1997) and consequently reduces inductions (Tunón *et al.*, 1996; NICE, 2008).

IOL for social reasons

Some women may wish to be induced without medical/post-dates indications. Midwives should discuss the risks of early/unnecessary IOL, but where resources allow, maternal request for IOL at term may be considered when there are reasonable psychological or social reasons and the woman is >40 weeks with a favourable cervix. Social induction is unlikely to be supported if there are contraindications to IOL or staffing/resource issues.

Induction for post-term pregnancy

NICE (2008) recommends offering IOL between 41 and 42 weeks to avoid the risks of prolonged pregnancy, stating that timing should take into account the woman's preferences and local circumstances.

Without IOL:

- by 40/40   58% will give birth
- by 41/40   74% will give birth
- by 42/40   82% will give birth
- 18% will remain undelivered after 42/40

The incidence of stillbirth increases with gestation around term (NICE, 2008):

- at 37/40   1:3000
- at 42/40   3:3000
- at 43/40   6:3000

There is no current evidence to suggest that IOL before 41/40 improves fetal or maternal outcomes, but IOL after this time has been found to marginally decrease rates of stillbirth and neonatal death in otherwise uncomplicated pregnancies (NICE, 2008). Cochrane review by Gulmezoglu *et al.* (2006) concludes that there is only a very slightly increased perinatal mortality beyond 41/40 and states 'the absolute risk is extremely small' and women should be counselled on both relative and absolute risks.

IOL versus expectant management for PROM at term

Premature rupture of membranes (PROM) at term:

- occurs in 8–10% of term pregnancies (NICE, 2008).
- 86% of women with PROM will go into spontaneous labour within 24 hours; the rate of spontaneous labour will then increase by 5% per day (NICE, 2008).
- NICE (2008) recommends IOL after 24 hours post-PROM.

Women induced after 24 hours were less likely than those managed expectantly to develop chorioamnionitis and endometritis, with no difference in instrumental/CS rates or adverse neonatal outcome (NICE, 2007). Neonatal infection rates were marginally reduced by early IOL in one study quoted by NICE. Women should be informed that neonatal outcomes are similar with either method (Dare *et al.*, 2006).

Assessing the cervix

The Bishop score is a subjective VE assessment, combining cervical effacement, consistency, position, dilatation and descent of the presenting part. A score of >6 is judged 'favourable' for IOL. Despite dilatation alone having been found to be a better determinant of successful IOL and vaginal delivery than the Bishop score (Williams *et al.*, 1997), it is still routinely used. Ultrasound scan has been shown to be of value in the prediction of successful IOL but is not widely used (Rane *et al.*, 2004).

Methods of induction

Natural methods

Women seem open to natural methods of inducing labour once their due date has arrived. Most natural methods have had little research into their effectiveness, but anecdotal reports show varying levels of success. Often women will combine several methods in the hope they can 'bring on labour' and avoid medical induction. Natural methods include the following:

- Breast/nipple stimulation: Kavanagh *et al.* (2005) state it is effective (also for treating postpartum haemorrhage) but recommends caution in high-risk groups.
- Sexual intercourse: a difficult and delicate area to study; research is inconclusive.
- Exercise, e.g. brisk walking.
- Eating fresh pineapple.
- Consuming a purgative, e.g. castor oil, or spicy foods, e.g. curry.
- Membrane sweeping.

NICE (2008) recommends membrane sweeping/stripping from term as a safe effective method of reducing post-term pregnancy in low-risk women. The midwife gently inserts a finger into the cervix and rotates it 360°, separating the membranes from the lower uterine segment. This aims to increase production of prostaglandins. Serial sweeping every 48 hours results in consistent reduction in post-term pregnancy regardless of Bishop score (Boulvain *et al.*, 2005). Women's satisfaction is generally high despite the procedure's discomfort, with most happy to accept it again in future (de Miranda *et al.*, 2006).

Complementary/alternative methods

Unless specifically trained in alternative methods, midwives would be wise to refer women to qualified practitioners, advising them to be cautious before using any of the methods discussed:

- Acupuncture/acupressure/moxibustion (also used for turning breeches)
- Reflexology
- Visualisation and meditation
- Hypnosis

- Herbal remedies
- Homeopathic remedies.

Cochrane reviews have examined some methods above; they generally conclude studies were too small or of poor quality to draw any conclusions. Numerous websites explore the use of alternative methods.

Surgical/pharmacological methods

- Amniotomy or artificial rupture of membranes (ARM)
- Prostaglandin
- IV oxytocin.

ARM

ARM involves a small degree of risk and constitutes a definite commitment to delivery. See Chapter 2 for risks, benefits and contraindications.

- Insufficient evidence supports ARM alone as an IOL method (Bricker and Luckas, 2007); even if the cervix is sufficiently dilated to allow ARM, it is good practice to give at least one dose of prostaglandin first, to ripen the cervix. However, some believe that multigravid women with a high Bishop score may respond favourably to ARM alone, preventing further intervention, so the decision should be individualised after discussion with the woman.
- CTG monitoring is **not** indicated, and water birth is **not** contraindicated following ARM induction once labour is established, if all appears normal.
- ARM plus IV oxytocin within one hour shortens any latent labour phase (Moldin and Sundell, 1996) although the optimal interval between ARM and Syntocinon is unclear.
- ARM is not automatically indicated following prostin administration if the woman is contracting and VE confirms progress.

Prostaglandins

- Prostaglandin (PGE$_2$) vaginal tablets, gel or controlled-release pessaries soften or 'ripen' the cervix. Costs vary but there does not appear to be a significant difference among the various types (NICE, 2008). Slow-release pessaries, e.g. Propess (see Table 19.1) have the advantage of removal from the vagina if hyperstimulation occurs.
- Oral prostaglandins have gastrointestinal side effects and lack evaluation, casting safety doubts, so are rarely used in the UK (Hawkins, 2000).
- Prostaglandins given prior to ARM increase its effectiveness (NICE, 2008).
- Prostaglandin alone reduces operative deliveries and increases likelihood of delivery <24 hours compared with oxytocin alone (Enkin *et al.*, 2000). The ability to remain mobile and upright in labour may play a part in this.
- Misoprostol is reported as a safe and effective IOL drug (Surbek *et al.*, 1997), but is currently unlicensed for obstetric use. NICE (2008) and Gaskin (2001) suggest risks are incompletely evaluated and it should only be offered following intrauterine death.

Table 19.1   Dinoprostone (Prostin E$_2$®)/Prostaglandin PGE$_2$/Propess.

Doseage for IOL: varies according to parity and cervical favourability. Prostin E$_2$ vaginal gel & vaginal pessary are not bioequivalent doses (JFC, 2012).

Prostin E$_2$ **Vaginal Gel:**	**Prostin E$_2$** **Vaginal Pessary (tablet):**	**Propess** **Vaginal Pessary (with retrieval device):**
Dinoprostone 400 mcg/ml: 2.5 ml (1 mg) £13.28.	Dinoprostone 3 mg price £13.27	Dinoprostone 10 mg price £30.00
800 mcg/ml: 2.5 ml (2 mg) £13.28	3 mg first dose	10 mg released over 24 hrs
1 mg or 2 mg (unfavourable primigravida 2 mg)	3 mg repeated after 6–8 hours if required	**Maximum Propess Dose:** Dose not to be repeated.
1–2 mg repeated after 6 hours if required	**Maximum Pessary Dose:** 6 mg (for all women)	Note: Remove tablet when cervical ripening adequate or 30 minutes before oxytocin.
Maximum Gel Dose: Primigravida 4 mg Multigravida 3 mg		Remove after 24 hours if not effective.

Route	Posterior fornix of vagina: avoid cervical canal.
Contraindications	Active cardiac, pulmonary, renal or hepatic disease.
	Placenta praevia, unexplained vaginal bleeding during pregnancy, major cephalopelvic disproportion, malpresentation.
	Ruptured membranes, fetal distress, grand multiparity, multiple pregnancy, previous CS or major uterine surgery (JFC, 2012). (*However, it is used judiciously in practice for some VBAC women.*)
Side effects	Nausea, vomiting, diarrhoea, fever, backache; vaginal symptoms (warmth, irritation, pain).
	Uterine hypertonus/severe uterine contractions, uterine rupture, placental abruption, fetal distress, cardiac arrest, low apgar score, stillbirth/neonatal death.
	Maternal hypertension, bronchospasm, pulmonary/amniotic fluid embolism (JFC, 2012).
Cautions	History of asthma, epilepsy, glaucoma/raised intraocular pressure, hepatic/renal impairment, hypertension, uterine scarring/rupture, risk factors for disseminated intravascular coagulation (DIC) (JFC, 2012).

- Once labour is established intermittent ausculatation (IA) is recommended, NOT continuous electronic fetal monitoring (EFM) unless there are other risk factors (NICE, 2008).

Oxytocin

- IV oxytocin (Syntocinon) is used to stimulate contractions if prostin and ARM have not achieved good labour progress.
- Administer via a controlled infusion pump/syringe driver with a non-return valve.
- Women who have had prostaglandins may respond dramatically to oxytocin and experience severe contractions. EFM is recommended during oxytocin induction to observe for uterine hypertonus, hypercontractility and/or fetal distress (NICE, 2008).

Care of a woman during IOL

Although IOL is a significant intervention in the normal process of labour, the midwife can do much to support the woman in her wish for a normal birth. Once the reason for IOL is understood and all agree that it is desirable, it is important to ascertain the woman's understanding of the process. Discuss how much she would actually like to know about the procedure (does she really want to see an amnihook?), and provide further explanation and written information if necessary. Be aware that the woman may be in a high state of anxiety, especially if IOL is indicated for a fetal concern.

Midwives can give reassurance and explanations about the length of time it may take to get labour established; sometimes several days. If IOL has to be postponed (sometimes after starting) due to a busy labour ward, further explanation and support will be needed for both women and partner. Midwives familiar with distressed women in antenatal beds who are well over their due dates and desperate to give birth recognise the need for sensitivity.

Include partners and birth supporters whenever possible so all members of the 'birthing team' can work together to achieve a satisfying experience for the woman. Familiarisation with the birth setting, advice regarding suitable clothing, refreshment, meals and rest will enhance the experience. Where possible, the woman should not be separated from her support; her midwife should give extra support if she is alone at any time.

IOL may be initiated on the labour ward for a high risk pregnancy, or for lower risk women on an antenatal ward (NICE, 2008) or as an outpatient.

General labour care applies as with spontaneous labour. Consent issues are just as important, and just because a woman has agreed to IOL, her consent for subsequent VEs and interventions is equally important. The midwife's documentation should show a clear plan of care, labour progress and drugs used in the IOL process.

Midwifery care for IOL

- Review notes/history to ascertain EDD, placental location and rule out contraindications.
- Discuss the procedure with the woman and partner(s) and gain consent. Make time to answer any questions and advise on coping mechanisms for 'prostin pains'/early labour, e.g. warmed wheatgerm bag, warm bath, TENS or going for a distracting walk.
- Ensure the IOL has been authorised and prostaglandin written up. Prostaglandins must be prescribed by a doctor although many units use patient group directions (PGDs) to ensure midwives can administer prostin for post-dates induction without a prescription. The midwife is responsible for ensuring the correct dose is administered safely.
- Ask the woman to empty her bladder.
- Ensure the woman's privacy.
- Commence CTG pre-procedure.
- Assess cervix and explain Bishop score.

- Administer appropriate dose of prostaglandin or ARM depending on Bishop score. Insert gel/pessary into posterior vaginal fornix. Local guidelines may apply, but NICE (2008) recommends:
  - one cycle of vaginal PGE_2 tablets or gel: one dose, followed by a second dose after 6 hours if labour is not established (up to a maximum of two doses).
  - one cycle of vaginal PGE_2 controlled-release pessary: one dose over 24 hours. Also see Table 19.1 for Propess dosage.
- Continue CTG until unequivocally normal (typically 30–60 min), but once labour is established intermittent auscultation is recommended following prostaglandin IOL in the absence of risk factors (NICE, 2008). Frustratingly the older NICE (2007) labour guidelines still state that induction of labour is an indication for continuous EFM – which will inevitably cause confusion.
- Ensure maternal and fetal surveillance is implemented, if IOL continuation is delayed.
- Warn the woman of side effects and advise reporting symptoms such as very strong, frequent, painful contractions, sudden nausea/vomiting or anything worrying her.
- Since intermittent monitoring is perfectly acceptable after normal initial CTG (NICE, 2008), labour in water is an option. Ensure labour is established first as early immersion can slow labour (see Chapter 7).
- Inform obstetrician of lack of progress or any concerns.
- Once in established labour, treat the woman as any other (see Chapter 1).
- Induced women are more likely to remain in semi-recumbent positions compared to non-induced labours: encourage mobilising and upright postures, which enhance contractions, shorten labour duration and reduce instrumental deliveries/CS (RCM, 2010).

Continuing IOL: care with IV oxytocin

If the woman has not established in labour despite IOL, she will naturally feel disappointed. She may have had several doses of prostaglandins over two/three days and be tired and despondent. The next option to discuss is oxytocin, which she still has the option to decline. Women have occasionally been known to go home and return several days later in spontaneous labour or for further IOL.

- Elicit the women's wishes and consent at every stage of the induction process. Clear explanations and support are vital.
- Ensure oxytocin is authorised and prescribed. Do not start <6 hours after prostaglandin due to combined uterotonic effects (NICE, 2008).
- Discuss analgesia prior to commencing IV oxytocin as it will probably be more painful: the woman may be happy to wait and see how she copes.
- Oxytocin regimes may vary among trusts. See Table 19.2. They **must** be monitored closely:
  - Site IV cannula.
  - Commence oxytocin infusion at recommended rate; increase at 30-min intervals (NICE, 2008).

Table 19.2   Oxytocin (Syntocinon®).

IV infusion for labour induction/ augmentation	1–2 mU/min, increased at 30 min intervals until contracting 3–4:10 mins.
	10–12 mU/min is often adequate.
	Maximum licensed dose 20 mU/min, but NICE (2008) states maximum dose 32 mU/min.
Do not confuse intrapartum and postpartum regimes – as doses vary widely	
Contraindications	Hypertonic uterine contractions, fetal distress.
	Avoid prolonged administration in oxytocin resistant uterine inertia, severe pre-eclampsia/cardiovascular disease (JFC, 2012).
Side effects	Nausea, vomiting, arrhythmia, headache.
	Uterine spasm (low doses) and uterine hyperstimulation (usually excessive doses) resulting in titanic contractions, uterine rupture, soft tissue damage, placental abruption, amniotic fluid embolism, fetal distress/asphyxia/death.
	Rarely rash, DIC, anaphylactic reaction (dyspnoea, hypotension, shock).
Caution	**Fetal:** heart rate abnormalities, asphyxia, intrauterine death. **Maternal**: mild/ moderate hypertension/cardiac disease. Women >35 years or previous CS.
	High dose and large volume infusion can cause water intoxication (JFC, 2012). Interactions can cause severe hypotension and arrhythmias when administered during anaesthetic (DoH, 2001).
	Oxytocics can potentiate prostaglandin effects: do not give within 6 hours of prostaglandins.
	Oxytocin should be stored in the fridge: heat may affect efficacy.

○ Use the minimum dose possible: aim for 4–5 contractions every 10 min. If over-contracting reduce infusion (NICE, 2008).

○ Continuous EFM recommended (NICE, 2008).

○ If severe hypercontractility or suspected fetal compromise: discontinue infusion immediately, suggest the woman adopts a left lateral position and summon an obstetrician. If the situation does not resolve tocolysis may be considered and/or delivery expedited. Although unlicensed for use in obstetrics, the beta-sympathomimetic drugs salbutamol (via inhaler) and terbutaline (0.25 mg sub-cutaneous), can be administered and are effective in reversing the effects of oxytocics (Hawkins, 2000).

Summary

- 20% of women experience IOL which many find stressful.
- Many women are open to trying natural/complementary IOL methods.
- Pharmacological/surgical IOL involves risk: it is never 'routine'.
- IOL can take several days and can be wearing for all involved.
- Informed choice throughout the IOL process is vital.
- Pharmacological IOL is usually more painful than spontaneous onset of labour.
- Main risks of prostaglandin and oxytocin are hypercontractility and fetal distress.
- IA is appropriate for prostaglandin IOL (after initial CTG) unless other concerns
- Continuous EFM during oxytocin IOL is recommended.
- Discontinue oxytocin infusion if hypercontracting or suspected fetal compromise.

Recommended reading

NICE (National Institute for Health and Clinical Excellence) (2008) *Clinical Guideline 70 – Induction of Labour*. London, NICE. http://publications.nice.org.uk/induction-of-labour-cg70/guidance

References

Boulvain, M., Marcoux, S., Bureau, M., Fortier, M., Fraser, W. (2001) Risks of induction of labour in uncomplicated term pregnancies. *Paediatric and Perinatal Epidemiology*, 15(2), 131–8.

Boulvain, M., Stan, C., Orion, O. (2005) Membrane sweeping for labour. *Cochrane Database of Systematic Reviews*, Issue 1.

Bricker, L., Luckas, M. (2007) Amniotomy alone for induction of labour. *Cochrane Database of Systematic Reviews*, Issue 4.

Dare, M., Middleton, P., Crowther, C, Flenady, V., Varatharaju, B. (2006) Planned early birth versus expectant management (waiting) for prelabour rupture of membranes at term (37 weeks or more). *Cochrane Database of Systemic Reviews*, Issue 1.

de Miranda, E., Van Der Bom, J. G., Bonsel, G. J., Bleker, O. P., Rosendaal, F. R. (2006) Membrane sweeping and prevention of post-term pregnancy in low-risk pregnancies: a randomised controlled trial. *BJOG: An International Journal of Obstetrics and Gynaecology*, 113(4), 402–8.

DoH (Department of Health) (2001) *Why Mothers Die, 1997–1999. The Fifth Report of the Confidential Enquiries into Maternal Deaths in the United Kingdom*. London, DoH, RCOG Press.

Ehrenthal, D. B., Jiang, X., Strobino, D. M. (2010) Labor induction and the risk of a cesarean delivery among nulliparous women at term. *Obstetrics and Gynecology*. 116(1), 35–42.

Enkin, M., Keirse, M., Neilson, J., Crowther, C., Duley, L., Hodnett, E., Hofmeyr, J. (2000) *A Guide to Effective Care in Pregnancy and Childbirth*, 3rd edn. Oxford, Oxford University Press.

Gardosi, J., Vanner, T., Francis, A. (1997) Gestational age and induction of labour for prolonged pregnancy. *British Journal of Obstetrics and Gynaecology* 104(7), 792–7.

Gaskin, I. M. (2001) The dark side of US obstetrics' love affair with misoprostol. *MIDIRS Midwifery Digest* 11(2), 205–9.

Gulmezoglu, A., Crowther, C., Middleton, P. (2006) Induction of labour for improving birth outcomes for women at or beyond term. *Cochrane Database of Systematic Reviews*, Issue 4.

Hawkins, D. F. (2000) Prescribing Drugs in Pregnancy. *A Guide to Preconception Counselling and Use of Medicines in Pregnancy, Labour and the Puerperium*. Euromed Communications.

Hodnett, E. D., Hannah, M. E., Weston, J. A., Ohlsson, A., Myhr, T. L., Wang, E. E., Hewson, S. A., Willan, A. R., Farine, D. (1997) Women's evaluations of induction of labor versus expectant management for prelabor rupture of the membranes at term. *Birth* 24(4), 214–20.

JFC (Joint Formulary Committee) (2012) *British National Formulary*. London, BMA and Royal Pharmaceutical Society of Great Britain, London.

Kavanagh, J., Kelly, A., Thomas, J. (2005) Breast stimulation for cervical ripening and induction of labour. *Cochrane Database of Systematic Reviews*, Issue 3.

Maslow, A. S., Sweeny, A. L. (2000) Elective induction of labor as a risk factor for caesarean delivery among low-risk women at term. *Obstetrics and Gynecology* 95(6), 917–22.

Moldin, P. G., Sundell, G. (1996) Induction of labour: a randomised clinical trial of amniotomy versus amniotomy with oxytocin infusion. *British Journal of Obstetrics and Gynaecology* 103(4), 306–12.

NICE (2001) *Clinical Guideline D: Induction of Labour*. London, NICE.

NICE (2007) *Clinical Guideline 55: Intrapartum Care*. London, NICE. http://publications.nice.org.uk/induction-of-labour-cg55/guidance

NICE (2008) *Clinical Guideline 70: Induction of Labour*. London, NICE. http://publications.nice.org.uk/induction-of-labour-cg70/guidance

Nuutulia, M., Halmesmaki, E., Hiilesmaav, E., Ylikorkala, O. (1999) Women's anticipation of and experiences with induction of labour. *Acta Obstetricia et Gynecologica Scandinavica* 78(8), 704–9.

Rane, S. M., Guirgis, R. R., Higgins, B., Nicolaides, K. H. (2004) The value of ultrasound in the prediction of successful induction of labour. *Ultrasound in Obstetrics and Gynecology* 24(5), 538–49.

RCM (Royal College of Midwives) (2005) *Campaign for Normal Birth*. http://www.rcmnormalbirth.org.uk

RCM (2010) *The Royal College of Midwives Survey of Positions used in Labour and Birth*. London, RCM. www.rcm.org.uk

RCOG (Royal College of Obstetricians and Gynaecologists) (2001) *Induction of Labour: Clinical Guideline 9*. London, RCOG.

Seyb, S. T., Berka, R. J., Socol, M. L., Dooley, S. L. (1999) Risk of caesarean delivery with elective induction of labor at term in nulliparous women. *Obstetrics and Gynecology* 94(4), 600–7.

Smith, G., Pell, J., Pasupathy, D., Dobbie, R. (2004) Factors predisposing to perinatal death related to uterine rupture during attempted vaginal birth after caesarean section. *British Medical Journal* 329, 375–7.

Surbek, D. V., Boesiger, H., Hoesli, I., Pavic, N., Holzgreve, W. (1997) A double-blind comparison of the safety and efficacy of intravaginal misoprostol and prostaglandin E2 to induce labor. *American Journal of Obstetrics and Gynecology* 177(5), 1018–23.

Tunón, K., Eik-Nes, S. H., Grøttum, P. (1996). A comparison between ultrasound and a reliable last menstrual period as predictors of the day of delivery in 15 000 examinations. *Ultrasound Obstet Gynecol* 8(3), 178–85.

Williams, M. C., Krammer, J., O'Brien, W. F. (1997) The value of the cervical score in predicting successful outcome of labor induction. *Obstetrics and Gynecology* 90(5), 784–9.

20 Pre-eclampsia

Annette Briley

Introduction

Pre-eclampsia is a condition peculiar to pregnancy, characterised by raised blood pressure (BP) and proteinuria. It can be associated with seizures (eclampsia) and multi-organ failure in the mother, while fetal complications include intrauterine growth restriction (IUGR) and placental abruption (Shennan and Chappell, 2001).

Pre-eclampsia leads to increased maternal and fetal mortality and morbidity. In the developed world it is a leading cause of maternal death, and in the UK most deaths have been consistently associated with suboptimal care, particularly by intrapartum care providers (CMACE, 2011).

See Box 20.1 for definitions of hypertension in pregnancy.

Underlying pathophysiology of pre-eclampsia

Pre-eclampsia is associated with abnormal implantation of the placenta and concomitant shallow trophoblastic invasion (Pijnenborg, 1994) leading to reduced placental perfusion. The maternal spinal arteries (also known as the uterine arteries) fail to undergo their normal physiological vasodilatation; blood flow may be further impeded by atherotic changes causing obstruction within the vessels.

The Midwife's Labour and Birth Handbook, Third Edition. Edited by Vicky Chapman and Cathy Charles.
© 2013 John Wiley & Sons, Ltd. Published 2013 by John Wiley & Sons, Ltd.

Box 20.1   Definitions of hypertensive disorders of pregnancy (NICE, 2011).

Mild hypertension: diastolic BP 90–99 mmHg, systolic 140–149 mmHg

Moderate hypertension: diastolic BP 100–109 mmHg, systolic 150–159 mmHg

Severe hypertension: diastolic BP ≥110 mmHg, systolic ≥160 mmHg

Gestational hypertension is new hypertension presenting after 20 weeks without significant proteinuria.

Pre-eclampsia is new hypertension presenting after 20 weeks with significant proteinuria.

Severe pre-eclampsia is pre-eclampsia with severe hypertension and/or with symptoms, and/or biochemical and/or haematological impairment.

This pathology causes increased resistance in the uteroplacental circulation with impaired intervillus blood flow resulting in ischaemia and hypoxia, manifested in the second half of pregnancy (Graham *et al.*, 2000).

A similar picture of inadequate trophoblastic invasion exists in pregnancies complicated by IUGR in women with no pre-eclampsia. This suggests that the maternal syndrome of pre-eclampsia must be associated with other features.

Incidence

The incidence of pre-eclampsia varies according to population characteristics and the definitions used to describe it (Davey and MacGillivray, 1988; Chappell *et al.*, 1999; Briley *et al.*, 2006).

- Pre-eclampsia is estimated at <5% in most populations. It may be 6–8% in some nations (Lain and Roberts, 2002; Rumbold *et al.*, 2006).

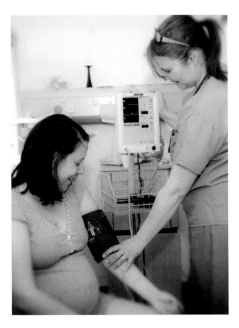

Fig. 20.1   Caution should be used with automated BP machines as most under-record pre-eclampsia BP. *Photo by Debbie Gagliano-Withers.*

- Gestational hypertension (elevated BP with no proteinuria and no pregnancy-related pathology) is approximately three times more common than pre-eclampsia (Shennan and Chappell, 2001).
- Up to 20% of all pregnant women will have some form of hypertension during pregnancy. Of these fewer than 10% will suffer serious disease.
- In the UK maternal death is rare: 22 women in England died of pre-eclampsia (including three due to acute fatty liver of pregnancy) in 2005–08: in 20 out of 22 care was sub-standard (CMACE, 2011). It is estimated that pre-eclampsia and eclampsia cause up to 25% of the 358 000 annual maternal deaths globally; with most avoidable (WHO, 2010, 2011).

Facts

- Pregnant women should be advised to seek advice if they experience pre-eclampsia symptoms (NICE, 2011; CMACE, 2011) – see Box 20.2.
- Pregnant women with a headache of sufficient severity to seek medical advice, or with new epigastric pain, should have BP measured and urine tested for protein, as a minimum (CMACE, 2011).
- Epigastric pain in the second half of pregnancy should be attributed to pre-eclampsia until proven otherwise (CMACE, 2011).
- Placental insufficiency is common in early-onset pre-eclampsia, and may lead to IUGR in 30% of pre-eclamptic pregnancies; sometimes also placental abruption and fetal demise (RCOG, 2006).
- In severe pre-eclampsia the main causes of maternal death are cerebral haemorrhage and acute respiratory distress syndrome (CMACE, 2011). Labour management therefore concentrates on BP control and fluid balance.
- Systolic BP is as important as diastolic (NICE, 2011; CMACE, 2011).

Box 20.2   Signs and symptoms of pre-eclampsia.

- Raised blood pressure (see Box 20.1)
- Proteinuria
- Severe headache
- Problems with vision, e.g. blurring or flashing before the eyes
- Severe pain just below the ribs (epigastric pain)
- Vomiting
- Sudden swelling of face, hands or feet

(NICE, 2011)

The diagnosis should also be considered in women with intrauterine growth restriction.

Associated risk factors

- First pregnancy.
- Subsequent pregnancy with new partner: risk returns to that of a primigravida (McCowan *et al.*, 1996), although miscarriages and terminations of pregnancy offer some protection (Strickland *et al.*, 1986).

- Paternal influence: risk is doubled if partner previously fathered a pre-eclamptic pregnancy (Need *et al.*, 1983; Dekker, 2002).
- Genetic link: a mother/sister with pre-eclampsia increases risk 4–8 times (Lie *et al.*, 1998).
- Assisted conception, particularly with donor gametes (Wang *et al.*, 2002).
- Multiple pregnancies (risk is doubled) (Duley *et al.*, 2001).
- Maternal age >35 years. Historically women under 20 were reported as increased risk, although Baker *et al.* (2009) refute this.
- Obesity (body mass index ≥30): risk increased fourfold (Poston *et al.*, 2006).
- Underlying maternal medical conditions, e.g. chronic hypertension, renal disease (Poston *et al.*, 2006), insulin resistance and glucose intolerance including gestational diabetes (Duley *et al.*, 2001; Ramsay *et al.*, 2006).
- The impact of multiple risk factors needs further research, but obesity and primiparity increase cumulative risk (Poston *et al.*, 2006; Smith *et al.*, 2007).

Signs and symptoms

Clinicians cannot rely on BP and proteinuria alone to diagnose pre-eclampsia. Just under 50% of all women presenting with pre-eclampsia will have had no previous hypertension or proteinuria (Douglas and Redman, 1994; Milne *et al.*, 2005).

See Box 20.2 for signs and symptoms of pre-eclampsia.

See Box 20.3 for signs and symptoms of **severe** pre-eclampsia.

Box 20.3   Signs and symptoms of severe pre-eclampsia.

BP
- Systolic >160 mmHg or diastolic ≥110 mmHg or MAP >125 mmHg (NICE, 2011).

Mean arterial pressure
- MAP between 125 and 140 mmHg for >45 min requires medical referral and treatment
- MAP ≥140 mmHg for >15 min requires **urgent** medical referral and treatment
- MAP >150 mmHg represents serious risk of cerebral autoregulatory dysfunction and subsequent risk of cerebral haemorrhage.

Significant proteinuria
- One 24 hour collection with total protein excretion ≥300 mg^a/24 hours, or;
- Two 'clean-catch midstream' or catheter specimens of urine collected ≥4 hours apart, measuring ≥ ++ on reagent strip, or;
- A spot urinary protein:creatinine ratio > 30 mg protein.

Other possible symptoms:
- Headache
- Visual disturbance
- Epigastric pain
- Brisk reflexes or clonus
- Platelet count <100 (× 10^9/l)
- Aspartate transaminase (AST) or alanine transaminase (ALT) >50 IU/l: there is significantly increased maternal morbidity above 150 IU/l (RCOG, 2006).

Traditionally midwives have worried about diastolic BP, but systolic hypertension $\geq$150 mmHg requires effective antihypertensive treatment; if >180 mmHg this is a medical emergency requiring urgent antihypertensive treatment (NICE, 2011; CMACE, 2011).

Fatal intracranial haemorrhage due to untreated systolic BP was the cause of several deaths CMACE (2011) investigated.

- **Blood tests** (see also 'Pre-eclampsia' under the heading 'Blood tests for specific conditions and blood pictures' page 374, Chapter 23).
  - **Full blood count.**
  - **Platelet count.** Endothelial dysfunction results in platelet dysfunction. If the platelet count is >50×10^9/l, haemostasis is likely to be normal.
  - **Clotting studies** are necessary because pre-eclampsia can cause disseminated intravascular coagulation.
  - **Uric acid or urate levels.** These are used to assess the severity of the disease and its progression. However, severe disease can occur in the presence of low, normal and high uric acid concentrations (Lie *et al.*, 1998).
  - **Plasma urea** and **creatinine** concentrations. Raised levels of these are generally associated with late renal involvement and serious disease. They are not a useful *early* indicator of disease severity, but should be obtained longitudinally to assess the progression of renal involvement.
  - **Liver function tests.** Pre-eclampsia can cause liver problems, e.g. subcapsular haematoma, rupture, hepatic infarction, and acute fatty liver of pregnancy (AFLP).

BP measurement

Care with BP measurement is essential. Evidence suggests it is often poorly performed.

- **Equipment.** Mercury sphygmomanometry remains the 'gold standard' for measuring BP. Many units no longer have these machines available, due to mercury safety concerns. Use a mercury sphygmomanometer for the first reading if possible, and if any uncertainty (CMACE, 2011; RCOG, 2006). If not available cross-check with another validated automated device for increased accuracy (RCOG, 2006). Some automated devices do not measure BP accurately if the pulse rate is irregular, so check the pulse first: if irregular, document and measure BP directly over the brachial using an aneroid device (NICE, 2011). Aneroid machines are commonly used and are reliable when maintained and regularly calibrated. Numerous automated devices are available although few are validated for pregnancy, and fewer for pre-eclampsia use. Most automated devices under-record pre-eclampsia BP.
- **Cuff size.** Always use the appropriate size cuff. The standard bladder (23 cm × 12 cm) is too small for at least 25% pregnant women. Undercuffing may overestimate BP by >10 mmHg leading to hypertension overdiagnosis. Overcuffing has the opposite (although smaller) effect by underestimating BP by up to 5 mmHg (Shennan *et al.*, 1996).
- **Maternal positioning.** Ensure the woman is sitting comfortably with her arm supported (NICE, 2011) (or per manufacturer's instructions for automated device). Where possible select an automated device that has been validated for use in

pregnancy. Do not talk, and discourage the woman from speaking during BP measurement.

- **Digit preference/digit avoidance.** Rounding the final digit of the BP to 0 occurs in >80% antenatal BP measurements. Operators also tend to avoid the digits requiring action, e.g. they record a diastolic of 88 rather than 90.
- **Korotkoff sounds.** During measurement deflate the cuff at 2–3 mmHg/second. This prevents overdiagnosis of diastolic hypertension. Korotkoff 4 (the fading or changing of sound) is *no longer recommended* due to problems with reproducibility. RCOG (2006) now recommends using Korotkoff 5 (the disappearance of sound).
- **Multiple readings.** This may be necessary as BP fluctuates naturally (RCOG, 2006).

Care during labour

> *'The number of deaths from pre-eclampsia/eclampsia has not fallen. The most pressing need, as before, is to treat hypertension (and especially systolic hypertension) quickly and effectively to prevent haemorrhagic stroke'* (CMACE, 2011).

Most units have a protocol for the management of the severely pre-eclamptic women in labour. It should be updated as new evidence becomes available. CMACE (2011) recommends the use of the modified early obstetric warning score (MEOWS) charts for all women who become unwell, as this will ensure speedy recognition and prompt treatment, reducing the risk of maternal morbidity. See page 258.

The decision to deliver will depend on maternal/fetal condition and gestational age. These factors will influence the place and mode of delivery, which ideally will take place in a consultant unit with neonatal facilities. Senior obstetric and anaesthetic staff should be involved in the care of women with moderate/severe pre-eclampsia/eclampsia (RCOG, 2006; NICE, 2011).

Multidisciplinary communication and documentation regarding the management of labour, test results and decisions are essential to ensure a high standard of care. It is important that the midwife caring for the woman should have experience in providing high-risk care, including drug regimes and the location and use of emergency/eclampsia/resuscitation equipment, and if not should be supported and supervised by a more experienced colleague.

Induction of labour is common: see Chapter 19.

Preterm birth

Pre-eclampsia is a major cause of (usually iatrogenic) prematurity, accounting for 15% of all preterm births, and 25% of all babies born at very low birth weights (<1.5 kg) (Macintosh, 2003). Therefore, many babies born to pre-eclamptic mothers will be admitted to a neonatal unit. If <34 weeks gestation, maternal corticosteroids should be administered to reduce neonatal respiratory problems (Brownfoot *et al.*, 2008).

If time allows, liaise with the woman and her family and the neonatal unit; this may include a visit or meeting the staff. Some women may require transfer to a specialist neonatal unit: this is likely to be very frightening for the woman and her family. If delivery is imminent and neonatal facilities not available, the baby may require urgent transfer soon after delivery. Take time to explain what is happening and why: this may offer some reassurance.

See Chapter 13 for more details on preterm birth.

Psychological support

Due to the intense surveillance and increased intervention during labour and birth, the midwife may easily focus on the woman's physical condition and forget about her emotional needs.

The woman may well be particularly disappointed if she has hoped for a labour with a more natural onset and minimal intervention, and/or had to change from home or midwife-led unit to an acute unit.

A relaxed environment may have a physiological as well as psychological effect, as stress will not help the woman's condition. Providing appropriate lighting and minimising noise can promote an atmosphere of calmness. There may still be choices that women can make if they are well enough.

Women with pre-eclampsia can become seriously ill very quickly, and this can be very frightening for them and those around them. They will need reassurance and a clear calm explanation of what is happening and what interventions are being offered. Whilst informed choice is not always possible in emergency situations, emotional support is essential.

Monitoring the maternal and fetal condition in moderate/severe pre-eclampsia

- Measure mild/moderate BP hourly, severe BP every 15 minutes.
- Many labour wards (and high dependency units) use mean arterial pressure (MAP) to guide management. See Box 20.3.
- Continue antenatal antihypertensive treatment.
- Carry out haematological and biochemical monitoring according to criteria from antenatal period, even if regional analgesia being considered.
- Do not routinely limit duration of second stage of labour if BP stable.

Fluid balance management

All women with moderate to severe pre-eclampsia should have an intravenous (IV) cannula sited for administration of fluids and medication.

Women with pre-eclampsia have leaky capillary membranes and a predisposition to low albumin levels; therefore if fluid administration is excessive or unmonitored they are prone to developing pulmonary oedema. General guidelines include:

- Maintain a strict fluid balance chart.
- Women who are severely ill are unlikely to want to eat in labour, but most will require oral fluids.
- Limit maintenance fluids to 80 ml/hour unless other ongoing fluid losses, e.g. haemorrhage (NICE, 2011).

- Catheterisation allows for precise urine output recording and clean testing for proteinuria.
  - Record hourly urine output: 100 ml over 4 hours is commonly said to be sufficient to maintain renal function, although RCOG (2006) states there is no evidence that maintaining a specific urine output prevents renal failure.
  - Oliguria is common in pre-eclampsia and should resolve as the condition improves (RCOG, 2006).

Biochemical/haematology tests. Further tests will be carried out in labour, using the same criteria as for the antenatal period (NICE, 2011). See page 374.

Antacids are usually recommended in labour in women with pre-eclampsia due to the increased risk of caesarean section.

Fetal heart (FHR) monitoring. Continuous CTG is recommended (RCOG 2006; NICE, 2007). Drugs such as antihypertensives and magnesium sulphate may affect the FHR, reducing variability and reactivity, thus a suboptimal trace is more likely.

Analgesia. General comfort measures include verbal reassurance, touch, massage and comfortable positions (within the restrictions of monitoring equipment). These simple non-invasive measures may promote a feeling of being supported and cared for which should help the woman cope with a medicalised labour and delivery. Epidural may be recommended because it causes vasodilatation which can lead to a reduction in BP and attenuate surges. An established effective epidural is also advantageous should an operative delivery be indicated. However, women with severe pre-eclampsia should not be preloaded with IV fluids before establishing low-dose epidural analgesia and combined spinal epidural analgesia (NICE, 2011).

The ultimate choice whether to have an epidural is the woman's, and if she makes an informed decision to decline epidural/spinal anaesthesia the midwife must support her in that decision. Policies vary between units, but if the woman's platelet count is considered low ($\leq$80), an epidural may be inadvisable.

Second stage

- Management will be determined by maternal and fetal condition. If both allow, a spontaneous vaginal delivery is the mode of choice. In moderate to severe pre-eclampsia there is a low threshold for intervention leading to instrumental delivery.
- Ensure that appropriate medical aid is available and that there are two midwives caring for the woman throughout the delivery.
- Monitor the BP closely: it may be unrealistic to check after each contraction, but in severe pre-eclampsia every 5–10 minutes is sensible.
- The duration of the second stage should not be automatically limited if the woman's blood pressure stays within target ranges (NICE, 2011).
- Involuntary pushing, whilst not discouraged, is not actively encouraged until the presenting part is visible on the perineum.
- Active pushing is contraindicated in moderate/severe pre-eclampsia as it involves directed, prolonged breath holding and bearing down which alters heart rate and increase stroke volume.

- Avoid the supine position: it compresses the distal aorta and reduces blood flow to the uterus and lower extremities (Sleep *et al.*, 2000). It also prolongs the second stage, causes a reduction in circulating oxytocin, reducing the frequency and strength of contractions and can lead to fetal heart rate abnormalities (Gupta *et al.*, 2012). Lateral and other alternative positions are preferable.
- In severe eclampsia if BP does not respond then operative birth is advised (NICE, 2011).
- General anaesthetic (GA) should be avoided because intubation causes hypertension and laryngeal oedema and risks maternal death. The anaesthetist should be given as much time as necessary to assess a woman for intubation and should not be pressured to go for a quick GA even if there appear to be pressing reasons to do so (CMACE, 2011). The mother's condition must take precedence over the baby.

Drugs used in the treatment of severe hypertension

Antihypertensive treatment should be started in women with a systolic BP >150 mmHg or a diastolic BP > 110 mmHg, but may be introduced at lower BP measurements in women with other symptoms of the disease. Drugs used in the acute management of severe hypertension include oral or IV labetalol, oral nifedipine or IV hydralazine.

In moderate hypertension, effective antenatal treatment may enable the continuation of the pregnancy, reducing some of the neonatal complications of prematurity. Any antenatally prescribed drugs should be continued through labour (NICE, 2011).

First line treatment: Labetalol

Labetalol has the advantage that it can be given immediately by mouth (siting a venflon and getting an infusion take time), is easily readministered, and gives a quick result. BP should reduce within 30 minutes.

- Initial oral dose 200 mg
- Second oral dose if necessary
- Bolus 50 mg IV over 1–5 minutes (works in 10 mins)
- Follow if necessary with IV infusion of undiluted labetalol 5 mg/ml at 4 ml/hr (i.e. 20 mg/hr): usual max 180 mg/hr. Double the rate every 30 minutes until BP stable.

NB: Can cause significant maternal bradycardia: treatment is IV atropine sulphate 0.6–2.4 mg in divided doses of 600 mcg.

Second line treatment: Nifedipine

- 10–30 mg orally (*not* sublingually as this can cause precipitous hypotension) repeated every 30 minutes to a maximum dose of 50 mg (Sibai, 2003; RCOG, 2006).
- Can be given in conjunction with labetalol.

- Nifedipine is a calcium channel blocker: can increase toxicity if given in conjunction with magnesium sulphate.

Third line treatment: Hydralazine

Hydralazine is used if labetatol or nifedipine are contraindicated, or fails to control the BP.

- Initial dose 5 mg IV in fluid
- 5 mg IV at 20 minute intervals
- Maximum cumulative dose of 20 mg (four doses of 5 mg IV over 80 min) (DoH, 2001).

Treatment to prevent or treat seizures: Magnesium sulphate

Magnesium sulphate has been demonstrated to reduce the risk of seizures (Duley *et al.*, 2002) and is the drug of choice either to prevent seizures (often along with a decision to deliver), or to treat actual seizures (eclampsia), even in the immediate postnatal period (RCOG, 2006). See page 329 for magnesium sulphate regime.

Care of a woman receiving drug treatment for severe hypertension

- Monitor closely, ensuring BP falls gradually. Rapid reduction will adversely affect the uteroplacental circulation and lead to fetal distress.
- Be aware FHR may react to the medication with reduced variability and reduced/absent accelerations ('flat trace').

Management of eclampsia

When pregnant women fit due to pre-eclampsia it is known as eclampsia. This may suggest that the convulsion itself is different from other sorts of convulsions, such as those due to epilepsy, but this is not the case. Therefore the basic principles of ABCD resuscitation apply (airway, breathing, circulation, drugs).

In the event of a fit it is important to stabilise the mother before delivering the baby. It is extremely important that the midwife explains everything that is happening to the woman and her partner/relatives.

Note: If a pregnant woman presents as semiconscious or drowsy, non-eclamptic conditions such as epilepsy are more likely to be the cause than eclampsia. However, if there is no history of previous convulsions always assume a fit in pregnancy is due to eclampsia.

Facts

- Fewer than 1% of women with pre-eclampsia have an eclamptic fit (Shennan and Chappell, 2001).
- 1.6% of women who have an eclamptic fit die; 35% have a major complications (RCOG, 2006).

Signs and symptoms preceding an eclamptic fit

The woman may experience:

- Feeling unwell
- Headache
- Epigastric pain
- Blurred vision
- Nausea/vomiting
- Confusion, irritability, disorientation.

However, often there is no warning.
Investigations may reveal:

- Signs of clonus (jerkiness) – but brisk tendon reflexes are not predictive of fitting (RCOG, 2006)
- Tender liver
- Abnormal liver enzymes (ALT or AST rising to >70 IU/l)
- Platelet count falling to $<100 \times 10^9/l$
- HELLP syndrome (see page 375).

Care during/following an eclamptic fit

Immediate action:

- Keep calm.
- Summon help, including medical aid; do not leave the woman alone.
- Pull the emergency bell if in hospital; dial 999 if at home.
- Think ABCD: airway, breathing, circulation, drugs.
- Ensure the woman is in a safe environment:
  - Remove obvious dangers
  - Do not try to restrain the woman or put anything in her mouth.
- Ensure that, once the fit has finished, the woman is in the left lateral position and administer oxygen via a face mask: these measures may maximise uteroplacental blood flow.
- Note the time and duration of the fit. Most fits are self-limiting but occasionally they are much harder to control, or recurrent.

Subsequent action:

- Maternal observations
  - Assess airway and breathing
  - Check pulse
  - BP
  - Pulse oximetry (if available)
  - Assess proteinuria (catheter sample if appropriate).
- **Gain IV access** (ideally two large bore IV cannulae) to enable IV drug administration and blood to be taken.
- **Monitor the fetus.** Expect initial poor FHR following a fit: perform a CTG if possible.
- **Catheterise** so urinary output can be accurately monitored.

- **Reassure:**
  - ○ Talk calmly and quietly to the woman through the fit and afterwards to reassure her, even though she may appear semiconscious.
  - ○ Reassure the woman's partner/relatives where possible; they will be very frightened.
- **Plan for delivery.** Once stabilised, unless there is a fetal bradycardia, there is no immediate urgency to deliver (RCOG, 2006), and a delay of several hours may occur to ensure the best care is available. The woman's condition must always take priority over the fetal condition.
- The third stage of labour should be actively managed with Syntocinon 10 units either IM or IV. Syntometrine and ergometrine should *not be given*, as these can further elevate BP.
- **Documentation.** Record accurately all events, including the details of the time and duration of the fit.

Drug treatment for eclampsia: magnesium sulphate anticonvulsant therapy

Magnesium sulphate is the therapy of choice to control seizures, as it reduces pneumonia, need for artificial ventilation and ITU admission compared with diazepam and phenytoin which should *no longer* be used as first-line drugs (Collaborative Eclampsia Trial, 1995; RCOG, 2006). The intravenous route is associated with fewer adverse effects.

- 4 g loading dose by bolus or infusion pump over 5–10 min, then;
- 1 g/hour infusion maintained for 24 hours after the last seizure or 24 hours after delivery.

Subsequent seizures should be treated (according to local protocol) with either:

- 2 g bolus, or;
- increase infusion rate to 1.5 g or 2 g/hour.

Subsequent seizures can also be treated with alternative agents such as diazepam or thiopentone, but only as single doses; the prolonged use of diazepam is associated with an increase in maternal death (Collaborative Eclampsia Trial, 1995).

If convulsions persist, intubation may be necessary to protect the airway and maintain oxygenation; in these cases the woman needs transfer to ITU where intermittent positive pressure ventilation is available (RCOG, 2006).

Care of the woman receiving magnesium sulphate infusion

Monitor for magnesium sulphate toxicity:

Fluid balance. Monitor urine output hourly. Magnesium sulphate is mostly excreted in the urine. If urine output less than 20 ml/hour stop infusion.

Reflexes. Magnesium sulphate toxicity causes loss of deep tendon reflexes. Stop infusion if patella reflexes absent.

Observe the woman for nausea, hot flushes, confusion, weakness, blurred vision and slurred speech.

Respiration. Monitor respiration rate hourly. If <14 breaths/min and/or pulse oximetry is <95% oxygen saturation, stop infusion. If respiratory depression occurs, calcium gluconate 1 g (10 ml) over 10 min can be given.

Blood levels. Take blood for magnesium levels 1 hour after commencing the maintenance dose and repeat 6-hourly. The therapeutic range is 2–4 mmol/l.

- If serum urea >10 mmol/l, or magnesium levels >4 mmol/l the dose needs to be *reduced.*
- If magnesium levels are <1.7 mmol/l the dose needs to be *increased.*

Postnatal BP management for women with pre-eclampsia or eclampsia

Women with severe pre-eclampsia or eclampsia need to be closely observed postnatally. CMACE (2011) state that BP is not always well monitored in the immediate postnatal period, and more deaths occurred postnatally than antenatally/intrapartum. Do not be complacent or assume that once the baby is born most of the danger is past.

Usually BP falls following delivery; however, it generally rises again around 24 hours postpartum. Up to 44% of eclampsia occurs postpartum, especially at term (Milne *et al.*, 2005) and it has been reported up to four weeks postnatally, although the incidence falls dramatically after the fourth postnatal day (RCOG, 2006). Most women with severe pre-eclampsia or eclampsia will need inpatient care for at least four days following delivery. The timing of transfer home needs to take account of the risk of late seizures.

- Women with untreated hypertension should have BP checked four times daily whilst in hospital and at least daily on days 3–5 postnatally. If BP is raised then recheck on alternate days until normal; commence antihypertensive drugs if BP >150/100 mmHg (NICE, 2011).
- If a woman has received antenatal antihypertensives then check BP four times daily whilst in hospital, then every 1–2 days until 2 weeks post delivery and patient is off treatment and BP normal (NICE, 2011).
- Any woman with pre-eclamptic symptoms in the postnatal period, even without any history of pre-eclampsia, must be carefully monitored and referred for investigation.

Currently, there is insufficient evidence to recommend any particular antihypertensive postnatally. Drugs prescribed for breastfeeding women may include labetalol, atenalol and nifedipine, either singly or in combination. Methyldopa is best avoided postnatally due to its link with depression and therefore should be stopped within 2 days of delivery (NICE, 2011).

HELLP syndrome

HELLP syndrome (H = haemolysis, EL = elevated liver enzymes, LP = low platelets) is a severe complication of pre-eclampsia. The severity of HELLP syndrome is not dependent on the severity of hypertension. HELLP syndrome has also been reported in normotensive women.

Incidence

- HELLP occurs in 0.2% of all pregnancies.
- It is more common in women with proteinuric hypertension (4–12% of women with pre-eclampsia or eclampsia).

Underlying pathophysiology

Impaired liver function is an element of HELLP syndrome (see page 375, Chapter 23).

Haemolysis. This is the breakdown of red blood cells causing the release of haemoglobin into the blood plasma. It is a normal process, as the life span of each red blood cell (RBC) is about 120 days. Normally the process is slow enough for RBCs to be removed by the liver, spleen and bone marrow. However, when the process occurs more rapidly and RBC production is unable to keep up, the resultant reduction in the number of circulating RBCs causes microangiopathic haemolytic anaemia.

Elevated liver enzymes. HELLP syndrome impairs liver function. Women commonly complain of epigastric pain caused by obstruction of blood flow in the hepatic sinusoids by intravascular fibrin deposition.

Low platelets. Platelets are the first line of defence against bleeding. They work by:

- Plugging holes in capillaries (primary haemostasis)
- Initiating coagulation
- As the blood escapes through bigger holes, eventually platelets become an integral part of most clots.

Thrombocytopenia is due to the increased consumption of platelets.

Signs and symptoms of HELLP

- HELLP syndrome is commonly diagnosed when the results of pre-eclampsia blood tests are reviewed.
- Women may complain of epigastric pain.
- Women may bleed excessively (for example, from cannula site) and the blood fails to clot.

Care of women with HELLP syndrome

Once HELLP syndrome is evident *urgent delivery* is required. However, this is problematic due to:

- Problems with low platelets, therefore regional blocks are contraindicated.
- The woman is a poor candidate for general anaesthesia as intubation increases BP.
- Risk of bleeding excessively at caesarean section.
- The woman already has a coagulopathy, with reduced intravascular volume; so a postpartum haemorrhage is particularly problematic.

Consequently management includes the following:

- Low threshold for CVP line.
- It is imperative to accurately record fluid balance.

Corticosteroids have been used in HELLP syndrome. There is evidence to suggest that they lead to a more rapid resolution of the biochemical and haematological abnormalities; however, there is no evidence that they reduce maternal morbidity (Clenney and Viera, 2004).

Summary

- Signs and symptoms of severe pre-eclampsia may include any of the following:
  - ○ BP ≥160/110 mmHg or MAP ≥125 mmHg
  - ○ Significant proteinuria
  - ○ Headache, nausea, confusion, blurred vision, epigastric pain, brisk reflexes and clonus
  - ○ Platelets $<100 \times 10^9/l$ and/or ALT/AST >50 IU/l.
- Drug treatment may include labetalol, nifedipine, hydralazine and magnesium sulphate.

First-stage labour care for severe pre-eclampsia

- BP check every 15–20 min in first stage, more frequently in second stage.
- Consider MAP instead of systolic/diastolic.
- Strict fluid balance chart:
  - ○ Hourly urine output (100 ml/4 hours)
  - ○ Limit fluid intake (approx 80 ml/hour).
- IV access, possibly.
- 4-hourly antacids.
- CTG recommended.
- Epidural/spinal may help lower BP, but don't preload with IV fluid.
- Psychological support for woman and birth partner(s).

Second-stage labour care for severe pre-eclampsia

- BP check every 5–10 min.
- Avoid active (sustained breath holding) pushing and supine position.
- Low threshold for instrumental delivery.
- Avoid general anaesthetic.

Eclamptic fit

- Eclampsia is an indication for urgent/accelerated delivery, but not as an emergency unless fetal compromise suspected.
- Action: get help, think ABC, give O_2, remove dangers; allow fit to pass.
- Post-fit: maternal observations, IV access, CTG and catheterise.
- The woman's condition always has priority over the baby's.

Useful resources

NICE (2011) *Hypertension in Pregnancy Guideline 107.* www.nice.org.uk

WHO (2011) *WHO Recommendations for Prevention and treatment of Pre-eclampsia and Eclampsia.* http://whqlibdoc.who.int/publications/2011/9789241548335_eng.pdf

ISSHP Guidelines Regarding Care of Women with Hypertensive Disorders in Pregnancy. www.isshp.org

Action on Pre-eclampsia (APEC) www.apec.org.uk

References

Baker, P. N., Wheeler, S. J., Sanders, T. A., *et al.* (2009) A prospective study of micronutrient status in adolescent pregnancy. *Am J Clin Nutr* 89(4), 114–24.

Briley, A. L., Poston, L., Shennan, A. H. (2006) Vitamin C and E and the prevention of pre-eclampsia. *The New England Journal of Medicine* 355(10), 1065.

Brownfoot, F. C., Crowther, C. A., Middleton, P. (2008) Different corticosteroids and regimens for accelerating fetal lung maturation for women at risk of preterm birth. *Cochrane Database of Systematic Reviews*, Issue 4.

CMACE (Centre for Maternal and Child Enquiries) (2011) Saving mothers' lives: reviewing maternal deaths to make motherhood safer: 2006–08. The Eighth Report on Confidential Enquiries into Maternal Deaths in the United Kingdom. *British Journal of Obstetrics and Gynaecology* 118 (Suppl. 1), 1–203. http://onlinelibrary.wiley.com/doi/10.1111/j.1471-0528.2010.02847.x/pdf

Chappell, L. C., Seed, P. T., Briley, A. L. Kelly, A. J., Lee, R., Hunt, B. J., Parmar, K., Bewley, S. J., Shennan, A. H., Steer, P. J., Poston, L. (1999) Prevention of pre-eclampsia by antioxidants: a randomised trial of vitamin C and vitamin E in women at increased risk of pre-eclampsia. *Lancet* 347, 810–16.

Clenney, T. L., Viera, A. J. (2004) Corticosteroids for HELLP (haemolysis, elevated liver enzymes low platelets) syndrome. *British Medical Journal* 329, 270–72.

CLASP Collaborative Eclampsia Trial (1995) Which anticonvulsant for women with eclampsia? Evidence from the collaborative eclampsia trial. *Lancet* 345(8963),1455–63; erratum in *Lancet*, 346, 258.

Davey, D. H., MacGillivray, I. (1988) The classification and definition of the hypertensive disorders of pregnancy. *American Journal of Obstetrics and Gynecology* 158, 892–8.

Dekker, G. (2002) The partner's role in the etiology of pre-eclampsia. *Journal of Reproductive Immunology* 57(1–2), 203–15.

DoH (2001) *Why Mothers Die, 1997–1999. The fifth annual report of the Confidential Enquiry into Maternal Deaths in the United Kingdom.* London, HMSO.

Douglas, K. A., Redman, C. W. G. (1994) Eclampsia in the United Kingdom. *British Medical Journal* 309, 1395–400.

Duley, L., Henderson-Smart, D., Knoght, M., King, J. (2001) Antiplatelet drugs for prevention of pre-eclampsia and its consequences: systematic review. *British Medical Journal* 322, 329–33.

Duley, L. and The MAGPIE Collaborative Group (2002) Do women with pre-eclampsia and their babies benefit from magnesium sulphate? The Magpie Trial: a randomised placebo controlled trial. *Lancet* 359, 1877–90.

Graham, C. H., Postovit, L. M., Park, H., Canning, M. T., Fitzpatrick, T. E. (2000) Adriana and Luisa Castellucci Award Lecture 1999: The role of oxygen in the regulation of trophoblast gene expression and invasion. *Placenta* 21, 443–50.

Gupta, J., Hofmeyr, G., Shehmar, M. (2012) Position in the second stage of labour for women without epidural anaesthesia. *Cochrane Database of Systematic Reviews*, Issue 5.

Lain, K., Roberts, J. (2002) Contemporary concepts of the pathenogenesis and management of pre-eclampsia. *Journal of the American Medical Association* 287, 3183–5.

Lie, R.T., Rasmussen, S., Brunborg, H., *et al.* (1998) Fetal and maternal contributions to risk of pre-eclampsia: population based study. *British Medical Journal* 316, 1343–7.

Macintosh, M. (ed.) (2003) *Project 27/28: an enquiry into quality of care and its effect on the survival of babies born at 27–28 weeks*. London, The Stationery Office.

McCowan, L., Buist, R.G., North, R. A., Gamble, G. (1996) Perinatal morbidity in chronic hypertension. *British Journal of Obstetrics and Gynaecology* 103, 123–9.

Milne, F., Redman, R., James Walker, J., Baker, P., Bradley, J., Cooper, C., de Swiet, M., Fletcher, G., Jokinen, M., Murphy, D., Nelson-Piercy, C., Osgood, V., Robson, S., Shennan, A., Tuffnell, A., Twaddle, S., Waugh, J. (2005) The pre-eclampsia community guideline (PRECOG). How to screen for and detect onset of pre-eclampsia in the community. *British Medical Journal* 330, 576–80.

NICE (National Institute for Health and Clinical Excellence) (2007) *Clinical Guideline 55: Intrapartum Care*. London, NICE.

NICE (2011) *Clinical Guildelines 107: Hypertensive Disorders of Pregnancy*. London, NICE.

Need, J. A., Bell, B., Meffin, E., Jones, W. R. (1983) Pre-eclampsia in pregnancies with donor insemination. *Journal of Reproductive Immunology* 5, 329–38.

Pijnenborg, R. (1994) Trophoblastic invasion. *Reproductive Medicine Review* 3, 53–73.

Poston, L., Briley, A. L., Seed, P. T., Shennan, A. H. (2006) Vitamin C and E in women at risk of pre-eclampsia (VIP trial): randomised placebo-controlled trial. *Lancet* 367(9267), 1534.

Ramsay, J., Greer, I., Sattar, N. (2006) ABC of obesity. Obesity and reproduction. *British Medical Journal* 333, 1159–62.

RCOG (Royal College of Obstetricians and Gynaecologists) (2006, reviewed 2010) *The Management of Severe Pre-eclampsia/eclampsia Guideline 10A*. London, RCOG.

Rumbold, A. R., Crowther, C. A., Haslam, R. R., Dekker, G. A., Robinson, J. A., for the ACTS Study Group (2006) Vitamins C and E and the risks of pre-eclampsia and perinatal complications. *New England Journal of Medicine* 354, 1796–806.

Shennan, A. H., Chappell, L. C. (2001) Pre-eclampsia. *Contemporary Clinical Gynaecology and Obstetrics* 1, 353–64.

Shennan, A. H., Gupta, M., Halligan, A., Taylor, D. A., de Swiet, M. (1996) Lack of reproducibility of korotkoff phase IV by mercury sphygmomanometry. *Lancet* 347, 139–42.

Shennan, C., Shennan, A. (1996) Blood pressure in pregnancy: the need for accurate measurement. *British Journal of Midwifery* 4(2), 102–8.

Sibai, B. (2003) Diagnosis and management of gestational hypertension and severe preeclampsia. *Obstetrics and Gynaecology* 102, 181–92.

Sleep, J., Roberts, J., Chalmers, L. (2000) The second stage of labour. In Enkin, M., Keirse, M. J. N. C., Neilson, J., Crowther, C., Duley, L., Hodnett, E., Hofmeyr, J. (eds) *A Guide to Effective Care in Pregnancy and Childbirth*, 3rd edn, pp. 289–99. Oxford, Oxford University Press.

Smith, G. C. S., Shah, I., Pell, J. P., Crossley, A., Dobbie, R. (2007) Maternal obesity in early pregnancy and risk of spontaneous and elective preterm deliveries: a retrospective cohort study. *American Journal of Public Health* 97(1), 157–62.

Strickland, D. M., Guzick, D. S., Cox, K., Grant, N. F., Rosenfeld, C. R. (1986) The relationship between abortion in the first pregnancy and development of pregnancy-induced hypertension in the subsequent pregnancy. *American Journal of Obstetrics and Gynecology* 154, 146–8.

Wang, J., Knottnerus, A., Schuit, G., Norman, R., Chan, A., Dekker, G. (2002) Surgically obtained sperm, and risk of gestational hypertension and pre-eclampsia. *Lancet* 359 (9307), 673–4.

WHO (World Health Organization) (2010) *Trends in Maternal Mortality 1998–2008.* www.wholib.doc/who.int

WHO (2011) *WHO Recommendations for Prevention and Treatment of Pre-eclampsia and Eclampsia.* http://whqlibdoc.who.int/publications/2011/9789241548335_eng.pdf

21 Stillbirth and neonatal death

Barbara Kavanagh and Cathy Charles

Introduction

Death is not the expected outcome of pregnancy, and parents can be left stunned. They have to face not only the loss of the baby they have created, but also of their hopes and dreams. They will undergo intense grief reactions, including shock, numbness, disbelief, emptiness, a sense of failure, anger and guilt. There may also be a recurrence of feelings related to any previous loss. Although every experience of grief is personal and intense, grieving for a lost baby is a normal healthy response to loss.

The midwife provides support in the very early stages of the grieving process, when denial, guilt and anger may be most in evidence (Butler, 2000). This is a difficult and demanding time: what professionals say and do is critically important. Their words and actions are frequently remembered by parents for years to come, and may influence their memories and their grieving.

The Midwife's Labour and Birth Handbook, Third Edition. Edited by Vicky Chapman and Cathy Charles.
© 2013 John Wiley & Sons, Ltd. Published 2013 by John Wiley & Sons, Ltd.

Definition

- A **stillbirth** is defined as a baby delivered without life after 24 weeks of pregnancy. The **stillbirth rate** is the number of stillbirths per 1000 births (CMACE, 2011).
- The Royal College of Obstetricians and Gynaecologists states that a baby known to have *died before* 24 weeks but *born after* 24 weeks (e.g. early death of a twin who is born later with its live sibling) should not be registered as a stillbirth (RCOG, 2005).
- The **perinatal mortality** rate is defined as the number of **stillbirths** and **early neonatal deaths** (those occurring in the first week of life) per 1000 births (CMACE, 2011).
- **Neonatal deaths** (NNDs) are deaths in the first month of life: they are divided into **early NND** (first 7 days) and **late NND** (7–28 days after birth).

Incidence and facts

- The UK (excluding Scotland) stillbirth rate was 5.2 per 1000 in 2009. NND rate was 5.4 per 1000 (CMACE, 2011): there were 4125 UK stillbirths (282 intrapartum) and 2511 NNDs (CMACE, 2011). Put more simply, 17 babies die every day.
- The NND rate for spontaneous vaginal birth is 3.2 per 1000 live births compared to 0.7 per 1000 live births for ventouse, 1.5 per 1000 live births for forceps and 3.8 per 1000 live births for caesarean section (CS) (CMACE, 2011).
- Overall UK perinatal and intrapartum-related deaths have shown a significant downward trend, although stillbirths rose marginally from 5.1 in 2008 to 5.2 in 2009 (CEMACE, 2011).
- The National Maternity Support Foundation has called on all trusts in England to provide a specialist bereavement midwife counsellor; currently fewer than half do so (NMSF, 2009; Henley and Schott, 2010).
- Women who miscarry in the second half of the second trimester should be cared for on the labour ward, not a gynaecology ward, so adequate support can be given (Henley and Schott, 2010).

Causes and predisposing factors for perinatal death

The main causes of stillbirth are broadly classified by CMACE (2011) as major congenital anomaly (9%), antepartum/intrapartum haemorrhage (11%), specific placental conditions (12%). At least 28% are unexplained. The overwhelming predisposing factor for neonatal death is prematurity. Other predisposing factors for perinatal death (see Box 21.1) are often complex. Maternal and fetal factors are often interrelated. Some are social and very hard to address. Others are disease specific and more controllable. Generally, however, predisposing factors have poor predictive value.

There is a very small increased stillbirth risk for planned primigravid homebirths (BECG, 2011), but most home stillbirths/NNDs delivered at home are sudden unplanned homebirths, usually preterm. Twenty-five per cent of unplanned homebirths are unbooked pregnancies (CEMACH, 2007) while others are due to rapid labour and inability to get to hospital in time.

There has been much focus on the fact that 10% of stillbirths occur in obese women (BMI >35), and great efforts are being been made to address this issue. What the benefits

Box 21.1   Predisposing/associated risk factors for stillbirth and neonatal death (CMACE, 2011).

Antenatal
- Maternal age <20 or >40
- Social deprivation, including drug/substance abuse
- Ethnicity: women of black and Asian origin have an increased risk. Women with refugee status may be three times more at risk (Lanchandani *et al.*, 2001)
- Placental problems, e.g. praevia, abruption and intrauterine growth retardation
- Maternal disorder, e.g. pre-eclampsia, infection, diabetes, cholestasis
- Prolonged pregnancy >41/40
- Multiple pregnancy
- Psychiatric disorder
- Isoimmunisation

Intrapartum
- Cord compression/accident
- Uterine rupture
- Haemorrhage/placental abruption

Newborn conditions
- Prematurity: by far the largest category
- Low birth weight
- Congenital malformation
- Respiratory disorder
- Birth trauma
- Infection
- Accident

N.B. Many stillbirths and neonatal deaths are *unexplained* and occur with no obvious predisposing factors.

will be, apart from stigmatising overweight women, remains to be seen. Obesity is another complex issue, related to socio-economic status, life stress and general health, and may prove resistant to intervention.

Diagnosing fetal death and decision making

The beginning of the grieving process

When a fetus or baby dies, parents should be told at once. Delay will inevitably cause greater stress. However, typically a stillbirth is suspected when the fetal heart cannot be heard by the midwife, sometimes in the community, and the woman may have to travel to a hospital for an ultrasound scan. The midwife may not wish to distress the mother unnecessarily, since this could be a false alarm, but honesty about any suspicions is usually the best policy. 'My fetal heart monitor may not be working properly' is not a good excuse.

Two doctors should be present for confirmation of intrauterine death and a skilled practitioner should perform real-time ultrasound (NICE, 2007a). Ideally both parents should be present. Staff attitudes and empathy at the outset of this traumatic experience will influence the grieving process, and the parents' memories.

Good communication and honesty are essential. Lovell (1983), cited by Moulder (1999), noted that some women criticised the handling of the diagnosis of intrauterine death or abnormality; a succession of different staff visited, some ill-prepared and unable to conceal their distress. On hearing that death has occurred, shock and numbness may temporarily prevent a mother from being overwhelmed by the full impact of the event (Jones, 1997). Some staff find it difficult to know what to say at this point. If a partner is present, it may be appropriate to give the couple a few moments alone before they are faced with painful decisions. A trained interpreter should be offered to women with limited English.

The father's distress is sometimes comparatively disregarded (SANDS, 2007). He may feel distraught with grief, angry, helpless, even guilty (Bennett *et al.*, 2005) and deeply disturbed by his partner's distress. He may suppress this, feeling he must not show the depth of his grief to staff, sometimes even his partner, fearing to further distress her. Acknowledge he too is a bereaved parent: ask him how he is and include him in all information-giving.

Planned termination for fetal abnormality may make it easier for staff to reconcile the death (Walpole, 2002) but it may not be easier for the parents. They are still bereaved parents, and guilt at having chosen to end their baby's life may compound their suffering.

Decision-making and choices

Supporting grieving parents to make important decisions at a time of unbearable sorrow and anguish is one of the most challenging roles undertaken by a midwife (Thomas, 1999). The midwife should have a caring, sensitive and non-judgemental attitude, acknowledging the importance of the loss. Basic counselling/listening skills are very helpful. It can be stressful to give control and choice to parents if their decisions differ from those that professionals would make on their behalf.

Due to the impact of overwhelming shock and disbelief, staff may have to repeat themselves as information is not always retained if given only once; this is especially true if the woman is in pain.

Mode of delivery

If possible, discuss in advance the options and support available for labour and birth. A woman whose baby has died in utero may be shocked to learn that she is advised to have a vaginal birth. It is a frightening thought to give birth to a dead baby. Her first reaction may be to request a caesarean. Take time to listen and discuss her worries about vaginal birth. Gently point out that CS may affect her physical and mental recovery, and perhaps her ability to identify and accept the loss of her baby.

Induction or expectant management

Unless the cause of the fetal death threatens the mother's life, late fetal death seldom poses a threat to maternal physical welfare (Howarth and Alfirevic, 2001). There is a small risk of disseminated intravascular coagulation (DIC) and postpartum haemorrhage (PPH) if the mother carries a dead baby for several weeks, but generally awaiting spontaneous labour is safe.

Radestad *et al.* (1996) noted increased anxiety in women induced more than 24 hours after diagnosis of intrauterine death, and suggested birth should occur as soon as feasible after diagnosis. Delaying birth, however, may give some parents time to come to terms, to some degree, with the situation: 'We felt blessed we were able to separate her birth from the numbing moment we were told her heart had stopped beating' (Smith *et al.*, 2011).

The decision of whether/when to induce rests with the parents and must be respected and supported.

At earlier gestations induction following intrauterine death may be more technically difficult (Howarth and Alfirevic, 2001). Sadly fetal well-being is no longer an issue, so side effects and complications relate only to the mother.

Place of birth

Whilst most women give birth in an obstetric unit following intrauterine death, they may choose otherwise, or a sudden adverse event may occur anywhere.

Women may deliberately choose home birth following diagnosis of intrauterine death (IUD): Thomas (1999) suggests that in the presence of an experienced midwife this sad event, occurring in the security of the home away from all the noise and intrusion of the hospital, can give parents positive memories and some sense of control over events.

Midwives in a stand-alone birth centre or at home may be less experienced in caring for a planned stillbirth, but in one sense the birth is like any other. Postnatally there is rarely any urgency, so blood samples and paperwork can usually be undertaken slowly. Consent for any post-mortem must be signed by a doctor, but this does not have to be done straight away. A supervisor of midwives can be an invaluable resource, and obstetric unit staff are often happy to give telephone advice.

If an *unexpected* stillbirth/NND occurs at home/birthing centre the woman will probably be transferred postnatally to an obstetric unit. However, the parents' choice remains paramount; transfer is not compulsory, however convenient this may be for the staff. Such events may be uniquely stressful for midwives who may be quite unprepared for the emotions (and paperwork) involved. Unexpected death will initiate an internal 'sudden untoward incident' (SUI) investigation. It is interesting how an unexplained death in an obstetric unit may result in much less instant uninformed criticism than a similar event at home/birthing centre.

A doctor or midwife will still need to certify death. Some GPs may be unwilling to be involved, particularly with an NND, since they are uncertain what to enter on the certificate as cause of death. Cases have been known where a GP feels obliged to report this technically 'unexplained death' to the police, and this can involve a lot of unnecessary bureaucracy and distress which an obstetric unit birth will avoid. Skin biopsies may need to be taken from the baby, which midwives may be inexperienced in performing.

These are just practical considerations, and should not discourage midwives from supporting women who choose to give birth at a stand-alone birth centre or at home.

The birth setting for an anticipated SB/NND, whether home, birth centre or obstetric unit, should be private and quiet, ideally well away from other birthing mothers. Only 55% of UK labour wards have such a facility (Henley and Schott, 2010).

Midwifery care in labour following intrauterine death

Compassion and individualised care

The woman needs sensitive care from a midwife who is not afraid of her or her baby, and who shows respect and regards the baby as a precious, delicate little person. Trust between the woman and her midwife is of key importance.

The diversity of women's needs must be understood. Touch, for example, may help some women during stillbirth, but not others (Butler, 2000). Cultural differences may affect reaction to loss; do not make assumptions (Schott and Henley, 1996; Nallon, 2007). The mother may be unwilling to see or hold her baby due to a specific religious or cultural prohibition against seeing a dead body. However, whilst she may technically belong to a religious group, she may hold ambivalent views and not wish to follow any rigid practice.

Observations

The parents may choose induction of labour: see Chapter 19 for observations and management.

If the fetus may have been dead some time, take maternal blood for full blood count and clotting, in case of DIC. One third of women with abruption and fetal demise develop some degree of coagulopathy (AAFP, 2012).

Once labour has commenced observations are as per normal labour (see Chapter 1).

Fetal heart monitoring is obviously not required. The absence of the baby's heartbeat serves as a painful and constant reminder to the mother and midwife that there is to be a tragic outcome to this labour.

Analgesia

Labour with a dead baby will be psychologically, and thus may be physically, more painful. Radestad *et al.* (1998) report that women undergoing stillbirth use more analgesia than other women and are more likely to describe their labour and birth as unbearably physically hard. Reassure the woman that support and pain relief are available to her at any time, although if infection/coagulopathy is suspected then epidural anaesthesia may be inadvisable (Swanson and Madej, 1997).

The birth of the baby

Giving comfort and support to the bereaved parents at this time of enormous sadness will help create a positive birth experience.

A slow gentle birth will minimise damage: the skin is often very fragile. A baby who has been dead for some time may be macerated: gently prepare parents for this possibility. Babies who have died often deliver slowly due to absent tone. Small premature breech babies can have a slow head delivery. These things can be very distressing. Clarify, preferably in advance, whether the mother wishes to have her baby given straight to her. If not, perhaps wrap it in a small towel (not paper, which can stick to skin) and then offer to the parents to hold if they wish. SANDS produce a pattern for 'angel pouches' for very small babies (see website).

Third stage of labour

If the dead baby has remained in utero for several weeks or if placental abruption is suspected, the mother has an increased PPH risk. Particular risk factors may also have been identified at confirmation of fetal death and by blood tests for infection and clotting studies. In such cases active management of the third stage is advised and a precautionary cannula may be advisable. Anecdotal accounts suggest that retained placenta or placental fragments are more common with very early gestation births.

Following birth, the placenta should be sent for histology following local guidelines. This varies between hospitals; some pathologists request the placenta is sent dry, others request it in formaldehyde.

Some parents may wish the placenta to be buried with their baby, requiring arrangements to be made for its return.

Neonatal death and unexpected death at/after birth

Expected death of a baby

Some women know while they are pregnant that their baby will die at or shortly after birth due to a recognised abnormality. They have the chance to plan for this immeasurably sad birth, preferably away from the sounds of new babies crying. All efforts should be made to minimise any interruptions, allowing the parents to have as much time with their baby as possible. If the baby is born alive some parents will value the midwife's continued presence, fearing their baby dying in their arms without anyone there. Others will simply want to be alone. Often a paediatrician or a neonatal practitioner (NNP) will be involved to some degree; parents may want the reassurance of being told by a specialist that their baby is not in pain or distress. Paediatricians and NNPs are often very skilled at supporting parents and staff when a baby is dying, as are chaplains and other religious advisors.

Low voices, gentle touch and great respect for the baby all help to ease the momentous pain of a baby passing. As with any death vigil, sometimes the end comes too quickly, and sometimes it drags on, prolonging the agony of all involved.

Unexpected stillbirth/NND

One of the most nightmarish scenarios is an unexpected intrapartum stillbirth/NND. It can be utterly devastating for everyone.

If the collapse is sudden, e.g. at the point of birth, the parents may have to watch the frantic efforts of staff to save their baby's life. If possible, assign one staff member to be with the parents while a baby is undergoing resuscitation attempts. It could be a maternity care assistant or student midwife if necessary – but be aware they may be very distressed themselves afterwards. Their difficult role is not to explain, but to be there for the parents. In the midst of a crisis parents often realise only too well that no-one can tell them much, and will often just watch wide-eyed as staff work on their baby. The baby may be transferred to a neonatal intensive care unit or may be declared dead in the birthing room there and then.

The shock of an unexpected death will affect everyone. It may be that the midwife who assisted at the birth also attempted the resuscitation, and must then support the parents in their grief. That is a tall order for any midwife and requires great strength of character.

The midwife may have to show great sensitivity to the distraught parents while dealing with the awful feeling (or indeed the absolute knowledge) that the care during the birth was in some way suboptimal. Remember, however, that staff often blame themselves (or each other) unnecessarily. The parents too may blame staff, rightly or wrongly, and may lose confidence in any or all staff connected with the death.

See page 361 on caring for parents following an adverse event.

Immediate care following stillbirth/NND: precious moments with the baby

The meeting with and parting from the baby is a unique time.

Attitudes to pregnancy loss have undergone a revolution in recent years. Many feel that it is good to offer the parents involvement with their dead baby (Matthews *et al.*, 2002; Hughes and Riches, 2003; SANDS, 2007). They should be aware that they can have as much time on their own with their baby as they wish. However, they should not be *forced* to view, hold, caress, or kiss the baby (SANDS, 2007; NICE, 2010). Hughes *et al.* (2002) found that holding their dead baby had a negative impact on some mothers and their next-born child, and suggested that parents should not be pressurised into holding the baby or be told that mourning will be more difficult if they do not. Unfortunately NICE (2007b) originally slightly misinterpreted Hughes *et al.*'s study, stating: 'it is now considered unhelpful for women to see and hold their babies (after stillbirth) unless they particularly wish to do so'. This was not a conclusion of the study; one of the researchers (Turton, 2008) later reiterated that some parents *did* value contact with their baby. In 2010, following careful negation with SANDS, NICE issued a clarification statement, stating that women should be treated on an individual basis, and should not be 'routinely encouraged' to see/hold their baby if they did not wish to. All a midwife can do is try to anticipate and respond to needs and wishes as far as they can be gauged. This is something of a no-win issue, as numerous anecdotal accounts suggest that many women regret not being given more information: 'Nobody sat down and spent just five minutes with me to inform me that one day I could regret not holding him' (Dimery, 2010).

If the parents wish to hold their baby, fears may be minimised by advising them beforehand how the baby will look and feel: e.g. it will feel initially floppy and may have some movement of the skull bones (Dyer, 1992). Later, sadly it may become more rigid as rigor mortis sets in.

If the baby is very macerated or appears very abnormal it may not be appropriate for parents to see him/her. This is 'a very fine judgement' (SANDS website) which has to be made on an individual basis. Sometimes parents will focus on one perfect feature of an otherwise very damaged baby and see beauty. Love does not always demand perfection.

Creating memories and mementos

'There will be no Christmases or birthdays or first day at school for these parents. All they have is now' (midwife, quoted by Henley and Schott, 2010).

Memories help to facilitate mourning. The problem is that parents have not had time to get to know their baby. Try to make the most of what is available to create special memories for them.

The SANDS form provides a helpful checklist (see Appendix) and SANDS also provide memory boxes/booklets, for mementos. Include locks of hair, footprints and handprints, name bands, cot card, tape measure and the baby's personal details, e.g. weight and measurements.

Photocopy the maternity notes for the parents so they have as much information validating their baby's existence as possible. Some staff are strangely reticent about photocopying CTGs, imagining some medicolegal consequence if all information is given to the parents to study. This is a ridiculous fear: women have a right to see their medical records and this up-front honesty is more likely to diffuse than provoke suspicion.

Most parents have a camera or mobile phone with them for the birth. If not, some units offer a camera for use by the parents. Photos should be taken carefully as they will be treasured for years (Randall, 2010). Hospital policy may recommend a photograph is placed in the mother's notes. Parents should be told that polaroid photos (rarely used these days) will eventually fade, especially if exposed to light.

Parents may wish to bathe and dress their baby in clothes they have chosen; this process may take a long time and should not be hurried. If parents wish, another family or staff member could do this.

The sensation of smell can be an emotional trigger. If parents wish, clothes, shawls and soft toys can be dusted with baby powder and placed in a plastic bag to preserve the smell for many years, providing powerful memories.

An entry in the hospital's book of remembrance can give the parents comfort: they can visit subsequently to view this in the hospital chapel.

Some parents may not wish to have mementos of their baby, for personal, cultural or religious reasons. Whilst these views would seem to be contrary to facilitating the grief process, they should not be viewed as abnormal or wrong (Schott and Henley, 1996). Unless there is an obvious cultural reason, it may be helpful to suggest that mementos are taken and filed away in the medical records, so that the parents could ask for them later if they wished. Some parents may take time to assimilate the experience and subsequently regret the absence of mementos.

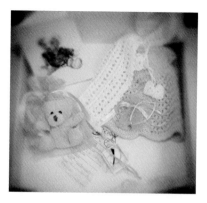

Fig. 21.1 A memory box, with cot card, a lock of hair and other mementos. *Photo by Debbie Gagliano-Withers.*

Other family members, e.g. siblings and grandparents, may wish to see the baby so they can create their own memories and say their own goodbyes. Parents need to be prepared for the honesty that children can show. This is a confusing time for them. They have often been looking forward to the birth of their baby brother/sister. They sometimes ask unexpected questions; honesty is usually best. Children are very accepting of death if they can participate and share the experience with their family (Dyer, 1992).

Ongoing postnatal care

Checklists, tests and paperwork

Various maternal tests can be undertaken to try to identify the cause of fetal death. Hospitals may vary in the blood tests offered (see page 376) Maternal and paternal genetic tests may also be offered, and possibly follow-up genetic counselling.

Checklists are helpful (see Appendix) but can sometimes be used inflexibly, as an end in themselves, rather than a way of ensuring that the parents' needs are met (Schott and Henley, 1996). Focusing on a checklist may be a way of depersonalising the situation and minimising the time spent with parents.

Post-mortem (autopsy)

Many parents want to know the cause of their baby's death, though the idea of a post-mortem is distressing. Staff may fear to approach the subject, although the urge to protect parents is often misplaced:

> *'The worst thing possible had happened – my baby had died. You couldn't tell me anything that was more upsetting than that'* (Henderson, 2006).

Since Alder Hey (Redfern, 2001) some parents are reluctant to allow a post-mortem on their baby, and the perinatal pathology service is experiencing recruitment and retention difficulties (Rose *et al.*, 2006). This unsatisfactory situation may lead staff to discourage parents from choosing this option. Post-mortems declined from 58% of deaths in 1993 to 39% of perinatal deaths and 25% of NNDs in 2008 (CMACE, 2011).

A coroner may order a post-mortem, particularly if the death is unexpected or resulted from an accident. Parents may expect that a post-mortem will give them the reason for their baby's death, but they should be aware that this is very often not the case: only around 20% yield a cause of death (CEMACH, 2007).

Post-mortem must be discussed very gently, giving clear unbiased information. Explanation of the procedure may help. The Department of Health has produced an information leaflet (DoH, 2003a). The NHS consent form (DoH, 2003b), revised following Alder Hey (DoH, 2003c) in trying to cover all eventualities, is very long and detailed; there is no perfect answer to the problem of giving full information and gaining full consent without overloading and distressing parents.

Post-mortem may be full or limited. Less invasive tests, e.g. X-rays, scans and tissue samples, may also be offered, although they yield less information. If parents wish to have a post-mortem or have any major tissue samples (e.g. brain biopsy) returned for burial with the baby, they should be warned that this may delay the funeral, possibly by some weeks.

It is also helpful if the midwife notes anything unusual noted after the birth in the notes and on the pathology request form, e.g. a true knot in the cord, a broken cord blood vessel and a pale baby's body with a very contused face (which might indicate a tight cord around the neck). Many such 'abnormalities' may be incidental, but observations at the time may be helpful. Do not assume that the pathologist will observe everything: they will appreciate comments made by clinicians at the time. By the time a placenta has been handled by pathology technicians, and perhaps a piece of placenta has been cut off for microscopic examination, a key diagnostic finding such as a small nick in a blood vessel may have been masked. Avoid, however, being drawn into speculation on the cause of the baby's death.

Registering the baby's death

Box 21.2 describes the various certification steps required for registering a baby's death prior to burial or cremation.

If a baby is born dead at less than 24 weeks gestation it cannot be registered at a register office. Most hospitals give a certificate of birth as a keepsake: a downloadable certificate is available from the SANDS website.

Box 21.2   Registering a baby's death and arranging the funeral.

Stillbirth

A **stillbirth certificate** is completed by the midwife or doctor who attended the birth. The parents take this to the *Registrar for Births Marriages and Deaths*.

- Within 3 weeks in Scotland
- Within 6 weeks in England and Wales
- Within 3 months in Northern Ireland

If the parents are married, either parent can register the stillbirth. If not, and the father wishes his name to be recorded, they must attend together or either parent can attend with a signed witnessed declaration by the other parent (see SANDS website).

Neonatal death

A **death certificate** is completed by a doctor or midwife. The parents take this to the registrar within 5 working days (8 working days in Scotland). They can register the birth at the same time.

If the birth has been previously registered, the death can be registered by one/both parents, whether married or not, another relative, someone else present at the death, or a health professional. If birth not previously registered see conditions for stillbirth above.

For both stillbirths and neonatal deaths the registrar will

- Issue a *Certificate for Burial or Cremation (CBC)* depending on the parents' wishes
- Place a stillborn baby's name on the stillbirth register.

The parents take the CBC to the hospital bereavement co-ordinator/chaplain or funeral director. Either can arrange the funeral. A stillborn baby's funeral is sometimes free, possibly including a memorial service conducted by a religious leader of choice or the hospital chaplain. Most hospital chapels have a book of remembrance.

For more information: www.uk-sands.org/Support/Certificates-and-registration.html

Spiritual beliefs and funeral arrangements

Formal burial or cremation is a legal requirement for all babies who are stillborn or die after birth, although a full service is not compulsory. For babies born dead <24 weeks a formal burial or cremation is not mandatory, but parents may desire it. A form must be provided to the funeral director from the hospital confirming that the baby was born before the age of viability and showed no signs of life.

A funeral can provide a focus for grieving families to mourn. Attendance at the funeral by staff involved with the baby's birth is often valued by both families and the staff themselves.

Many parents may have had little or no contact with death and have never had to think about making funeral arrangements. Rajan (1992) reports women being deeply hurt when asked how they would like the baby 'disposed of'. This is such a sensitive issue and it should be handled with great respect.

The spiritual and religious outlook of individuals often takes on more importance during bereavement (Jones, 1997). Asking the bereaved couple if they wish to see a hospital chaplain, or other religious person if appropriate, may help them reach decisions and gain spiritual support. This may include having the baby baptised and/or named although this may not be suitable for every faith and culture. Hospital chaplains are usually a wonderful source of information and support. Most are extremely sensitive and will not dwell on religious matters if the parents do not wish it. However, even the most atheist parents may wish to speak some words over their baby to say goodbye. A few formal words spoken by a chaplain may help parents to have some sense of a rite of passage, and encourage tears to fall, such as: 'We cry for James today, for the life he will not have and the hopes we had for him. We are so sad to say goodbye to this beautiful boy.'

Staying in hospital

Naturally many women find it painful to see newborn babies and mothers or pregnant women. Many may wish to leave hospital within a few hours of stillbirth/NND. Radestad *et al.* (1998) suggest that the length of stay after a baby's death may depend on the mother's opinion of the maternity hospital environment.

If a mother wishes to stay, or is too unwell to leave, if possible let her choose the kind of postnatal room she would like. Most will want a single room. Around 75% of UK postnatal wards have a secluded dedicated room (Henley and Schott, 2010); ideally this should have an en-suite bathroom and a double bed so that the father can stay. Parents should be able to spend as much time as they want with their baby. A mortuary fridge on the maternity unit would make this easier, but fewer than half UK units have this (Henley and Schott, 2010).

The option of taking the baby home

It is important to offer choice. Parents may not realise that they can take their baby home before the funeral, allowing them to spend precious time together as a family before saying goodbye. Midwives may be uncomfortable with this option and resist discussing it with the parents. Nevertheless, the issue should not be avoided. The SANDS website has a downloadable form for taking a baby home (see 'Useful contacts') to avoid misunderstandings.

Going home

On discharge from hospital, give appropriate information to the parents, including funeral options, and support groups, e.g. SANDS. Reassure them they can return to see their baby whenever they wish before the funeral. Give them a contact number. Often the hospital chaplain is the ideal contact, and he/she will often be the source of most information.

Inform the Bounty Pack organiser to cancel postnatal mailings (Henley and Schott, 2010). Inform the mother she is entitled to eight weeks of child benefit and ensure she has a claim form. SANDS (website) have a benefits leaflet for bereaved parents.

Inform the GP, health visitor and community midwife. Tell the parents you have done this, and that the community midwife will contact them the next day. The community midwife is often in an ideal position to support the parents, giving them time to retell the story and express their grief in the privacy of their home.

Inform mothers that they will probably have the normal sensation of full breasts a few days after the birth, which can continue for some weeks. It is distressing to produce milk with no baby to feed. Drugs like bromocriptine are hardly ever used these days as they are poorly effective and have unpleasant side effects. Suggest simple analgesia and minimal stimulation.

Arrange a consultant obstetrician appointment for about 6 weeks' time. Tell parents this is a discussion about the baby's death and does not normally include a physical examination of the mother. A gynaecology rather than maternity clinic appointment avoids the mother waiting with pregnant/postnatal mothers. A longer (often double length) appointment is appropriate.

In any contact with bereaved parents, whether before, during or after birth, avoid the urge to comment unnecessarily. Listening is the most help you can give. Bereaved families recount repeatedly that they valued staff who could just 'be with' them, rather than those who tried to explain or make sense of the event. Unhelpful statements include:

- 'You can always have another'
- 'He was so young you hardly got to know him'
- 'At least you have other children'
- 'You'll soon get over it'
- 'You will never get over it' (FSID, 2009).

Planning for a future pregnancy

'A new layer of grief surfaces when parents become pregnant and then again when they see their baby' (O'Leary, 2004).

The subject of contraception should be approached with tact and sensitivity. A woman may ask about the timing of a future pregnancy, the risks involved and the chances of a live healthy baby. Gently inform her that difficulties can arise if she becomes pregnant while she is still mourning, or has not been able to mourn, for her lost baby. The new pregnancy can hinder the completion of the grieving process, as it deprives the mother of time and space to mourn (Greaves, 1994). It can be worse if the baby is born near the anniversary of the lost baby. However, some parents are keen to try for another baby as soon as possible. This is a very personal decision, and up to the couple.

Midwives should be aware of the special needs of parents undergoing a subsequent pregnancy. A SANDS teardrop sticker on the maternity notes, if the woman wishes, is a helpful reminder to all staff that a woman has experienced a previous loss.

Bear in mind:

- Parents (and staff) may be more anxious in pregnancy and labour; more intervention is likely.
- Women with uncomplicated subsequent pregnancies are often classified 'high-risk' because of their previous loss, and offered/request frequent scans and/or early induction or elective CS. These (often clinically unnecessary) interventions may feel right for them, but paradoxically may reinforce their perception that their pregnancy is fragile.
- The birth may intensify, not diminish, grieving for the previous baby: joy coexists with a sense of loss. Parents may even feel numb/emotionally flat. It can be especially hard if the babies are the same sex.
- Grief for a lost baby does not go away, and the baby can never be 'replaced'.

Staff should acknowledge the previous baby, use his/her name and ask about similar characteristics, just as they would with a previous live child.

SANDS (website) have a leaflet 'The next pregnancy: guidance for parents' which is very helpful.

Supporting staff

Midwives may feel emotionally unsupported, just as grieving mothers were 30 years ago:

- Midwives want more training in perinatal bereavement (Henley and Schott, 2010).
- They often feel guilty when a baby dies, even if it is not their fault (Cowan and Wainwright, 2001).
- They feel their ability to give good care is hampered by lack of time (Kaunonen *et al.*, 2000).
- A midwife's personal circumstances may affect how s/he will cope (Cowan and Wainwright, 2001).
- Midwives report conflict in moving from a perinatal death to the next client expecting a happy birth (Henley and Schott, 2010). They value 'time out' to recover before rushing into the next birth.
- Students usually want to be involved in perinatal death (Mitchell and Catron, 2002) although often trained staff think they should be protected (Nallon, 2007).
- Staff value the support of their colleagues, but also should be able to access professional support/counselling (SANDS, 2007; Henley and Schott, 2010) including debriefing (Nallon, 2007).

SANDS have created a bereavement network specifically for practitioners: http://bereavement-network.rcm.org.uk/login/

Finally the words of a retired hospital chaplain:

'I have not lost a child at birth, but I have had other losses in my life and I have experienced . . . trying to be efficient in an acute grief situation. At least I have learned this – there should be no such thing as trying to be efficient in acute grief. Allow the feelings to be there. Allow yourself the same freedom as you would allow others. That is my message to myself and others' (Anderson, 2012).

Summary

- What staff do and say following perinatal death can affect the grieving process.
- Midwives should have a sensitive non-judgemental approach, with good listening skills.
- Give parents clear information; be prepared to repeat it.
- Parents may wish to touch or hold their baby, but do not force them.
- Respect personal, cultural and religious beliefs.
- Memories and mementos will help parents mourn.
- A new birth can open up old scars.
- Caregivers need emotional support and time for debriefing.

Useful contacts

Child Bereavement Charity www.childbereavement.org.uk
Stillbirth and Neonatal Death Society (SANDS) www.uk-sands.org
Downloadable form for taking a baby home: www.uk-sands.org/Improving-Care/Resources-for-health-professionals/Forms-and-certificates-to-download.html
The Miscarriage Association www.miscarriageassociation.org.uk

References

AAFP (American Academy of Family Physicians) (2012) *Advanced Life Support in Obstetrics. Course Syllabus Manual.* Leawood, Kansas, AAFP.

Anderson, A. (2012) Life is a constant negotiation with loss. *MIDIRS* 22(1), 28–31.

(BECG) Birthplace in England Collaborative Group (2011) Perinatal and maternal outcomes by planned place of birth for healthy women with low risk pregnancies: the Birthplace in England national prospective cohort study. *British Medical Journal* 343. www.npeu.ox.ac.uk/birthplace or http://www.bmj.com/content/343/bmj.d7400

Bennett, S., Litz, B., Lee, B., Maguen, S. (2005) The scope and impact of perinatal loss: current status and future directions. *Professional Psychology: Research and Practice* 36(2), 180–87.

Butler, M. (2000) Facilitating the grief process: the role of the midwife. *The Practising Midwife* 3(36), 37.

CEMACH (Confidential Enquiry into Maternal and Child Health) (2007) *Perinatal Mortality 2005 England Wales and Northern Ireland.* London, RCOG Press. www.cemach.org.uk

CMACE (Centre for Maternal and Child Enquiries) (2011) Perinatal Mortality 2009: UK. CMACE www.rcog.org.uk/files/rcog-corp/Perinatal%20Mortality%20Report%202008.pdf

Cowan, L., Wainwright, M. (2001) The death of a baby in our care: the impact on the midwife. *MIDIRS Midwifery Digest* 11(3), 313–6.

Dimery, M. (2010) Creating Memories. *RCM* Dec, 38–9.

DoH (Department of Health) (2003a) *A Guide to the Postmortem Examination Procedure Involving a Baby or Child*. London, DOH. www.doh.gov.uk

DoH (Department of Health) (2003b) *Consent to a Hospital Postmortem Examination on a Baby or Child*. London, DoH. www.doh.gov.uk

DoH (Department of Health) (2003c) *Families and Post Mortems: A Code of Practice*. London, DoH. www.doh.gov.uk

Dyer, M. (1992) Stillborn – still precious. *MIDIRS Midwifery Digest* 2(2), 341–4.

Gardner, J. (1999) Perinatal death: uncovering the needs of midwives and nurses and exploring helpful interventions in the United States, England, and Japan. *Journal of Transcultural Nursing* 10(2), 120–30.

FSID (Foundation for the Study of Infant Deaths) (2009) *Guidelines for Health Visitors and Midwives when a Baby Dies Suddenly and Unexpectedly*. http://fsid.org.uk/Document.Doc?id=89

Greaves, J. (1994) Normal and abnormal grief reactions: midwifery care after stillbirth. *British Journal of Midwifery* 2(2), 61–5.

Henderson, N. (2006) Communicating with families about post-mortems: practical guidance. *Paediatric Nursing* 18(1), 38–40.

Henley, A., Schott, J. (2010) Bereavement Care Report 2010: survey of UK maternity units and the care they provide to parents whose baby dies before, during or shortly after birth. SANDS www.uk-sands.org

Howarth, G. R. and Alfirevic, Z. (2001) Induction of labour following late fetal death (age 24 weeks) (protocol for a Cochrane Review). *The Cochrane Library*, Issue 4.

Hughes, P., Riches, S. (2003) Psychological aspects of perinatal loss. *Current Opinion in Obstetrics and Gynaecology* 15(2), 107–11.

Hughes, P., Turton, P., Hopper, E., Evans, C. (2002) Assessment of guidelines for good practice in psychosocial care of mothers after stillbirth: a cohort study. *Lancet* 360(9327), 114–8.

Jones, M. (1997) Mothers who need to grieve: the reality of mourning the loss of a baby. *British Journal of Midwifery* 5(8), 478–81.

Kaunonen, M., Tarrka, M. T., Hautamaki, K., Paunonen, M. (2000) The staff's experience of the death of a child and of supporting the family. *International Nursing Review* 47(1), 46–52.

Lanchandani, S., Shiel, O., MacQuillan, K. (2001) Obstetric profiles and pregnancy outcomes of immigrant women with refugee status. *Irish Medical Journal* 94(3), 79–80.

Lovell, A. (1983) Some question of identity. *Social Science and Medicine* 17(11), 755–61.

Matthews, M., Kohner, K., Kersting, A., Fish, S., Baez, E., McCabe, A., Ambuehl, E., Brooks, D., Hughes, P., Turton, P., Hopper, E., Evans, C. (2002) Psychological care of mothers after stillbirth. *Lancet* 360(9345), 1600–602.

Mitchell, M., Catron, G. (2002) Teaching grief and bereavement: involving support groups in educating student midwives. *Practising Midwife* 5(8), 26–7.

Moulder, C. (1999) Late pregnancy loss: issues in hospital care. *British Journal of Midwifery* 1, 244–7.

Nallon, K. (2007) Midwives' needs in relation to the provision of bereavement support to parents affected by perinatal death. Part two. *MIDIRS* 17(1), 109–12.

NICE (National Institute for Health and Clinical Excellence) (2007a) *Clinical Guideline 55: Intrapartum Care*. London, NICE.

NICE (2007b updated 2010) *CG45 Antenatal and Postnatal Mental Health: Understanding NICE Guidance*. London, NICE. http://guidance.nice.org.uk/CG4

NMSF (National Maternity Support Foundation) (2009) *Who Cares when you Lose a Baby? A comprehensive study into bereavement midwife care across NHS Trusts.* www.rcm.org.uk/ EasySiteWeb/getresource.axd?AssetID=122350&servicetype=Attach

O'Leary, J. (2004) Grief and its impact on prenatal attachment in the subsequent pregnancy. *Archives of Women's Mental Health* 7(1), 7–8.

O'Leary, J. (2005) The baby who follows the loss of a sibling: special considerations in the postpartum period. *International Journal of Childbirth Education* 20(4), 28–30.

Radestad, I., Steineck, G., Nordin, C., Sjogren, B. (1996) Psychological complications after stillbirth – influence of memories and immediate management: population based study. *British Medical Journal* 312, 1505–508.

Radestad, I., Nordin, C., Steineck, G., Sjogren, B. (1998) A comparison of women's memories of care during pregnancy, labour and delivery after stillbirth or live birth. *Midwifery* 14, 111–7.

Rajan, L. (1992) 'Not just me dreaming': parents mourning pregnancy loss. *Health Visitor* 65, 354–7.

Randall, L. (2010) A midwife's guide to bereavement photography *MIDIRS* 20(3): 384–8.

Redfern, M. (2001) *The Royal Liverpool Children's Enquiry Report.* London, The Stationary Office.

Rose, C., Evans, M., Tooley, J. (2006) Falling rates of perinatal post-mortem examination: are we to blame? *Archive of Diseases in Childhood – Fetal Neonatal Edition* 91(6), F465.

RCOG (Royal College of Obstetricians and Gynaecologists) (2005) *Registration of Stillbirths and Certification of Pregnancy Losses before 24 Weeks of Gestation.* Good practice no 4. London, RCOG.

Schott, J., Henley, A. (1996) Childbearing losses. *British Journal of Midwifery* 4(10), 52.

Smith, R., Homer, C., Homer, A., Homer, D. (2011) Learning about grief and loss though Harper's story. *MIDIRS* 21(1), 19–22.

Stillbirth and Neonatal Death Society (SANDS) (2007) *Pregnancy Loss and the Death of a Baby: Guidelines for Professionals.* London, SANDS. www.uk-sands.org

Swanson, L., Madej, T. H. (1997) The febrile obstetric patient. In Russell, I. F., Lyons, G. (eds) *Clinical Problems in Obstetric Anaesthesia*, pp. 123–31. London, Chapman and Hall.

Thomas, J. (1999) A baby's death – helping parents make difficult choices. *The Practising Midwife* 2(7), 16–19.

Turton, P. (2008) To see or not to see: should parents hold their stillborn? *Midwives* April/May, 16.

Walpole, L. (2002) Perinatal loss: qualitative and quantitative explorations of midwives' experiences. In *Proceedings of the International Confederation of Midwives Conference 2002.* The Hague ICM, Vienna.

Appendix: Checklist following a pregnancy loss after 24 weeks

This is an example of a checklist that can be used following delivery of a stillbirth or neonatal death. Many maternity units will have devised their own form, which can be ticked, signed and dated as appropriate.

Mother's Name . . . .   Partner's Name . . . .

Unit No. . . . .   Telephone No. . . . .

	Please tick, sign and date where appropriate
1. Both parents informed of stillbirth/death by:	Name: . . . .
2. Consultant Obstetrician and Supervisor of Midwives informed:	. . . . Consultant . . . . Supervisor
3. Parents given opportunity to see/hold the baby	
4. Mementos offered to parents (please tick): Photographs: Other: Taken ☐ Lock of hair ☐ Accepted by parents ☐ Cot card ☐ Kept in notes ☐ Name band ☐ Foot/hand print ☐	
5. Religious advisor notified (if desired by parents). Baptism or other religious ceremony offered	
6. Consent for post-mortem requested? Consent given: Yes ☐ Declined ☐	
7. Inform mortician as soon as possible that consent for post-mortem has been obtained	
8. Date and time of post-mortem given?	
9. Post-mortem form completed by **medical staff**?	
10. GP informed: By telephone ☐ By letter ☐	
11. Notice of death form completed?	
12. Community midwife informed on day of discharge: By telephone ☐ By discharge letter ☐	
13. Health visitor informed?	
14. Apply 'teardrop' sticker to mother's notes?	
15. Anti-D given? Yes ☐ No ☐	
16. Rubella/MMR vaccination arranged/given? Yes ☐ No ☐	

Contd.

17. Bloods taken for investigation? 　　　　　　　　　Yes ☐　　No ☐ (Note: not listed as may vary between hospitals)	
18. Mother given information regarding lactation?	
19. Contact groups discussed (if appropriate)? 　　– SANDS 　　– ARC 　　– Miscarriage Association	
20. Parentcraft/Relaxation classes cancelled?	
20. At discharge, have TTO drugs been given? 　　　　　　　　　Yes ☐　　No ☐ (TTO – to take out)	
22. Inform Consultant's Secretary of need for appointment as 　　soon as possible and attach 'proforma' to notes 　　　　　　　　　Yes ☐　　No ☐ 　　　　　　　Date of appointment	
23. Genetic counselling appointment made (if appropriate) 　　　　　　　　　Yes ☐　　No ☐	
24. Death or Stillbirth certificate completed, explained and 　　given to parents. Print name of Certifying Officer on 　　counterfoil.	
25. Information on funeral arrangements given and 　　discussed.	
26. Parents' decision on funeral arrangements: 　　Hospital: 　　Burial ☐　　Cremation ☐　　Informal service ☐ 　　Private: 　　Burial ☐　　Cremation ☐	
27. Chapel service requested 　　　　　　　　　Yes ☐　　No ☐	
28. Parents given information about The Book of 　　Remembrance?	
29. Notify Bereavement Co-ordinator	
30. CMACE form completed	

When completed retain this checklist in mother's notes

22 Risk management, litigation and complaints

Cathy Charles

Introduction

The idea that something may go wrong with a birth and/or that a woman may choose to complain or sue is anathema to those midwives who believe in the process of normal birth and who base their relationships with women on trust. Many midwives are uncomfortable with the concept of risk management, and there is a widespread belief that midwives are being pressured into practising defensively which is at odds with a caring attitude.

The mental distress caused to the injured individual and their family following an adverse event can be immense. It is easy, however, to forget the staff involved. A bad outcome can occur however well a midwife has practised. It is even more distressing if someone realises they have made a mistake.

This chapter is, however, intended to both inform and reassure. If midwives practise safely with a good knowledge base, communicate well with colleagues and women

The Midwife's Labour and Birth Handbook, Third Edition. Edited by Vicky Chapman and Cathy Charles.
© 2013 John Wiley & Sons, Ltd. Published 2013 by John Wiley & Sons, Ltd.

and keep good records, they will minimise their chances of an adverse outcome. An understanding of the principles of basic maternity clinical risk management will help all midwives to reflect on their care.

Incidence and facts

- In England 62 746 maternity-related incidents were reported in one year (Kings Fund, 2008):
  - Two thirds caused no harm to mothers or babies
  - 21% caused 'low harm'
  - 1.5% caused 'severe harm'.
- Medical negligence claims are increasing, diverting funds from client care; alleged cardiotocograph (CTG) misinterpretation is the most common claim.
- Around 25% of NHS litigation cases are maternity-related, but they account for 70% of total NHS litigation payments (Hepworth, 2003).
- A severely brain-damaged child may be awarded over £5 million costs.
- In 2009/10 there were 2844 maternity complaints in England; 12% were about staff attitude (NHSIC, 2011).

Clinical risk management: learning from adverse events

At national level there are a number of Confidential Enquiries which collate serious adverse events, e.g. The Centre for Maternal and Child Health (CMACE) which publishes maternal and perinatal death summaries, highlights some anonymised individual cases, and makes recommendations. Learning is shared nationally, however, and information is not fed back to individual trusts. At local level all trusts now have clinical risk management (CRM) teams to analyse and learn from adverse events. CRM is a way of identifying critical incidents and adverse outcomes, to establish if, why and where things went wrong. Root cause analysis can help distinguish individual mistakes by staff from 'latent failures' of the organisation. Lessons learned can help reduce the likelihood of recurrence.

Trusts increasingly expect staff to automatically report certain types of incident, either in paper form or electronically. Failure to report, particularly for serious incidents, may incur severe criticism.

Many midwives believe that CRM exists primarily to minimise the chances of litigation. While this may be the driver for trusts to invest money in CRM (Symon, 2001), it should not make midwives cynical about risk management in principle. Whatever the reason for its evolution, CRM encourages a willingness to learn from our mistakes in a logical and analytical way, hopefully in a 'fair blame' (not a 'no blame') environment. This can help midwives to give better care to women, surely something that everyone can relate to.

Unfortunately, CRM in some trusts has been clumsily implemented by weak managers who are quick to leap to simplistic solutions and blame staff. It is vital to implement CRM in a supportive way, involving supervisors of midwives, and not to simply make it part of a hierarchical way of controlling midwives. If not, risk management simply becomes another means of enforcing compliance with medicalised policies and protocols and eroding individual clinical judgement. Interpretation of national guidelines (e.g. NICE/RCOG) can become very prescriptive, and midwives may feel they have 'transgressed' in failing to follow what are, after all, only guidelines, not mandatory practice. Although the midwifery voice is getting louder, the obstetric voice is very much the lead on most national guideline development.

The process of event analysis

Most adverse events occur for not just one but several reasons. The clinician giving the care may be simply the last link in the chain of small events which have led to the incident. The midwife who links up an intravenous infusion to an epidural catheter may have done so for several different reasons. It is helpful to look at the unit workload, common working practices in that area, drug administration procedures, training and updating opportunities, as well as the individual's competence (is this just a one-off aberration for that midwife?) and any obvious ill health issues. It would also be simple to make a practical change that would reduce the chances of a recurrence despite all these factors, e.g. making sure that epidural tubing is a different colour from intravenous tubing and labelled with 'epidural' stickers. Good incident investigators avoid coming to easy conclusions, but always remain vigilant for simple steps like this to reduce risk.

It is helpful to use a systematic approach to analyse adverse events. The National Patient Safety Agency (NPSA) (www.npsa.nhs.uk) has developed a Root Cause Analysis (RCA) toolkit, which can be supplied free to NHS staff, and a training programme to assist staff in analysis. Ideally all staff involved in an adverse event should meet to review what happened. Often if the case involves many different professionals, this is not practicable unless the outcome was particularly severe, e.g. maternal death.

A well-managed incident review can be a very positive experience. Staff may be able to dispel unfounded guilt, realise what went well or did not, express distress and benefit from the support of colleagues. Real insights into what, if anything, went wrong, and what might be learned to prevent a recurrence or mitigate its effects can improve care in future situations. Conversely, a poorly reviewed case can compound guilt, set staff against each other and fail to prevent a recurrence since little has been learned.

All staff can contribute to effective care review in many different ways. It is good to be involved in multidisciplinary case review, but informal methods are often underrated. Anecdotal discussion, including the ubiquitous 'coffee room chat', as staff offload their thoughts about recent cases, can be a rich source of insight, support and learning.

Most maternity units also have regular multidisciplinary open meetings to discuss interesting cases/near misses. These tend sometimes to be obstetric led, but midwives increasingly attend and present cases. Such meetings can provide good learning and enhance interprofessional understanding. They are, however, only a broad overview, not a systematic process. The danger is that the most assertive voice may dominate and inaccurate conclusions result. In serious incidents there is no substitute for calm methodical analysis of the notes, statements and verbal accounts.

The NHSLA have produced a toolkit: Improving Safety in Maternity Services (Kings Fund, 2012) to encourage a more proactive approach to safe practice.

Litigation

It is unfortunate that much maternity care is based on fear of litigation. Obstetric decision making in particular often tries to contain risk by taking the 'safest' line, i.e. intervene early before things go wrong, instead of giving the best care to a woman in labour. Midwives are affected by this fear too, but have overall as a profession somehow managed to resist, to an extent, this overwhelming pressure. This brings them into inevitable conflict with obstetricians at times. This generalisation does not of course take into account the fact that there are many intelligent supportive obstetricians and risk-averse unsupportive midwives.

Dissatisfaction with their birth may be partly due to women's rising expectations, but it may also be due to genuine unhappiness at unjustified opposition to their wishes. Whereas some parents may be unhappy with insufficient action, litigation may also, conversely, arise from women denied the normal birth they expected due to unnecessary intervention (RCM, 2005). If this were to become commonplace, it might refocus the interventionist approach that currently erodes much maternity care.

CTGs are a real source of difficulty in litigation, as even experts disagree when interpreting traces. This is of course outside a midwife's control. What is within our control is to ensure we are as competent as we can be in the somewhat grey area of CTG interpretation. Regular CTG training is now mandatory in most trusts and is a Clinical Negligence Scheme for Trusts (CNST) requirement. (Refer to Chapter 3 for CTG records and storage.)

It is commonly said that it is not so much *if* but *when* a midwife will have to stand up in court to explain his/her actions. This is nonsense. Fewer than 2% of medical negligence claims actually go to court (NHSLA website) so most midwives will never have the experience of a court appearance. Whilst of course parents may need money to care for a disabled child, sometimes an injured party's initial impulse to sue may be part of a process of grieving and not always based on true negligence. Many want simply an explanation of what happened, an apology, and to prevent a recurrence (Vincent *et al.*, 1994). Other means, e.g. the complaints procedure, may serve these people better. Despite a widely held belief that people will litigate for the most minor issues, and that 'no win no fee' legal firms have fuelled this culture, in fact only a very tiny proportion of people sue. No solicitor wants to take on a case that has no chance of success. Consequently, most cases that get further than a preliminary letter have genuine issues to be addressed.

This chapter is not intended to document the process of litigation. There are many other resources which will do this: the NHSLA website has a brief guide for clinicians on clinical negligence litigation with a simple diagram showing the process of a claim.

Vicarious liability of employer

NHS employees are covered by vicarious liability, by which the law can hold one person or institution liable for the actions of another. So in theory a woman who chooses to sue for the negligent actions of an NHS midwife will in fact sue the trust which employs the midwife, not the individual midwife. Concerns exist as to whether a trust board may try to recover part of the costs from the negligent employee, since this is possible in law, although extremely unlikely.

It is not possible, as is widely believed, for an employer to shirk vicarious liability when a midwife has worked later than the nominated shift. The midwife is still performing the work for which he/she is contracted, and staying on duty when responding to a particular need (e.g. a woman who gives birth just after the end of a shift period) is practising flexibly and sensitively (Jenkins, 1995). However, voluntarily grossly exceeding sensible working hours is more of a grey area; this is unwise for all kinds of reasons, and midwives who work excessive hours make themselves very vulnerable.

The liability position for independent midwives (IMs) is different, since they are self-employed and therefore personally responsible for obtaining professional indemnity insurance (PII). Controversially in 1994 the Royal College of Midwives withdrew its PII for independent midwives after a member's ballot (Anderson, 2007). The last commercial insurance provider for IMs withdrew in 2002. IMs therefore have no choice but to practise without insurance and have to inform their clients of this before they are engaged.

Clinical risk management organisations

- The NHS Litigation Authority (NHSLA) for England and Wales has a litigation 'risk pooling' scheme, i.e. trusts pay into a central scheme which then meets the cost of any litigation. Without this scheme, one big litigation case could bankrupt a service.
- The NHSLA administers the CNST for England and Wales. CNST publishes Maternity Clinical Risk Management Standards (CNST, 2012) to assess the way CRM activities are organised. They focus on communication, clinical care and staffing levels.
- Scotland has the Clinical Negligence and Other Risks Scheme (CNORIS) which operates very similarly to CNST.
- Trusts are assessed by CNST/CNORIS 1–3 yearly: those who demonstrate good practice get a discount on their contributions. Such contributions can be over £1 million: a significant dent in the maternity budget.
- CNST/CNORIS standards are largely common sense and do not necessarily conflict with the desire of midwives to give flexible individualised care, although they are very policy/protocol driven. It is very important that midwives are involved in their trust's policy development groups to ensure that workable, sensible, flexible and evidence-based protocols are developed.

Records

The old maxims 'if you didn't write it down it didn't happen' or 'you are only as good as your written records' have some truth, as records are a key factor in demonstrating care.

- Records should be clear, accurate and readable when photocopied or scanned.
- Entries must be dated (use the 24-hour clock) and signed, with the writer's name and position printed clearly alongside.
- Any error should be scored with a single line so it is still readable, and the correction dated, timed and signed.
- Records should be written as contemporaneously as possible. Any later entry should be clearly dated, timed and signed.
- Any consultations/referrals should be documented.
- Refer to Chapter 3 for CTG documentation.
- Try to avoid unnecessary detail: sometimes it can be almost impossible to extract relevant information from notes full of random wandering prose.
- Patients have a right to access their own records under the Data Protection Act 1998.

- For a list of midwifery abbreviations visit http://www.studentmidwife.net/fob/common-abbreviations.531/ or to search for the meaning of abbreviations visit http://www.all-acronyms.com/tag/midwife
- Records must be retained for 25 years. Community and independent midwives will need to securely store their diaries and records for 25 years, or pass them on to their employer or local supervising authority (NMC, 2004; Griffiths, 2007).

However, remember that records are only part of the picture. What will carry great weight in court is what the woman perceived, i.e. interactions with staff, verbal explanations given to her at the time and her *understanding* of what was happening during the incident. Remember: you may write 'VE with consent' in the maternity notes, but if the woman has not given express consent, and explains this articulately in court, then the record may give scant protection. 'Poor practice and lack of communication are likely to be the underlying factors in litigation – and no amount of documentation will ever cover that up' (Morris, 2005).

Complaints

Many more midwives are likely to be involved in some way with a formal or informal complaint than litigation. Symon (2006) reminds us however: 'We should not conclude that complaints lurk around every corner. Given the number of women having babies in Britain the incidence of complaints is comparatively low.'

Sidgewick (2006) suggests that complaints tend to have four recurrent factors:

- Poor communication with client/family
- Poor communication between professionals
- Poor staffing
- Staff attitude.

Complaints should be treated positively, as showing that people believe that the organisation should know about their concerns. The process can, however, be very upsetting: even the best midwives may at some point in their career have to read a distressing letter from someone they have cared for, cataloguing an unhappy experience. This can come as a real shock.

Most people tend to forgive well-intentioned mistakes when everyone is honest about what happened. A home visit from a manager and opportunity to retell the story may reassure many women that someone is listening, and that changes are being made to improve the experience for other mothers. However, the Parliamentary and Health Service Ombudsman for England (HSOE, 2003) has noted that people may become more, not less, angry if a complaint is investigated clumsily, and this dissatisfaction may lead to litigation (Symon, 2006).

For the NHS complaints procedure, go to the Department of Health website www.dh.gov.uk .

Writing a statement

It may feel intimidating to be asked to provide a statement to a supervisor, manager or the risk management team. It is normal procedure, however, to collect statements from clinicians involved in an adverse event, as a proactive way of gathering facts for case investigation. Most statements are only used for this purpose, although they are kept on file for any possible future litigation. In the unlikely case that litigation ensues, the trust's solicitor will sit down and prepare a formal statement with the clinician. Original statements written without such help may be a useful aide memoir for this process, but are rarely used in court.

The Royal College of Midwives has produced guidance on statement writing (RCM, 1997).

Caring for the mother or father following an adverse event

This is a challenge for all involved. Any support will obviously depend on the nature of the adverse event: it is not possible to be prescriptive about this. If the baby has died, refer to Chapter 21 for how to support parents.

If you fear there may have been some error or omission which contributed to the outcome, you are in an awkward position. Honesty is of course normally the best policy with parents, but until you know the facts it is usually best to avoid speculation. Staff may feel guilty quite unjustifiably: a bad outcome does not necessarily mean that someone has done something wrong. It is natural that parents may feel they have to blame someone. It is possible to be supportive without lying: 'None of us at the moment know why this has happened' is often the honest truth.

Parents may feel angry towards staff following an adverse outcome, behaving in a distressed and hostile way. They may feel rejected or abandoned by staff: indeed this may not be paranoia, it may be actually happening. Midwives need to deal with their own feelings and resist the urge to avoid parents who may be expressing negative thoughts.

The midwife who feels he/she may be even partly responsible for any adverse event is in a particularly difficult position. Whilst it is natural and helpful to give parents the opportunity to ask questions about the birth, be aware that by 'explaining' what happened, midwives may, consciously or unconsciously, attempt to justify their own actions or those of others. Fear of the consequences of admitting blame may change the interaction too. There are no answers to these difficult dilemmas: midwives can only be aware of the problems and attempt to navigate their way through this difficult territory.

The Patient Advice and Liaison Service (PALS) can provide support and advice to parents who have experienced an adverse event.

Midwives who need a confidential ear may wish to access staff support services for non-judgemental listening, e.g. RCM counselling service. See also 'Supporting staff' in Chapter 21.

Conclusion

Midwives face a challenge in offering competent, sensitive and responsive care to women without practising defensively. Adverse events can shake our faith in midwifery. We can only do our best in trying to minimise them and learn from them. Despite everyone's best efforts, occasional bad outcomes will occur; the secret is to keep a sense of balance.

Summary

- There need be no conflict between woman-centred care and awareness of risk management issues.
- Adverse events distress everyone: staff can feel victims too.
- Almost everyone will have to write a statement at some point.
- Good analysis of adverse events can enable helpful learning.
- Very few staff will actually appear in court.
- NHS midwives are covered by their employer's vicarious liability. Independent midwives practise without insurance cover.
- Complaints may be a good sign of willingness to express dissatisfaction.
- Parents need sensitive, not defensive, supportors following an adverse event.

Useful contacts

CMACE (Centre for Maternal and Child Enquiries) (2011) Perinatal Mortality 2009: United Kingdom. CMACE: London. www.rcog.org.uk/files/rcog-corp/Perinatal% 20Mortality%20Report%202008.pdf

CMACE (Centre for Maternal and Child Enquiries) (2011) *Saving Mothers' Lives: reviewing maternal deaths to make motherhood safer: 2006–2008*. The Eighth Report of the Confidential Enquiries into Maternal Deaths in the United Kingdom *BJOG* 118, (suppl.1), 1–203. http://onlinelibrary.wiley.com/doi/10.1111/j.1471-0528.2010.02847.x/pdf

Clinical Negligence Scheme for Trusts (CNST). www.nhsla.com

Clinical Negligence and Other Risks Scheme (CNORIS). www.cnoris.com

Complaints procedure (Department of Health). www.dh.gov.uk

National Patient Safety Agency (NPSA). www.npsa.nhs.uk

NHS Litigation Authority (NHSLA). www.nhsla.com

Patient Advice and Liaison Service (PALS). www.dh.gov.uk. For details of local services contact local hospital, clinic, GP or NHS Direct 0845 46 47.

Root Cause Analysis (RCA) toolkit. www.npsa.nhs.uk

Royal College of Midwives (RCM). 24-hour counselling service. Telephone: 0845 605 00 44.

References

Anderson, T. (2007) Is this the end of independent midwifery? *Practising Midwife* 10(2), 4–5.

CNST (2012) *Maternity Clinical Risk Management Standards*. NHS Litigation Authority. www.nhsla.com

Griffiths, R. (2007) Record keeping: midwives and the law. *British Journal of Midwifery* 15(5), 303–4.

Health Service Ombudsman for England (HSOE) (2003) *Annual Report* 2002–3. London, HMSO.

Hepworth, S. (2003) Clinical cases by speciality. *NHS Litigation Authority Journal* 2, 4.

Jenkins, R. (1995) *The Law and the Midwife*. Oxford, Blackwell Science.

Kings Fund (2008) *Safe Births: Everybody's Business. An independent inquiry into the safety of maternity services in England*. London, Kings Fund. www.kingsfund.org.uk

Kings Fund (2012) *Improving Safety in Maternity Services; A toolkit for teams*. London, Kings Fund. www.nhsla.com/NR/rdonlyres/BBC3242C-552E-40A0-AE5A-87204817E000/0/ImprovingSafetyinMaternityServicesAtoolkitforteams.pdf

Morris, S. (2005) Is fear at the heart of hard labour? *MIDIRS Midwifery Digest* 15(4), 508–11.

NHS Confederation (2001) *Building a Safer NHS for Patients*. London, NHS Confederation Publications.

Nursing and Midwifery Council (NMC) (2004) *Midwives Rules and Standards*. www.nmc-uk.org

NHSIC (NHS Information Centre) (2011) *Data on Written Complaints in the NHS* 2010–11 www.ic.nhs.uk

Royal College of Midwives (RCM) (1997) *Statement Writing*. www.rcm.org.uk/college/support-at-work/workplace-advice/statement-writing/?locale=en

Royal College of Midwives (RCM) (2005) RCM annual conference (guest speaker Janine Wynn-Davies). *Midwives* 9(6), 231.

Sidgewick, C. (2006) Everybody's business: managing midwifery complaints. *British Journal of Midwifery* 14(2), 70–1.

Symon, A. (2001) *Obstetric Litigation from A to Z*. London, Quay Books.

Symon, A. (2006) Are we facing a complaints and litigation crisis in the health service? *British Journal of Midwifery* 14(3), 164–5.

Vincent, C., Young, M., Phillpips, A. (1994) Why do people sue doctors? *NHSLA Journal* 2, 4.

23 Intrapartum blood tests

Vicky Chapman and Julie Davis

Blood tests

This chapter describes blood tests relevant to labour and includes practical information on taking blood.

Maternal reference ranges

Normal reference ranges for blood results vary between different hospitals/laboratories, studies and authors, and are normally based on non-pregnant population studies. The changing haemodynamics of pregnancy present a different blood picture to the non-pregnant population and this picture changes more dramatically with advancing gestation. This should be remembered when evaluating reference ranges for pregnant and labouring women. Some examples are given in Table 23.1.

Taking a blood sample

Explain why you want to take blood and gain the woman's consent. Ensure she knows when the result will be communicated to her.

- Cleanse/swab skin.
- Apply tourniquet: loosen within a minute as prolonged application causes stasis and haemoconcentration, invalidating some blood results (Pagana and Pagana, 2008).

- Learn to 'feel' for the vein with gloves on – veins feel resilient, bouncy and refill when depressed. Avoid potential infusion sites.
- Insert needle at 30–45° to the vein holding the syringe steady; click vacuum tube into syringe. The needle will pierce the tube; it will fill automatically.
- Additives can affect some biochemistry results and can interfere with coagulation times, so draw in the correct order (Table 23.1a).
- Regardless of additive type, gently invert all tubes (do not shake) to ensure thorough mixing of blood (BD Diagnostics, 2010).
- Do not resheath needle; dispose of it in sharps container.
- Label samples, send to lab and document in the woman's notes.
- For urgent specimens ensure the lab is expecting the sample.

Tips for tricky veins

'I increasingly use a butterfly in the back of the hand for tricky customers, as it accesses a smaller vein easily, and once it's in and taped then it is less easily dislodged by sudden jerks!' (Midwife).

'I tend to aim where I feel the vein lies hidden and just go in a little deeper than usual: I am usually successful' (Midwife).

Deep veins

Apply the tourniquet, encourage the woman to clench and unclench her fist and tap or pat the veins: they usually become palpable and raised. Go for the 'feel', not just what you see. Veins that are deep and not visible can be felt by rolling the fingertips over the vein, like feeling for a guitar string. Deep veins require slightly deeper insertion of the needle at the location you 'feel' the vein.

Slow bleeder

Release tourniquet, let the arm dangle, encourage the woman to clench and unclench her fist, to help 'pump' the blood.

Nervous or needle phobic women

Consider the use of local anaesthetic cream (e.g. EMLA): apply one hour prior to procedure to several potential sites to avoid access problems. Very phobic women usually respond well to a second person distracting them, focusing on conscious breathing and relaxing. If working alone, encourage the woman to lie on the couch (in case she faints!) and to look away while you take her blood. Work quickly and talk calmly throughout.

Biochemistry

Biochemists usually work with *serum* or *plasma* to test for components or chemicals in the blood, e.g. blood sugar, hormones and lipids.

Table 23.1a   Blood reference ranges in pregnancy*

Table 23.1a Blood Reference Ranges	Non-Pregnant / General population	First Trimester	Second Trimester	Third Trimester
Clotting studies (BLUE-Sodium citrate tubes)				
APTT (secs)	26.3 - 39.4		during pregnancy 22.6 - 38.0	
PT (secs)	12.7 - 15		during pregnancy 9.5 -13.5	
Fibrinogen g/L	2.3 - 5	2.4 - 5.1	2.9 - 5.4	3.7 - 6.2
Electrolytes (GOLD-serum separating tube (Lithium heparin tubes))				
Sodium (mmol/L)	136 -146	133 -148	129 -148	130 - 148
Potassium (mmol/L)	3.5 - 5	3.6 - 5	3.3 - 5	3.3 - 5.1
Renal function tests (GOLD-serum separating tube (Lithium heparin tubes))				
Creatinine (µmol/L)	44 - 80	35 - 62	35 - 71	35 - 80
Uric acid (mg/dL)	2.5 - 5.6	2 - 4.2	2.4 - 4.9	3.1 - 6.3
Urea (mmol/L)	2.5 - 7.1	2.5 - 4.3	1.1 - 4.6	1.1 - 3.9
Liver function tests (GOLD-serum separating tube (Lithium heparin tubes))				
ALT (U/L)	7 - 41	3 - 30	2 - 33	2 - 25
AST (U/L)	12 - 38	3 - 23	3 - 33	4 - 32
ALP (U/L)	33 - 96	17 - 88	25 - 126	38 - 229
Bilirubin (µmol/L)	5.1 - 22.2	1.7 - 6.8	1.7 - 13.7	1.7 - 18.8
Albumin (clotted sample) g/L	41 - 53	31 - 51	26 - 45	23 - 42
Other biochemistry tests				
Serum bile acid (µmol/L) (GOLD/SST)	0.3 - 4.8	0 - 4.9	0 - 9.1	0 - 11.3
Serum ferritin (ng/mL) (GOLD/SST)	10 -150	6 - 130	10 - 230	10 - 166
C-reactive protein (mg/L) (GOLD/SST)	0.2 - 3	unknown	0.4 - 20.3	0.4 - 8.1
Glucose (fluoride tube)	Non-fasting: 3.6 - 6 mmol/L		Labour 4 - 7mmol/L (72-126 mg/dL)	
(PURPLE - EDTA tubes)				
Hb (g/dL)	11 - 15	10.6 - 13.3	9.7 - 13.5	9.5 - 14.2
Platelets (x 10⁹/L)	165 - 415	-	-	115 - 350
WBC (x10⁹/L)	1.5 - 6	3 - 10	3 - 10	6 - 16
Haematocrit / PCV %	36 - 48	31 - 39	31 - 40	32 - 42
MCV (fl)	79 - 93	85 - 96	85 - 97	83 - 98

Table 23.1b Bloods tests for specific conditions: bottle colour and order of draw

Test	Pre-Eclampsia	HELLP syndrome	Disseminated Intravascular Coagulation DIC	Infection	Intra-hepatic Cholestasis	Intrapartum Haemorrhage	Postpartum Haemorrhage	Emergency Caesarean	Stillbirth (NB: tests vary)
ORDER OF DRAW - for multiple samples: 1.Blood Culture Bottles 2.Coagulation Tubes - *invert sample 3-4 times* 3.Non-Additive Tubes - *invert sample 5-6 times* 4.Additive Tubes -*invert sample 8-10 times* (BD Diagnostics, 2010) **Blood cultures**				✓					
Clotting studies *(BLUE-Sodium citrate tubes)*	✓	✓	✓		✓	✓	✓		✓
Blood group / Cross matching *(PINK - EDTA tubes)*			✓			✓	✓	✓	
Electrolytes *(GOLD-serum separating tube (Lithium heparin tubes))*	✓	✓							
Renal function tests *(GOLD-serum separating tube (Lithium heparin tubes))*	✓	✓							✓
Liver function tests *(GOLD-serum separating tube (Lithium heparin tubes))*	✓	✓			✓				✓
Kleihauer *(PURPLE - EDTA tubes)*									
Full blood count *(PURPLE - EDTA tubes)*	✓	✓	✓			✓	✓	✓	✓

*Pregnancy reference ranges vary between laboratories, studies and authors. Interpret bloods according to the laboratory where you work. These pregnancy ranges have been compiled and adapted mainly from the work of www.perinatology.com and Abbassi-Ghanavati *et al.* (2009) (U&Es); Ramsay (2010) (Haematology); Bacq (2011) (LFTs)

Electrolytes

(GOLD serum separating (lithium heparin) tube)

- **Sodium (Na): 129–148 mmol/L.** Sodium is involved in regulation of water volume which affects blood pressure and a number of critical body functions. It is regulated by the kidneys and adrenal gland.
- **Potassium (K): 3.4–5.2 mmol/L.** Potassium regulates water balance and acid base. It is vital for normal cardiac electrical activity; very high or low concentrations are associated with cardiac electrical abnormality, e.g. ventricular fibrillation or asystole.

Renal function tests

(GOLD serum separating (lithium heparin) tube)

- **Creatinine: 35–80 μmol/L.** Creatinine is a nitrogenous waste product of muscle metabolism. It is filtered by the glomeruli in the kidney, so the renal clearance rate provides an approximate measurement of the glomerular filtration rate and indication of renal function.
- **Uric acid: 2.0–6.3 mg/dL.** Uric acid is the end product of protein metabolism. Elevated uric acid levels may reflect decreased renal blood flow caused by vasoconstriction.
- **Urea: 2.5–4.6 mmol/L.** Urea is a waste product of metabolism which is excreted via the kidneys.

Glucose

(GREY fluoride tube)

- **Fasting glucose: 3.5–5.9 mmol/L (63–106 mg/dL)**
- **1 hour post-prandial <7.8 mmol/L (141 mg/dL) (NICE, 2008)**
- **Diabetic women in labour glucose maintenance levels: 4–7 mmol/L (72–126 mg/dL)**

Glucose is the primary source of energy for the body's cells. Glucose is absorbed via the gut, into the circulation where the pancreas secretes insulin-enabling liver cells to remove glucose from the blood and produce glycogen. Diabetes is a metabolic disease where a person has a high blood sugar either because they do not produce insulin (type 1 or insulin dependent diabetes (IDD)) or because cells do not respond to the insulin produced (type 2 or insulin resistant). Gestational diabetes is triggered by pregnancy, and usually (but not always) resolves once the baby is born. Gestational diabetes is usually type 2, and can be controlled by diet changes and/or oral medication but can sometimes require insulin control.

Diabetic glycaemic control during labour and birth

Poor intrapartum glycaemic control is associated with adverse neonatal outcomes, particularly neonatal hypoglycaemia and respiratory distress, so NICE (2008) recommend:

- Hourly blood glucose
- Maintain levels at **4–7 mmol/L**

- In women whose blood glucose is not maintained or those with type 1 diabetes consider intravenous dextrose and sliding scale insulin infusion.

Post-birth

- Women with insulin-treated pre-existing diabetes should reduce their insulin immediately after birth and monitor their blood glucose levels carefully to establish the appropriate dose.
- Diabetic women are at increased risk of hypoglycaemia postnatally, especially when breastfeeding.

Newborns of diabetic mothers

Maintain glucose levels >2.0 mmol/L

Women with diabetes should aim to feed their babies as soon as possible (within 30 minutes of birth) and then at frequent intervals (2–3 hours) until pre-feeding blood glucose levels are maintained at 2 mmol/L or more. Hypoglycaemia is a possibility and NICE (2008) advise blood glucose testing should be carried out in babies of women with diabetes 2–4 hours after birth.

Liver function tests

(GOLD-serum separating tube)

Abnormal liver function tests in pregnancy may be caused by hyperemesis gravidarum, cytomegalovirus, hepatitis, fatty liver of pregnancy, pre-eclampsia/HELLP syndrome or liver disease (e.g. alcoholic hepatitis; intrahepatic cholestasis).

Pregnancy liver enzyme ranges are lower than non-pregnant reference ranges often used; physiological haemodilution alone results in lower values for alanine transaminase (ALT), aspartate transaminase (AST) and bilirubin (Bacq, 2011).

- **Alanine transaminase/ALT: 2–30 U/L; aspartate transaminase/AST: 3–33 U/L.** ALT and AST are useful for the routine diagnosis of liver problems/diseases during pregnancy. Any increase in serum ALT or AST levels should be considered pathological and requires further evaluation (Bacq, 2011).
- **Alkaline phosphatase: 40–229 U/L** (raised in pregnancy +++). Alkaline phosphatase (ALP) is produced by the placenta from the first trimester onwards: by the third trimester it is so greatly raised that it has virtually no diagnostic value in pregnancy.
- **Bilirubin: 1.7–17 µmol/L.** Bilirubin is a pigment removed from the blood during haemoglobin destruction; it is conjugated in the liver and excreted in the bile. During a normal pregnancy levels do not usually rise. However, in liver disease, bile duct blockage or in HELLP syndrome (**H**aemolysis, **E**levated **L**iver enzymes, **L**ow **P**latelets) levels can increase.
- **Total albumin: 23–50 g/L** *(NB: requires a clotted blood sample)*. Albumin is the protein that transports bilirubin; it is synthesised in the liver so is indicative of liver function (Bacq, 2011).

Serum bile acid

(GOLD serum separating (lithium heparin) tube)

Serum bile acid: 0.3–11.3 μmol/L

In a healthy pregnancy serum bile acid rises slightly with gestation. Obstetric cholestasis or intrahepatic cholestasis of pregnancy (ICP) is a condition of biliary impairment, characterised by maternal pruritus; 10–15% of women also suffer from jaundice (Geenes and Williamson, 2009). It usually occurs around the third trimester. ICP increases the risk of adverse fetal outcome relative to maternal serum bile acid levels: mild cholestasis 20 μmol/L carries a small risk, while severe cholestasis > 40 μmol/L carries the greatest risk of intrauterine death (Glantz *et al.*, 2004).

Serum ferritin

(GOLD serum separating (lithium heparin) tube)

Ferritin levels range: 15–250 μg/mL. Levels <10 μg/L require treatment

Ferritin is a protein inside the cell that stores iron for future use. Serum ferritin levels demonstrate how much iron the body has stored, and is therefore a more accurate (but more expensive) test for anaemia than haemoglobin estimation, which is affected by haemodilution.

C-reactive protein

(GOLD serum separating (lithium heparin) tube)

Normal pregnancy levels <20 mg/L (2 mg/dL)

C reactive protein (CRP) is a protein that is produced by the liver and circulated in the blood. It forms part of the body's early defence system against infection. Levels rise dramatically in response to infection or inflammation, typically within 2–6 hours of an acute inflammatory stimulus, peaking at 48 hours. In pregnancy the *normal range* of circulating CRP can be much higher than in the general population, and elevates further in labour.

Haematology and coagulopathy

Haematology tests *whole blood* to perform full blood counts, films and other specialised tests. Coagulopathy forms a sub-section of haematology and receives *citrated* blood samples to analyse blood clotting times and coagulation factors.

Full blood count

(PURPLE Ethylenediamine-tetra-acetic acid (EDTA) tube)

Haemoglobin (Hb): 9.5–13.5 g/dL (104–135 g/L)

Haemoglobin (Hb) is the pigment contained in the red blood cells which enables them to transport oxygen around the body. Anaemia may cause tiredness and dyspnoea: it has little effect on labour itself but can potentiate the effect of any haemorrhage at birth.

There are no definitive ranges for Hb and there is variance in the literature over optimal Hb. Pregnant women are often falsely diagnosed as anaemic. Red cell mass increases by around 10–20% in pregnancy, but since plasma volume increases 20–80% by mid pregnancy, the red blood cells become diluted ('haemodilution') which causes Hb levels to appear to drop (Ramsay, 2010). Interpret the Hb in the light of the full blood picture, i.e. mean corpuscular volume (MCV), mean cell haemoglobin (MCH) and haematocrit (HCT). If the haematocrit is low, and the MCV and MCH are normal, anaemia is unlikely; low MCV with low Hb indicates iron deficiency anaemia (requiring iron supplementation).

Cochrane found that taking preventative iron supplementation maintained Hb levels, preventing anaemia but had no detectable benefit on maternal or fetal outcomes (Pena-Rosaa and Viteri, 2009). Another Cochrane review highlighted a lack of good quality trials and poor monitoring of side-effects resulting from iron supplementation/overloading (Hb>13.0 g/dL) (Reveiz *et al.*, 2011).

NICE (2008) has a low threshold for iron supplementation, recommending it if Hb <11 g/dL at booking, or <10.5 g/dL after 28 weeks.

A raised Hb >13.5 is abnormal and suggests inadequate plasma volume, which can be associated with pre-eclampsia and poor fetal growth (Ramsay, 2010).

Platelets: 115–350 x 10^9/L

Platelets are cells which 'plug' up holes to prevent bleeding and form part of the body's coagulation system. There is evidence of platelet hyperdestruction during pregnancy, particularly during the third trimester. In some women platelets decrease notably and the lower limit of 'normal' at term is considered 115 $\times$ 10^9/L (Ramsay, 2010). Platelets may be abnormally reduced <100 $\times$ 10^9/L in pre-eclampsia and in HELLP syndrome (Ramsay, 2010). High levels suggest other conditions such as thrombocytopenia, enlarged spleen or the effect of some drugs, e.g. heparin.

White blood cells (WBC): 6–16 $\times$ 10^9/L

WBC or leucocytes protect the body from infection and foreign material. There are several types with distinct and different actions. During pregnancy neutrophils increase significantly, monocyte count is higher and lymphocyte count lower. WBC count increases throughout pregnancy and peaks just after birth.

A WBC >16 $\times$ 10^9/L during pregnancy or >25 $\times$ 10^9/L soon after delivery is considered abnormal (Ramsay, 2010) and may indicate infection. Acute infection requires prompt action to prevent septicaemia.

Haematocrit or packed cell volume (PCV): 30–42%

The term hematocrit means 'to separate blood' and haematocrit is the percentage of red blood cells within the plasma. In a non-pregnant woman this is 36–48%. Any increase or decrease in plasma volume affects the hematocrit. As mentioned earlier, the haematocrit decreases in pregnancy, since plasma volume increases by 20–80% while red blood cells only increase by 10–20%, resulting in diluted red blood cells (haemodilution).

Mean corpuscular volume (MCV): 83–98 fL

MCV is the average volume of a single red cell. Slightly raised MCV with low Hb is typical in pregnancy (Ramsay, 2010). MCV is regarded as the most sensitive red cell index for the identification of iron deficiency. Values below 70 fL occur only with iron deficiency anaemia or thalassaemia minor (Kirkpatrick and Alexander, 1996).

Mean corpuscular haemoglobin (MCH): 27–33 pg

MCV is the amount and volume of haemoglobin inside the red blood cell and should be relatively unchanged in pregnancy.

Clotting screening

(*BLUE sodium citrate tube*)
   Samples must be tested as soon as possible on the day of collection.

Prothrombin time (PT): 9.5–13.5 seconds (s)

Prothrombin is a plasma protein produced by the liver. Clotting is caused by a series of chemical reactions, including the conversion of prothrombin to thrombin.

Activated partial thromboplastin time (APTT): 22.6–38 s

APTT is a measure of the functionality of the intrinsic common pathways of the co-agulation cascade. Proteins are activated sequentially along either the extrinsic (tissue related) or intrinsic (blood vessel related) pathways. The branches of the pathway then converge and complete their task with the formation of a stable blood clot. The APTT test measures the length of time (in seconds) for clotting to occur when reagents are added to plasma in a test tube.

Fibrinogen

(*BLUE sodium citrate tube*)

Fibrinogen: 2.4–6.2 g/L

Fibrinogen is a protein present in plasma; levels increase as gestation advances (Ramsay, 2010). During tissue injury it is activated by thrombin to form fibrin, a fibrous mesh that impedes blood flow, arresting haemorrhage. Fibrinolysis is the enzymatic breakdown of the fibrin in blood clots; this action is generally suppressed during pregnancy, with maximum suppression during labour (Ramsay, 2010).

The D-dimer test

(BLUE sodium citrate tube)

D-dimer normal adult values <433 μg/L, increase in pregnancy 300–1700 μg/L

D-dimers are degradation products of fibrin derivatives; and indicate fibrin clot break-down, which occurs in pulmonary embolism, deep vein thrombosis, disseminated intravascular coagulation, renal or liver disease. Raised fibrin degradation products (FDP) and D-dimer have poor prognostic value in pregnancy as elevated levels may reflect natural increased fibrin generation and degradation in the placental circulation rather than increased fibrinolytic activity (Ramsay, 2010).

Blood bank (immunohaematology)

This department determines blood group, rhesus status, and any antigen or antibodies. It also prepares blood components, derivatives and transfusion products.

Kleihauer

(Maternal blood sample 6 ml in PURPLE EDTA tube)
   If the mother is Rhesus (Rh) negative and the baby is Rhesus (Rh) positive, the mother can produce antibodies against the Rhesus D antigen on her baby's red blood cells, usually as a result of fetomaternal transfusion (FMH). This antigen can cause destruction of RhD-positive fetal red blood cells leading to the development of Rh disease, with subsequent fetal/neonatal morbidity including hydrops fetalis, and in severe cases death.
   Following birth, or a sensitizing event in pregnancy, the Kleihauer test can be used to detect if fetal haemoglobin has entered the maternal circulation, the degree of FMH and thus the correct dose of anti-D immunoglobulin for the mother. IgG anti-D (anti-RhD) antibodies bind to and lead to the destruction of fetal RhD-positive red blood cells that have passed from the fetal to the maternal circulation. Studies have shown that 99% of women will have a FMH of less than 4 ml at delivery, requiring the standard dose of 500 IU. For each millilitre over 4 ml a further 125 micrograms (100 IU) of anti-D will be required (RCOG, 2011).

Direct Coombs test (DCT)

(Umbilical cord sample 5 ml in PURPLE EDTA tube)
   Blood is taken from any vessel in the baby's umbilical cord for DCT, which detects if the baby has developed antibodies to the mother's blood. This sample is also tested to determine the baby's blood group.

Group and save

(*PINK EDTA tube*)

This determines blood group and rhesus status. The serum is saved for 5–7 days. Antibody screening is also carried out. This may be done prior to caesarean section (CS), or if a woman presents with an antepartum haemorrhage, placenta praevia, intrauterine death or a medical/obstetric problem that may necessitate a blood transfusion.

Cross-matching

(*PINK EDTA tube*)

The donor's red and white blood cells are mixed with the recipient's serum to confirm if the donated blood will be compatible with the potential recipient. Routinely performed preoperatively, also performed urgently, e.g. serious haemorrhage.

Blood tests for specific conditions and blood pictures

Pre-eclampsia

- FBC
- Electrolytes
- Renal function tests (including uric acid)
- Liver function tests
- Clotting studies

Pre-eclampsia is a syndrome which may reduce perfusion of all maternal organ systems, primarily kidneys, liver, placenta and brain. The vascular system undergoes raised peripheral resistance, reduced plasma volume, reduced cardiac output and sometimes haemolysis. The renal system has a reduced uric acid clearance, renal blood flow and glomerular filtration rate. As the liver is put under stress, liver enzymes increase and the clotting system tends towards coagulation in severe cases. See Table 23.2.

Table 23.2   Blood picture for pre-eclampsia.

Sample	Level
Electrolytes	Unchanged
Hb	May increase
PCV	May increase
Platelets	May decrease
Clotting time	May be normal or prolonged in severe stages
Creatinine	May increase
Uric acid	Increased
Urea	May increase
Liver enzymes	Increased except for bilirubin (unchanged unless HELLP syndrome)

HELLP syndrome

- FBC
- Electrolytes
- Clotting
- Liver function tests
- Renal function tests

HELLP syndrome is characterised by **H**aemolysis, **E**levated **L**iver enzymes and **L**ow **P**latelets, and is a serious, potentially fatal pregnancy complication. It is usually found in conjunction with severe pre-eclampsia: pathophysiological changes result in vascular system injury with hypoxic liver changes. Arterial vasospasms damage small blood vessels forming lesions. These allow platelet aggregation and fibrin network formation. As red cells are forced through the network under pressure, haemolysis results. As the haemolytic process continues, haematocrit levels fall and bilirubin levels rise (Poole, 1988). Diagnosis is aided by laboratory findings, and early diagnosis is essential to prevent further complications of disseminated intravascular coagulation, hepatic and renal failure (refer to HELLP syndrome in Chapter 20). See Table 23.3.

Table 23.3   Blood picture for HELLP syndrome.

Sample	Level
Hb	May decrease
MCV	Decreased
Platelets	Decreased
PT/APTT	Unchanged
Fibrinogen	Increased
Creatinine	Increased
Uric acid	Increased
Urea	Increased
Liver enzymes	Increased

Adapted from Poole (1988).

Disseminated intravascular coagulation (DIC)

- FBC (platelets)
- Clotting studies (PT, APTT, fibrinogen, fibrin degradation)
- D-dimer

Disseminated intravascular coagulation (DIC) is a pathological activation of blood clotting mechanisms. It results most commonly from eclampsia and HELLP syndrome, but occasionally from placental abruption, intrauterine death, amniotic fluid embolism, PPH and infection. DIC is a contradictory process of coagulation and anticoagulation: initially there is widespread activation of blood coagulation, and subsequent fibrin formation, which leads to blood clots in small- and mid-sized vessels throughout the body. These clots disrupt blood flow to organs and also consume coagulation products resulting in widespread haemorrhage. See Table 23.4.

Table 23.4   Blood picture for DIC.

Sample	Level
Platelets	Decreased
PT	Increased
APTT	Increased
Fibrinogen	Decreased in acute DIC
	May be normal in chronic DIC
D-dimer	Increased

Stillbirth

Local practice may vary but the following are usually taken:

- FBC
- Group and save
- LFT and serum bile acid
- Clotting studies
- Infection screen: parvovirus and TORCH: i.e. **T**oxoplasma gondii, **O**ther viruses (HIV, measles and more), **R**ubella, **C**ytomegalovirus and **H**erpes simplex.
- Auto-immune antibodies (e.g. lupus, anticardiolipin)
- Kleihauer

If the cause of fetal death is known and a maternal disorder has contributed, then relevant bloods will obviously be needed. Genetic testing of both parents may be indicated, but this will require counselling and is unlikely to be performed in the immediate postnatal period. If the baby has been dead for some time there is a small increased DIC risk. See Table 23.1.

Severe haemorrhage

- FBC
- Group and save
- Clotting studies
- Kleihauer (ante or intra-partum haemorrhage only)
- Cross match and **order blood products urgently**

Each unit should have a multidisciplinary massive haemorrhage protocol; liaison with the haematologist is essential (CEMACH, 2004; CNST, 2006). Urgent platelet and fresh frozen plasma infusion may be required - especially if coagulopathy is present. See Table 23.1a and Chapter 16.

Fetal blood tests

Fetal blood pH sampling and lactate testing

Fetal blood pH sampling (FBS) tests fetal capillary blood (intrapartum) or umbilical cord blood (post-partum) to assess pH values and acid-base status (Table 23.5)

Table 23.5   Fetal blood pH and action required.

Fetal blood pH	Recommended action
≥7.25	No action at present: repeat FBS in 1 hour if FHR concern persists
	If later FBS stable and FHR unchanged, defer further FBS unless further FHR abnormalities develop
7.21–7.24	Repeat FBS in 30 minutes if FHR concern persists
	If later FBS stable and FHR unchanged, defer further FBS unless further FHR abnormalities develop
<7.20	Urgent birth is indicated

If a third FBS is contemplated or after an abnormal FBS result, consultant obstetric opinion should be sought (NICE, 2007).

Adapted from NICE (2007).

Since the 1990s FBS has become an integral adjunct to electronic fetal monitoring in the UK. It has been recommended by NICE since 2001 to help identify both fetuses at risk, and, significantly, those *not* at risk, reducing unnecessary interventions such as CS and instrumental delivery. However, while it has assumed considerable importance the evidence for its use is weak (Mahendru and Lees, 2011). Cochrane review suggests that the use of FBS with CTG reduces instrumental deliveries but not CS and makes no difference to neonatal outcome (Alfirevic *et al.*, 2006):

> '*FBS remains an invasive procedure: obtaining an adequate blood sample can be difficult and the pH results are affected by handling of the sample, aerobic contamination and processing. In the light of the existing evidence, the role of intrapartum FBS as a diagnostic technique is unproven.*'

Lactate is an alternative test to pH sampling during labour, and has similar or better predictive value than testing for pH. It requires a smaller sample and has a higher sample success rate than pH analysis. Cochrane refrains from advocating its widespread use until more studies on its clinical benefit, use and safety are available (East *et al.*, 2010).

Fetal blood sampling procedure and maternal consent

Informed consent should be obtained and the woman should be aware of the implications of an abnormal result. However, since FBS appears to have little little advantage over CTG alone in diagnosing hypoxia (Alfirevic *et al.*, 2006) it is not easy to present the facts to the woman in labour. If we are entirely honest we should say that FBS is invasive, often painful, can take 10 minutes or longer and may need repeating at 30-minute intervals, will involve cutting the baby's skin and may not be very accurate (also that the midwife's focus may be distracted from the woman to the process of obtaining and testing the blood sample). However, despite evidence to the contrary, FBS is regarded by many as a gold standard and midwives may find it difficult to challenge it, even with the evidence of a Cochrane review behind them.

Contraindications to FBS

- The woman does not give consent
- Maternal infection (e.g. HIV, hepatitis, *active* herpes)
- Prematurity <34 weeks
- Fetal bleeding disorders, e.g. haemophilia
- If during second stage of labour the CTG is pathological and there is clear evidence suggestive of acute fetal compromise (NICE, 2007). Instrumental or operative delivery is indicated at this point.

FBS procedure

- The woman will require good emotional support: offer Entonox if required.
- The cervix must be adequately dilated to gain access to the head, and membranes ruptured.
- The woman should be in the left lateral position to prevent aortocaval compression.
- An amnioscope is passed into the vagina and, once visualised, the presenting part cleaned and dried.
- Ethyl chloride may be sprayed on.
- A thin layer of liquid paraffin is usually applied to help give a good blood droplet.
- A small incision is made and the blood collected in a dry heparin-coated glass capillary tube for analysis.

Cord blood sampling

Cord blood analysis may be required to aid neonatal management, for medical audits and for litigation and legal purposes. There is no evidence to suggest that routine cord blood analysis should be the norm after all births and NICE (2007) advises against it.

Practices may vary between units. Selective reasons may be as follows:

- Abnormal fetal heart rate (FHR) in labour
- Instrumental delivery
- Caesarean birth
- Low Apgar score
- Preterm birth
- Any other situation where suspected fetal compromise has occurred.

When carrying out umbilical cord samples after delivery, particularly for presumed fetal distress, normally both the artery and the vein are sampled (Tables 23.6 and 23.7). Firstly, this will ensure that the umbilical artery value can be recognised (the

Table 23.6 Umbilical venous blood analysis.

Venous blood	Normal range	Median
pH	7.17–7.48	7.35
pCO$_2$	3.5–7.9 kPa	5.3
Base deficit	−1.0 to 8.9 mmol/L	2.4 mmol/L

Adapted from Westgate *et al.* (1994).

Table 23.7 Umbilical arterial blood analysis.

Arterial blood	Normal range	Median
pH	7.05–7.38	7.26
pCO$_2$	4.9–10.7 kPa	7.3
Base deficit	–2.5 to 9.7 mmol/L	2.4 mmol/L

Adapted from Westgate *et al.* (1994).

artery has a lower O$_2$ tension and saturation, lower pH, greater base deficit and higher CO$_2$ tension). Secondly, as the umbilical artery represents fetal circulation and the umbilical vein blood shows the influence of the placenta, the balance between fetal acid production and placental oxygen can be assessed by comparing both samples. However, opinions differ, and some suggest a single arterial sample is sufficient (Tong *et al.*, 2002).

References

Abbassi-Ghanavati, M., Greer, L. G., Cunningham, F. G. (2009) Pregnancy and laboratory studies: a reference table for clinicians. *Obstetrics and Gynecology* 114(6), 1326–31.

Alfirevic, Z., Devane, D., Gyte, G. M. (2006) Continuous cardiotocography (CTG) as a form of electronic fetal monitoring (EFM) for fetal assessment during labour. *Cochrane Database of Systematic Reviews* 19, 3.

Bacq, Y. (2011) *The Liver in Normal Pregnancy. Madame Curie Bioscience Database: 2010–11.* www.ncbi.nlm.nih.gov/books/NBK6005/

BD Diagnostics (2010) *Pre-anaylytical Systems* (online). www.bd.com/ukm

CEMACH (2004) *Why Mothers Die 2000–2002. The Sixth Report of Confidential Enquiries into Maternal Deaths in the United Kingdom.* London, RCOG Press.

CNST (Clinical Negligence Scheme for Trusts) (2006) *Maternity Clinical Risk Management Standards.* NHS Litigation Authority.

East, C. E., Leader, L. R., Sheehan, P., Henshall, N. E., Colditz, P. B. (2010) Intrapartum fetal scalp lactate sampling for fetal assessment in the presence of a non-reassuring fetal heart rate trace. *Cochrane Database of Systematic Reviews* 17(3), CD006174.

Geenes, V., Williamson, C. (2009) Intrahepatic cholestasis of pregnancy. *World Journal of Gastroenterology* 15(17), 2049–66.

Glantz, A., Marschall, H. U., Mattsson, L. A. (2004) Intrahepatic cholestasis of pregnancy: Relationships between bile acid levels and fetal complication rates. *Hepatology* 40, 467–74.

Kirkpatrick, C., Alexander, S. (1996) Antepartum and postpartum assessment of haemoglobin, haematocrit and serum ferritin. In Wildschut, H., Weiner, C. P., Peters, T. J. (eds) *When to Screen in Obstetrics and Gynaecology*, pp. 80–95. London, WB Saunders.

Mahendru, A. A., Lees, C. C. (2011) Is intrapartum fetal blood sampling a gold standard diagnostic tool for fetal distress? *European Journal of Obstetric and Gynaecolical Reproductive Biology* 156(2), 137–9.

NICE (National Institute for Health and Clinical Excellence) (2001) *The Use of Electronic Fetal Monitoring: The use and interpretation of cardiotocography in intrapartum fetal surveillance'* (Inherited clinical guideline C). This guideline is now withdrawn and replaced with (2007) *Intrapartum Care: Clinical Guideline 55:* see below:

NICE (2007) *Intrapartum Care: Clinical Guideline 55.* London, NICE www.nice.org.uk/cg55

NICE (2008) *Diabetes in Pregnancy: Clinical guideline 63.* London, NICE. www.nice.org .uk/cg63

Pagana, K., Pagana, T. (2008) User guide to test preparation and procedures. *Mosbys Diagnostic and Laboratory Tests Reference*, p. xiv. Mosby. 9th Edition.

Pena-Rosas, J. P., Viteri, F. E. (2009) Effects and safety of preventative oral iron or iron + folic acid supplementation. *Cochrane Database of Systematic Reviews.* (4), CD004736.

Poole, J. H. (1988) Getting a perspective on HELLP syndrome. *American Journal of Maternal and Child Health* 13, 432–7.

Ramsay, M. (2010) Normal hematatological changes during pregnancy and the puerperium. In Pavord, S., Hunt, B. (eds) *The Obstetric Haematology Manual* pp.3–11. Cambridge, Cambridge University Press.

RCOG (Royal College of Obstetricians and Gynaecologists) (2011) *The Use of Anti-D Immunologloglobulin for Rhesus D Prophylaxsis. Green Top Guideline no 22.* www.rcog.org.uk

Reveiz, L., Gyte, G. M. L., Cuervo, L. G., Casasbuenas, A. (2011) Treatments for iron-deficiency anaemia in pregnancy. *Cochrane Database of Systematic Reviews I*, Issue 10.

Tong, S., Egan, V., Griffin, J., Wallace, E. M. (2002) Cord blood sampling at delivery: do we need to always collect from both vessels? *BJOG* 109:1175–1177.

Westgate, J., Garibaldi, J. M., Greene, K. R. (1994) Umbilical cord blood gas analysis at delivery. *British Journal of Obstetrics and Gynaecology* 101, 1054–63.

24 Medicines and the midwife

Vicky Chapman

Introduction

'A practising midwife shall only supply and administer those medicines, including analgesics, in respect of which she has received the appropriate training as to use, dosage and methods of administration' (NMC, 2004).

This chapter presents the midwife's position regarding the supply and administration of medicines.

Facts

- Midwifery practice is subject to legislation:
  - The Medicines Act 1968
  - The Misuse of Drugs Act 1971
  - Midwives Rules and Standards (NMC, 2004)
  - Standards for Medicines Management (NMC, 2007).
- Midwives should expect their supervisor of midwives (SOM) to audit their drug administration records periodically (NMC, 2004).
- Independent midwives should seek advice from their SOM regarding any matters related to the supply, administration, storage, surrender and destruction of controlled drugs and other medicines (NMC, 2004).
- Independent midwives often use supply orders provided by their SOM to enable them to acquire controlled drugs. They also need to have an agreement in place

The Midwife's Labour and Birth Handbook, Third Edition. Edited by Vicky Chapman and Cathy Charles.
© 2013 John Wiley & Sons, Ltd. Published 2013 by John Wiley & Sons, Ltd.

with a local pharmacist from whom they can purchase medicines, which they can supply to their clients.
- Despite being covered by midwife exemptions to supply drugs like ferrous sulphate, there is no national system enabling community midwives to obtain these drugs other than by obtaining a GP prescription.
- There is no requirement for midwives to receive formal training or updates on medicines they use in everyday practice; most simply learn 'on the job'.

Midwife exemption orders

Certain health care professionals are exempt from the general rules governing sale, supply and administration of medicines; hence the term 'exemptions'.

Within everyday practice, registered midwives can *supply* and *administer*, on their own initiative, certain medicines specified under **midwife exemption orders (MEOs)**. To do this they *do not* require a prescription, patient group direction or patient specific direction. Most drugs given by the midwife are listed under MEOs.

MEOs include a broad group of medicines that are specific to midwifery practice: see Table 24.1. However, midwives and managers are often confused about the nature and scope of MEOs (Forrester and Homeyard, 2011; NES, 2011).

Table 24.1   Midwife Exemption Orders.

	Midwives can supply and administer the following:
General sales list (GSL)	A medicine normally obtainable from retail outlets, e.g. supermarkets.
Pharmacy (P)	No prescription required, but medicine can only be bought from a pharmacy under a pharmacist's supervision.
Certain Prescription Only Medicines (POM)	Medicines only sold or supplied with a prescription. In 2010 legislation came into force which expands and updates the range of POMs that may be sold, supplied or administered by registered midwives in the course of their professional practice (NMC, 2010). For a list of POMs the midwife can administer see Table 24.2.

Many bodies offer information on MEOs, e.g. the Nursing and Midwifery Council (NMC), the Medicines and Healthcare Products Regulatory Agency (MHRA), employers and NHS trusts. However, no-one holds overall responsibility for ensuring issues are clear and workable in practice. The British National Formulary (BNF) are considering including a section for MEOs, but at present there is no comprehensive list of medicines covered by MEOs and the NMC will not use brand names (by which many are known) for fear of 'showing a preference for a particular brand'. This leaves midwives without a centralised, valid source of reliable information. Individual trusts sometimes provide information on which medicines midwives can administer under MEOs, but many trusts still mistakenly believe that a patient group direction (PGD) is required for a MEO medicine.

NHS Education for Scotland (NES) are proactively addressing this issue; creating a National Formulary for midwives to include medicines commonly used by midwives in practice, highlighting those supplied/administered under MEOs. NES (2011) suggests that this should clarify midwife powers and provide national and professional consistency across Scotland. In addition NES (2011) have produced *Midwives and Medicines* which every UK midwife should read, as it makes up for shortfalls in information elsewhere.

On 1 June 2010 new legislation came into force which expanded and updated the range of prescription only medicines that may be sold, supplied or administered by registered midwives in the course of their professional practice (NMC, 2010).

What does this mean for midwives in clinical practice?

Supply

A practising midwife can *supply* GSL, P or POM medicines.

Example: The midwife can *supply* a course of ferrous sulphate for treatment of anaemia to a woman who is anaemic, e.g. in the community antenatally or on discharge from the postnatal ward (TTOs) for the woman to take home and use.

Documentation: It is the midwife's duty to label the medicine with clear instructions and to document according to local arrangements (usually in the woman's hand-held notes) that these drugs have been supplied.

A problem for some community midwives is that there is not always an NHS supply system that enables them to access medicines.

Administration

A practising midwife can *administer* medicines listed under MEOs: these include all GSL and P medicines and certain listed POMs and intravenous (IV) fluids.

Example: The midwife may administer pain relief in labour such as entonox (P) or controlled drugs such as pethidine (POM) or morphine (POM). The midwife is covered under MEOs to administer these on his/her own initiative.

Documentation: Medicines administered must be documented according to local arrangements, usually in the woman's hand-held notes and/or drug chart/kardex if an inpatient. If administered during labour these should also be recorded on the partogram.

Controlled drugs have an additional requirement; they need to be checked and counted and signed for in controlled drugs book.

There are many medicines that the midwife is covered under MEOs to give on his/her own authority (see Table 24.2) but this list is not exhaustive and medicines such as antibiotics are not covered. In such instances the midwife will commonly refer to a doctor for a prescription; or the medicine may be available through a PGD (see below).

Aren't midwives prescribing?

Exemptions are distinct from prescribing. Prescribing requires the involvement of a pharmacist in the sale or supply of the medicine (MHRA, 2012).

NMC spokespersons on midwife exemptions (Forrester and Homeyard, 2011) highlight 'widespread existing confusion around midwives' responsibilities for medicines management. The great majority of midwives do not prescribe medicines, essentially because it is not necessary for them to do so in their role. However, it has become

Table 24.2   Midwife Exemption Orders: examples of medicines covered.

- All medicinal products on a General Sale List (GLS)
- All Pharmacy (P) medicines
- Prescription Only Medicines containing any of the following:

  Diclofenac
  Hydrocortisone acetate
  Miconazole
  Nystatin

- Prescription Only Medicines for parenteral administration containing any of the following substances:

  Adrenaline
  Anti-D immunoglobulin
  Cyclizine lactate
  Diamorphine
  Ergometrine maleate
  Hepatitis B vaccine
  Hepatitis immunoglobulin
  Lidocaine (lignocaine)/Lidocaine hydrochloride
  Morphine
  Naloxone hydrochloride (narcan®)
  Oxytocin, natural and synthetic
  Pethidine hydrochloride
  Phytomenadione (vitamin K)
  Prochloperazine (stemetil®)

Examples of some common medicines midwives can administer under MEOs

Analgesics	Diamorphine
	Diclofenic (Voltarol)
	Entonox
	Paracetamol
	Pethidine
Anti-emetics	Cyclizine lactate
	Prochloperazine (stemetil®)
Antacids	Aluminum hydroxide (Maalox)
	Ranitidine (Zantac)
Apperients	Glycerine suppositories
	Micro-enema
	Lactulose
Emergency drugs	Adrenaline 1:1000
Local anaesthetic (only while attending woman in childbirth)	Lidocaine (lignocaine)/Lidocaine hydrochloride
Oxytocis (for the third stage)	Syntometrine
	Syntocinon
Oxytocics (for post-partum haemorrhage)	Syntometrine
	Syntocinon
	Ergometrine maleate
	Carboprost (hemabate®)
Rhesus disease	Anti-D immunoglobulin
Others	Anusol-HC
	Ferrous sulphate
	Miconazole 2%
	Hepatitis B vaccine
	Hepatitis immunoglobulin
Neonatal	Naloxone hydrochloride (narcan®)
	Phytomenadione (vitamin K)
	Nystatin
IV fluids	Haemaccel, Gelofusine, Hartmann's solution
	Sodium Chloride 0.9% (also for use as an IV bolus flush).

'When supplying or administering medicines under midwives exemptions, midwives must ensure their practice is evidence based. Midwives must be familiar with current guidance published in the British National Formulary and British National Formulary for Children, including the use, side effects and contra-indications of the medicines' (NMC, 2010).

apparent that many midwives are under the impression that they do prescribe, when in fact they are administering'.

Only midwives who have completed an NMC approved programme and recorded this in the NMC register can prescribe. They can then prescribe from the agreed formulary linked to their recorded qualification (NMC, 2006). There are currently only 685 midwives (<0.6% midwives) with a recorded prescriber qualification (Forrester and Homeyard, 2011).

Student midwives

Recent amendments to MEOs clarify that student midwives can administer drugs listed under MEOs (except controlled drugs) providing they are under the direct supervision of their sign-off mentor.

Standing orders

Many midwives work in units that provide standing orders. However, there is no legal definition for standing orders and they do not exist under any medicines legislation (NMC, 2007). The NMC recommend that the term 'standing orders' is no longer used.

Patient group directions (PGDs)

PGDs provide for the supply and administration of medicines by certain health professionals without a prescription. These medicines are approved for supply/administration by local doctors and pharmacists for patients in pre-identified clinical situations. An example of a useful PGD for midwives is the administration of prostaglandins. Women pre-identified as requiring induction of labour (IOL) can be admitted and the midwife (if named in the PGD) can commence IOL by administering the prostaglandins without a prescription or written doctor's instruction.

PGDs can be a complex topic and there is much confusion about midwives' involvement. Part of the confusion is due to the fact that PGDs are intended for all health professionals, not just midwives. Another area of confusion is when PGDs are used incorrectly and contain medicines midwives can already supply/administer under MEOs. This 'demonstrates a lack of knowledge and/or understanding of the operationalisation of exemption orders especially in relation to GSL and P medicines' (NES, 2011). The NMC also acknowledge this as a problem and recommend MEO substances be removed from PGDs (Forrester and Homeyard, 2010).

- PGDs are not a form of prescribing, and while midwives should ideally be involved in drawing up and signing off PGDs, a PGD must be signed off by a doctor and pharmacist involved in the PGD development (NMC, 2007).
- PGDs can only be administered by midwives named in each PGD document: PGD administration cannot be delegated, even to a student.

Documentation and drug errors

Midwives are required to keep accurate, detailed records of the supply/administration of all medicines. Below are the guidelines for best practice adapted from the NMC.

Safety and good practice

- Correctly identify the woman/baby to whom the medicine is to be administered.
- Check the person is not allergic to the medicine before administration.
- Check dosage, method of administration, route and timing in the context of the woman's condition and any co-existing therapies.
- Check that the prescription, and/or the label on the medicine dispensed by a pharmacist, is clearly written and unambiguous.
- Check expiry date.

Documentation

- Document immediately all medicines administered; avoid abbreviations.
- Ensure written entries are clear, legible, accurately dated, timed and signed with the signature printed alongside the first entry.
- Clearly countersign the signature of any student supervised in the administration of medicines.

Some suggest the midwife should document if s/he has administered a medicine under MEOs. Local policy will dictate if/how this is done but Forrester (personal correspondence, 2012) advocates using a section on a medication chart to record medicines administered under MEOs: 'We are very keen to get a clear message out that midwives do not prescribe, and completing the prescription chart, for example in the "once only" section often confuses this message'. In practice it is not always possible to document 'MEO' as space is limited on the drug kardex/chart, there is not always a specific section for midwives to do this. In addition, drug errors have been known to occur when documentation is in separate places.

Avoiding and reporting drug errors

NMC (2007) states it is unacceptable to prepare substances for injection in advance of their immediate use and that a practitioner should not administer a medication drawn up by another practitioner when not in their presence. Also that a second *registered professional* checks any complex drug calculation (for example see Box 24.1).

Box 24.1   Example of drug calculation.

Formula for liquids:

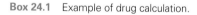

$$\frac{\text{What you want}}{\text{What you have}} \times \text{volume} = \text{dose to be administered}$$

Example:

100 mg penicillin is prescribed; it comes as a preparation of 125 mg of penicillin in 5 ml solution:

$$\frac{100\ \text{mg}}{125\ \text{mg}} \times 5\ \text{ml} = 4\ \text{ml}$$

If a midwife makes or identifies an error in the administration of a drug, it should be reported immediately to the prescriber and the line manager/employer. A practising midwife should also inform their named SOM (RCM, 2006; NMC, 2007). Any error or near miss should be reported to the local risk management team.

The NMC supports the use of critical incident procedures for clinical errors but urges managers, when considering disciplinary action in relation to the administration of medicines to distinguish between *'those cases where the error was the result of reckless or incompetent practice or was concealed, and those that resulted from other causes, such as serious pressure of work, and where there was immediate, honest disclosure in the patient's interest'* (NMC, 2007).

Common abbreviations

Internationally recognised units and symbols are used in the BNF where possible: the Joint Formulary Committee (JFC, 2012) recommends that directions should be in English without abbreviation; however, they acknowledge that often abbreviations are used. The back page of any BNF lists Latin abbreviations deemed acceptable. Midwives should be able to use and interpret abbreviations (see Tables 24.3 to 24.5 for abbreviations and units).

Table 24.3   Abbreviations for route and administration.

Route of administration		Frequency of administration	
Abbreviation	Route	Abbreviation	Frequency
IM	intramuscular	stat	immediately
IV	intravenous	od (*omni die*)	once a day
sc	subcutaneous	bd (*bis die*)	twice a day
po/per oram	oral	tds (*ter die sumendus*)	three times a day
pr/per rectum	rectal	qds (*quater die sumendus*)	four times a day
pv/per vaginum	vaginal	nocte	at night
buccal	between cheek & gum	prn (*pro re nata*)	as needed

Table 24.4   Units of measurement.

Abbreviation	Unit
μg or mcg	microgram
mg	milligram
g	gram
kg	kilogram
ml or mL	millilitre
l or L	litre
IU	international units
mU	milliunits

Table 24.5   Unit multiples.

1000 nanograms (ng) =	1 microgram (μg or mcg)
1000 micrograms (μg or mcg) =	1 milligram (mg)
1000 milligrams (mg) =	1 gram (g)

Useful contacts

BNF (The British National Formulary). Information about medicines in UK, published twice a year. www.bnf.org

Medicines and Midwives. NHS Education for Scotland (NES) *Clarifying Midwives Role Regarding Medicines.* www.nes.scot.nhs.uk

MHRA (Medicines and Healthcare Products Regulatory Agency). www.mhra.gov.uk/ Howweregulate/Medicines/Availabilityprescribingsellingandsupplyingofmedicines/ ExemptionsfromMedicinesActrestrictions/Midwives/index.htm

References

Forrester, M., Homeyard, C. (2010) Changes to midwives' exemptions. *Midwives* August, 28–9.

Forrester, M., Homeyard, C. (2011) Aren't midwives prescribing? *RCM Midwives/feedback.* Issue 3. www.rcm.org.uk/midwives/your-views/feedback-issue-3-2011/

Forrester, M. (2012) personal correspondence regarding midwife exemptions.

JFC (Joint Formulary Committee) (2012) *British National Formulary,* 63rd edn. London, BMJ Group and Pharmaceutical Press.

MHRA (The Medicines and Healthcare Products Regulatory Agency) (2012). http://www. mhra.gov.uk/Howweregulate/Medicines/Availabilityprescribingsellingandsupplying ofmedicines/ExemptionsfromMedicinesActrestrictions/Midwives/index.htm

NHS Education for Scotland (NES) (2011) *Midwives and Medicines,* 2nd edn, Vance, M. (ed.) NES.

NMC (Nursing and Midwifery Council) (2006) *Standards of Proficiency for Nurse and Midwife Prescribers.* London, NMC.

NMC (2004) *Midwives Rules and Standards.* London, NMC.

NMC (2007) *Standards for Medicines Management.* London, NMC.

NMC (2010) *Changes to Midwives' Exemptions.* London, NMC. www.nmc-uk.org/Docu ments/Circulars/2010circulars/NMCcircular06_2010.pdf

RCM (Royal College of Midwives) (2006) *Midwifery and Medicines Legislation: An Information Paper.* London, RCM. http://www.rcm.org.uk/info/pages/recentDocs.php

The Medicines Act 1968. http://www.legislation.gov.uk/ukpga/1968/67

The Misuse of Drugs Act 1971. http://www.legislation.gov.uk/ukpga/1971/38

Index

Boldface page numbers refer to key citations.

The Midwife's Labour and Birth Handbook, Third Edition. Edited by Vicky Chapman and Cathy Charles.
© 2013 John Wiley & Sons, Ltd. Published 2013 by John Wiley & Sons, Ltd.